BRITISH MEDICAL BULLETIN

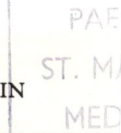

BRITISH MEDIC

British Medical Bulletin is published four times each year, in January, April, July and October.

Subscriptions and single-copy orders should be sent to: Longman Group UK Ltd, Subscriptions Department, Fourth Avenue, Harlow, Essex CM19 5AA.

Subscription rates for 1989 are: £70 (UK) or £87.50/$157.50 (overseas)

Single copies will be available at £25.00 (UK) or £31.50/$49.25 (overseas)

NEXT ISSUE

Volume 45 No. 1   DIABETES   January 1989

Scientific Editor: R D G LESLIE

Introduction	D A Pyke
Molecular structure of insulin	G Dodson, J & U Derewenda
Synthesis and secretion of insulin	S Howell
Possible mechanisms of auto-immune damage	G Bottazzo
Aetiology of insulin dependent diabetes	R D G Leslie & O. Vergani
Aetiology of insulin dependent diabetes	R Taylor
Insulin treatment	P Home
Diabetic neuropathy	J D Ward
Diabetic nephropathy	P Watkins, P Drury, G-C Viberti and J Walker
Glycosylation	L Kennedy
Genetics of diabetes	G Hitman
Microcircultion and diabetes	J Tooke
Islet transplantation	P Morris
Diabetic emergencies	K G M M Alberti
Insulin action	M Houslay
Lipids and arterial disease	J Betteridge

CHURCHILL LIVINGSTONE, Medical Division of Longman Group U.K. Limited. Typeset and printed by H Charlesworth & Co Ltd, Huddersfield

Distributed in the United States of America by Churchill Livingstone Inc., 1560 Broadway, New York, NY 10036, and by associated companies, branches and representatives throughout the world. This journal is indexed, abstracted and/or publishd online in the following media: Current Contents, Scientific Serials Review, Excerpta Medica, USSR Academy of Science, Biological Abstracts, UMI (Microform), BRS Colleague (full text), Index Medicus

© The British Council 1988

All rights reserved. No part of this publication may be reproduced, stored in a retrieval system, or transmitted in any form or by any means, electronic, mechanical, photocopying, recording or otherwise, without either the prior written permission of the copyright owner, or a licence permitting restricted copying in the United Kingdom issued by the Copyright Licensing Agency Ltd, 33-34 Alfred Place, London WC1E 7DP.

(Copyright in all materials published in *British Medical Bulletin* prior to 1981 rests with the individual contributors and not with the British Council.)

ISSN 0007-1420   ISBN 0 443 04040 0

BRITISH
MEDICAL BULLETIN

VOLUME FORTY-FOUR
1988

CHURCHILL LIVINGSTONE
EDINBURGH, LONDON, MELBOURNE AND NEW YORK

CHURCHILL LIVINGSTONE
Medical Division of Longman Group UK Limited

Distributed in the United States of America by Churchill Livingstone Inc., 1560 Broadway, New York, NY 10036, and by associated companies, branches and representatives throughout the world.

© The British Council 1988

All rights reserved. No part of this publication may be reproduced, stored in a retrieval system, or transmitted in any form or by any means, electronic, mechanical, photocopying, recording or otherwise, without the prior written permision of the copyright owner, or a licence permitting restricted copying in the United Kingdom issued by the Copyright Licensing Agency Ltd, 33-34 Alfred Place, London WC1E 7DP.

ISSN 0007-1420
ISBN 0 443 04040 0

The Very Immature Infant—Less than 28 Weeks Gestation

Scientific Editors: *A Whitelaw & R W I Cooke*

Introduction *D Hull*	821
Physiology of the mid-trimester fetus *C H Rodeck and U Nicolini*	826
Extreme prematurity: The aetiology of preterm delivery *P R Bennett and M G Elder*	850
Epidemiology of birth before 28 weeks gestation *A Macfarlane, S Cole, A Johnson and B Botting*	861
Lung development in the second trimester *J S Wigglesworth*	894
Adaptation of the respiratory system *A D Milner and A Greenough*	909
Surfactant therapy for very premature babies *C J Morley*	919
Development of renal function *N Modi*	935
The immature skin *N Rutter*	957
Thermal control in very immature infants *D Hull*	971
Growth and nutrition of the very preterm infant *J C L Shaw*	984
The gastrointestinal tract *P J Milla and W M Bissett*	1010
Cardiovascular adaptation in the very immature infant *A R Wilkinson*	1025
Development of immunity *A Whitelaw and J Parkin*	1037
New non-invasive methods for assessing brain oxygenation and haemodynamics *E O R Reynolds, J S Wyatt, D Azzepardi, D T Delpi, E B Cady, M Cope and S Wray*	1052
Neurophysiological assessment of the immature central nervous system *J A Eyre*	1076
The immature visual system and premature birth *A R Fielder, M J Moseley and Y K Ng*	1093
Clinical issues *N McIntosh*	1119
Outcome and costs of care for the very immature infant *R W I Cooke*	1133

1988 Vol. 44 No. 4

Professor Hull chaired the committee which included Dr A Whitelaw, Dr R W I Cooke and Mr N McIntosh that planned this number of the *British Medical Bulletin*. We are grateful to them for their help, and particularly to Dr Whitelaw and Dr Cooke who acted as Scientific Editors for the number.

British Medical Bulletin is published by Churchill Livingstone for The British Council, 10 Spring Gardens, London SW1A 2BN

Introduction

David Hull
Department of Child Health, Queen's Medical Centre, Nottingham, UK

With modern neonatal care, the majority of infants born at or after 28 weeks of gestation live to leave the nursery in good condition. This is due in the main to the provision of a controlled and protecting environment, the early supply of fluid and food which are given intravenously if necessary, the careful monitoring of respiration and the administration of ventilatory support when appropriate, and the liberal use of antibiotics to control infections.

Not many years ago, infants born before 28 weeks gestation were considered to be non-viable, this was based on the general experience that in practice none of them survived. As a consequence they were given little attention either before, during or after birth. They were recorded in national statistics as abortions. Despite the inattention, some of them did show signs of life, a weak heart beat, or a few fruitless gasps. There is however, no biological characteristic which clearly distinguishes between the infant born before 28 weeks gestation and one born after. With the increasing success of neonatal care, it was inevitable that some of these 'pre-viable' infants would live, initially for a few hours, then for a few days and then finally break free from the sophisticated support needed to keep them alive over the first few days after birth. As a consequence of some surviving, more and more of these very immature infants began to receive attention both before and immediately after birth and more survived so that definitions had to change; an infant is now considered 'pre-viable' before 24 weeks gestation. Such definitions are important within legal settings; they also, in part, determine clinical management and influence clinical management, but there is also no clear biological event that separates a 24 week infant from one born before that time, and there are already some claims that infants of 22 weeks gestation can live given appropriate care. It is interesting that it was thought that an infant born before 28 weeks gestation could not survive because the lungs could not open sufficiently to provide an adequate supply of oxygen, the same reasons are now being proposed for the 24 week cut off.

Infants born in the 24 to 28 weeks gestation band do differ in a number of ways from more mature infants; they are creatures of the late 20th century, designed for intra-uterine existence but surviving without it by virtue of high technology. Like newly hatched tortoises born on a sandy beach, some make it to the sea and others do not, some are damaged in the attempt and do not survive, others make the sea but are left with permanent damage which leaves them at a serious disadvantage. The numbers are given by Dr Alison McFarlane and the present position with respect to mortality and handicap is the subject of Dr Richard Cooke's chapter.

If we are to give them better attention so that more live and fewer are damaged by their initial experiences we need to know far more about their nature. Only then will we be able to develop our skills and technology to meet their requirements. In this edition of the British Medical Bulletin leading clinicians skilled in the care of very immature infants have been asked to write of what they know of the structure and function of most of the major biological systems at this stage in development and how they perform when challenged by premature birth. They were given a difficult task, and they each give reasons why they found it to be difficult. One is that 24 to 28 weeks is an artificial band and whilst in some systems dramatic and step wise changes occur for example in skin permeability, in others the changes were more gradual. The second was that there is little or no information. Infants of this gestation have a very tentative grasp on life, they are surrounded by life supporting systems which severely restrict any attempts to make independent careful observations, and the systems themselves influence or may even determine the way the infant responds. The temptation is to extrapolate from data collected from more mature infants which whilst it may be the best that we have, can be misleading. There are no animal models which can be used, most other mammals if born a day or so before term do not and cannot be made to survive. What is perhaps remarkable is that the human infant can emerge after only 2/3 of the usual span of intra-uterine life and survive. In many ways it is the infant in the 24–28 week gestation band which most resembles other mammals born a day or so early, at least in respect to cardio-respiratory responses.

Professor Charles Rodeck sets the scene by discussing the physiology of the mid-trimester fetus. Studying them once they are born is of theoretical interest as well as practical value. How do the developing body systems at this stage in intrauterine life adapt to changing requirements imposed by birth? Does the brain for instance develop best in a warm, wet but dark environment? What happens to the developing eye if it does receive light signals so early in its development? We do know that the growth of the retina can be severely disordered. This is a fascinating topic and more than justifies a separate chapter and no doubt in the not too distant future will require a whole edition. What Professor Alistair Fielder and his colleagues have written is just a foretaste.

The unique biological characteristics of the 'independent fetus' obviously opens up the possibility of new approaches to care. For example the permeable skin not only has implications for temperature control and fluid balance, it also might permit fluid and drug administration, and perhaps most dramatic and maybe the most critical, gaseous exchange. Dr Nick Rutter outlines the possibilities in his chapter but the phenomenon is mentioned in a number of others.

Creating a world for the very immature infant which is similar to that the fetus enjoys in the uterus, whilst quite a challenge, is perhaps one of the easier problems. The intra-uterine environment is held at a near constant temperature, and is wet, dark and sterile. The technical challenge is to 'incubate' the child whilst allowing access for the care which the infant needs. The control of the thermal environment and its adjustment as the infant's own thermoregulatory mechanisms mature is the topic of my own chapter. It is interesting to read a previous Medical Bulletin on Perinatal Research in 1975, we have moved a long way since then. There is no reason why we cannot control the thermal environment with authority and to tune it to the individual needs of each infant just as we would to an older child or an adult.

The intra-uterine environment is usually sterile, rarely do organisms penetrate the fetal envelope. Whilst every attempt is made to avoid infections in neonatal nurseries they do not, nor is it currently intended that they should, provide a sterile environment. So inevitably the infant will be colonized with organisms. The hope is that these will be friendly and non-invasive. Our current strategy is to attack them if there is the slightest possibility that they have entered the infant's body at sites in which they can cause damage. Just how vulnerable the infant of 24 to 28 weeks gestation is to infection is discussed by Dr Andy Whitelaw and Dr Jacqueline Parkin. If the environment is not sterile, if the physical protective structures are not in place, if life support systems involve invasive techniques then reinforcing the infant's own biological defence systems makes sense.

The major challenge of birth to the infant's systems is adjusting to life without the placenta. An immediate response is required from both the heart and circulation, and from the respiratory system. Both have great difficulty. Dr Andrew Wilkinson describes the cardio-vascular responses in Chapter 12. It is the opening of the lungs and the establishment of effective gaseous exchange which is the most critical, and it has received a lot of attention both in research and in clinical practice. Professor Jonathan Wigglesworth considers the structure and Professor Tony Milner the function of lungs and Dr Colin Morley deals with the question of surfactant. There are many good reasons why the lungs of such immature babies may not be effective, most of them we can do little about. A relative deficiency of surfactant may be open to remedy.

As clinicians the authors inevitably are primarily concerned with supporting the infant's fragile existence. Expert bodies when considering the appropriate nutrition for *term infants* recommend breast milk, and in the absence of any evidence to the contrary suggest that artificial feeds should resemble human milk in so far as that is technically possible. We now have a fair amount of information on the nutrition requirements of prematurely born infants over 28 weeks gestation and know that for them human breast milk alone is often not sufficient. But we know very little about the nutritional requirements of the infant born in the last third of the second trimester. Dr Jonathan Shaw states the current position and the grounds for his current practice, and Drs Milla and Bisset describe what adaptions the infant's bowel has to make to get the goodness out of the feed.

During the mid trimester of pregnancy the brain grows and develops rapidly, one might imagine that it was at its most vulnerable, and it seems reasonable to ask the question as to whether it is feasible to support the 24 week infant sufficiently to meet the moment to moment needs of the brain so that its long term performance is not compromised. So the study of the brain, its structure, function and development is of the greatest importance. This is for the infant's and the family's sake. It is also central to decisions on therapeutic approaches, the clinical provision, and the allocation of resources. A damaged child not only lives an incomplete life, and places extra demands on those who love and care for him or her, but also make demands on health, educational and social resources. It is right and proper that they should receive such support, but it is more important that every attempt is made to minimize the need for them. So the investigation of the function of the brain of the 24 week infant in its strange new environment justifies the engagement of the most able minds with the most appropriate tools. Some of these are remarkably sophisticated and Professor Osmond Reynolds and his colleagues review the position. One way of studying the performance of the brain is by recording its electrical activity, and there has been much interest in the use of evoked responses, so that it is particularly appropriate that this technology should be used to explore the development of brain activity in the most immature. This is the topic of the chapter written by Dr Janet Eyre.

Of course the ideal solution for the infant would be to remain a fetus, and for the premature birth to be avoided altogether. Hopefully that will ultimately be achieved, though from the chapter by Professor Elder and Mr P Bennet there seems little reason to anticipate that this will be in the foreseeable future. So the challenge will remain of how to care for these infants whilst expanding our understanding of their nature so that we can care for them more effectively.

It all too easy to forget that they are new beings with rights, families and friends and that birth is as major a social event to them as it is for infants born at term. There might be an argument for placing the very immature infant into an isolated environment and treating it like an artificial womb until the infant can emerge independent and free and enjoy more his or her 'birth'. Professor Neil McIntosh deals with this human interface and emphasizes the infant's personal needs in Chapter 17.

The emphasis has been on the biology of these infants born too early, but there are clearly major social and ethical issues related to the way we receive them into our world. We will have to accept that as we understand them better so we will increase our appreciation of the needs and how to address them of infants born at an even earlier gestation and they no doubt will be the subject of a future issue.

Physiology of the mid-trimester fetus

C H Rodeck
U Nicolini
Royal Postgraduate Medical School, Institute of Obstetrics and Gynaecology,
Queen Charlotte's Maternity Hospital, London, UK

> Ultrasound, cardiotocography, Doppler blood flow studies of the fetal and placental circulation, fetal blood and tissue sampling have provided in recent years completely new information on fetal physiology during gestation.
> The present knowledge of the physiology of the mid-trimester fetus has been reviewed and is summarized in the following subjects: fetal growth, amniotic fluid, cardiovascular system, acid-base balance, lungs, kidneys and fetal blood.

The introduction of new methods of direct and indirect investigation of the human fetus has provided a new body of information which previously could only be achieved through data obtained from newborns and from animal studies. Moreover, the interrelationship between maternal, placental and fetal physiology can now be dynamically assessed. Real-time ultrasound, cardiotocography, Doppler blood flow study of the fetal and placental circulation and fetal blood and tissue sampling by needling are among the techniques which have allowed better understanding of the physiology of the mid-trimester fetus.

This knowledge constitutes the basis for prenatal diagnosis of congenital defects and for the diagnosis and management of fetal disorders which are intimately connected with the pathology of the second and third trimester and the neonatal period.

The present and future possibilities of fetal therapy also require a thorough understanding of the physiology of the second trimester, which is the period when major developments occur in preparation for postnatal life.

FETAL GROWTH

The biological phenomenon of fetal growth in the human has mainly been described in the past from measurements obtained in aborted fetuses or newborn infants. Since the introduction of ultrasound in obstetrics, several growth charts of different parameters relating to the head or body size have been published (Table 1).[1-10]

Only recently have fetal anthropometric variables been regarded as a possible means of investigation of the process of intrauterine growth. Different mathematical models describing this process have been proposed, the commonest being a polynomial model. It cannot however reflect growth throughout the whole of pregnancy, as it is not suitable to describe the period from conception to the early second trimester when ultrasonic measurements are lacking. The whole matter has been extensively investigated in recent years by analysis of both transverse and longitudinal studies.[11,12] Various mathematical models have been tested to satisfy both the best adherence to experimental data and the requirement that the fitting curve starts at a point which is at or somewhat later than conception, depending on when the investigated parameter is considered to become measurable.

In summary, polynomial functions used in different studies are generally similar, indicating that the process of fetal growth is also very similar in different populations. The other applied mathe-

Table 1 List of some of the most popular ultrasonic growth charts for the most widely used fetal parameters

Parameter	Author(s)	Year of publication
Head		
Biparietal diameter	Campbell & Newman[1]	1971
Head circumference	Hadlock et al.[2]	1982
Cerebellum	Smith et al.[3]	1986
Eye	Mayden et al.[4]	1982
Trunk		
Thoracic circumference	Chitkara et al.[5]	1987
Heart volume	Jeanty & Romero[6]	1984
Abdominal circumference	Campbell & Wilkin[7]	1975
Kidney circumference	Grannum et al.[8]	1980
Limbs		
Femur	Hohler & Quetel[9]	1982
Humerus		
Radius-Ulna	Queenan et al.[10]	1980
Tibia-Fibula		

matical models, however different, all have shown that the growth rate in early pregnancy is higher for the fetal head than for the trunk, whereas the opposite is true in the last trimester (Fig. 1).[13] Moreover, the flex point of growth (i.e. when the rate of growth reaches its maximum) is around 16 weeks for the head and 20 weeks for the abdomen.[14] The well known phenomenon of a slower growth rate in the third trimester, described by the typical S-shaped curve of newborn weight versus gestational age has its origin, therefore, much earlier than was previously thought. This may be related to the availability of substrates and oxygen to the fetus through the placenta and suggests that after 20 weeks this gradually becomes limited. Placental weight and DNA content are in fact no longer increasing in the last part of the pregnacy but fetal supplies are maintained by the continuous increase in the area of exchange on the villous surface, by placental transfer and by maternal and fetal blood flow (see below). An alternative explana-

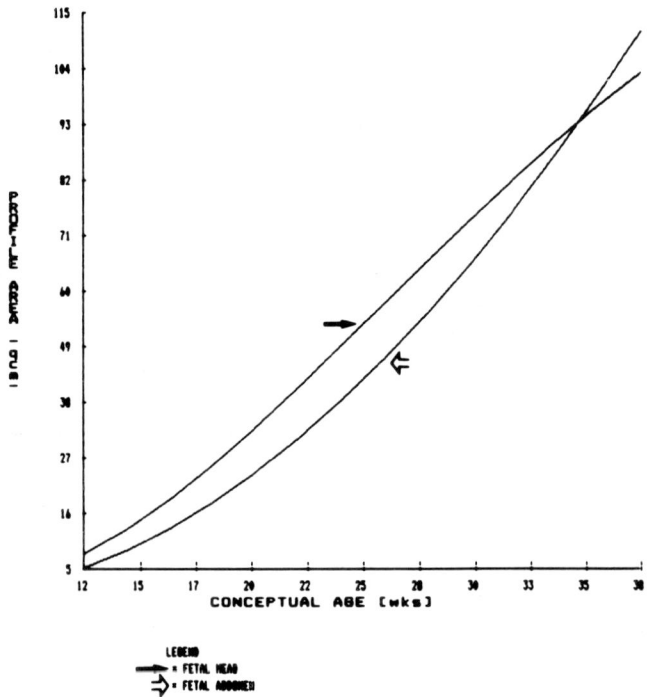

Fig. 1 Average longitudinal growth curves for the fetal head and abdominal profile areas.[13] From: Rossavik IK et al: Journal of Clinical Ultrasound 1987; 15:31. By kind permission of the authors and the publishers.

tion is that the earlier phase of fetal growth is one of cell multiplication (hyperplasia) and the later of increase in cell size (hypertrophy).

AMNIOTIC FLUID

The amniotic fluid has been the principal source of information for several aspects of fetal physiology until direct access to fetal tissues, especially blood, became available more recently. Although they are also dependent on maternal factors, the quantity and components of the amniotic fluid are mainly related to fetal variables. Fetal urine production and swallowing are the main factors involved in the production and removal of amniotic fluid. At 18 weeks the fetus voids 7–17 ml per day and swallows 4–11 ml per day.[15] These figures rise in the late third trimester respectively to 600–700 ml[16] and 200 ml.[17] Thus, any pathology which alters the efficiency of these processes is reflected in a diminution or an increase of the quantity of amniotic fluid, which is on average equal to 240 ml at 15–16 weeks,[18] increases by 10–13 ml per day at 18 weeks[15] and is equal to 670 ml at 25–26 weeks (Fig. 2). The turnover of amniotic fluid has been estimated to be as high as 500 ml per hour,[19] but considerable criticism has been raised[20] about this figure which was derived from measurements of isotopic water transfer between mother, fetus and amniotic fluid. A precise, non-invasive method of estimation of the volume of amniotic fluid is not presently available, but qualitative or semi-quantitative evaluation by ultrasound can easily detect major changes.

Examples of clinical use of amniocentesis for biochemical and cytological analysis are innumerable. From spectrophotometry of amniotic fluid for the evaluation of the severity of Rh alloimmunization, to L/S ratio for assessment of lung maturity, from detection of fetal chromosomal abnormalities to prenatal diagnosis of metabolic disorders, amniotic fluid provides invaluable, though indirect, data on fetal physiology and pathology. Early in pregnancy the amniotic fluid is considered to be equivalent to isotonic extracellular fluid in equilibrium with maternal and fetal compartments across tissue layers largely impermeable to protein. After 20 weeks, when fetal skin keratinization develops, isotopic water and most solutes cannot be exchanged between fetus and amniotic fluid through fetal skin; thereafter the kidneys, lungs and the gastrointestinal tract mainly determine the characteristics and biochemistry of the amniotic fluid. However, fetal skin remains

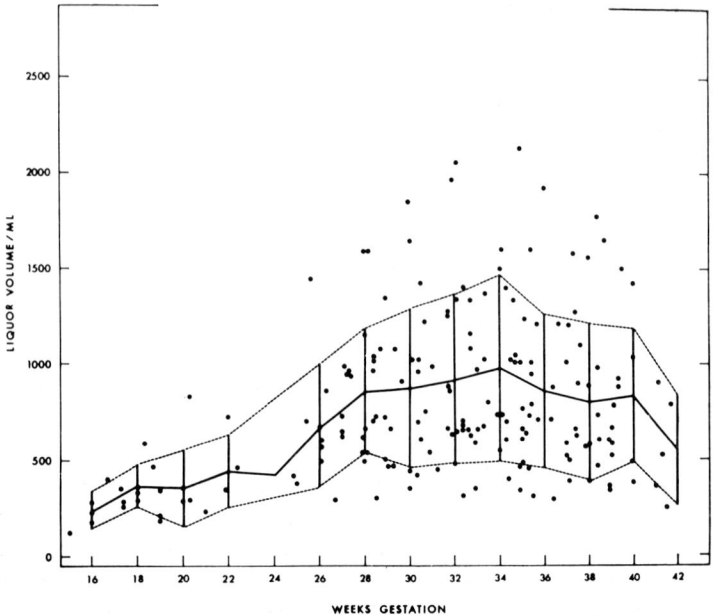

Fig. 2 Amniotic fluid volume throughout gestation. (mean +/− 1 SD).[18] From: Queenan JT et al: American Journal of Obstetrics and Gynecology 1972; 114:34. By kind permission of the authors and the publishers.

permeable to small lipophilic compounds such as oxygen and carbon dioxide, the latter having been shown to be parallel in the amniotic fluid to changes in fetal P_{CO_2}.[21] Another possible source of exchange between the fetal compartment and amniotic fluid is the fetal surface of the placenta which is easily crossed by water, sodium, chloride, urea and creatinine.[22]

The normal biochemical and hormonal constituents of amniotic fluid throughout gestation have been reviewed extensively.[23]

CARDIOVASCULAR SYSTEM

Heart rate

Apart from fetal heart rate, other aspects of the physiology of the cardiocirculatory system in the human have, in the past, only been extrapolated from animal studies.

Cardiotocography and simultaneous real-time observation of fetal activity (breathing movements and body movements) have allowed interesting observations to be made about physiological changes which occur with advancing gestational age. Mean fetal heart rate decreases significantly from 143 beats per minute (bpm) at 19–24 weeks to 132–137 in the last trimester, there being no difference between the sexes.[24] Fetal heart rate is known to be related to maternal heart rate in term fetuses,[25] but this has not been demonstrated in the second trimester. The influence of gestational age on fetal heart rate can also be seen in the percentage of reactive nonstress tests, which rises from 17% between 23 and 27 weeks to 94% at term.[26] This is due to a positive association between gestational age and number and amplitude of fetal heart rate accelerations. Moreover, fetal body movements in the second trimester tend to be associated with a low-amplitude type of acceleration rather than with accelerations above 15 bpm.[27] The mean number of fetal body movements appears to decrease with gestational age, while fetal breathing activity increases and the response to a rise in fetal glycaemia, as it occurs after a maternal meal in the third trimester, cannot be recorded before 26 weeks.[27] Thus, given the relationship between fetal activity and heart rate, the changes in fetal heart rate with gestational age are at least partly due to the modification in the patterns of fetal activity. This is relatively uncoordinated in the second trimester, while a precise organization in cycles of fetal rest and activity becomes evident in the third trimester. The phases of high fetal heart rate variability and those of low variability also increase in length with gestational age, resulting in a reduction of the number of active/quiet cycles per hour in older fetuses.[28]

Blood flow

Direct measurements of the cardiac output are lacking in the human fetus. Measurements of blood flow velocity in different fetal vessels have been performed using the pulsed Doppler technique. However, a quantitative estimate of flow requires measurement of the diameter of the vessel and of the angle between the ultrasonic beam and the axis of the vessel; neither can be precisely estimated. Analysis of the waveform of the Doppler shift has been more reliably used to evaluate changes in flow velocity throughout pregnancy in normal and pathological conditions in the umbilical artery, aorta, cerebral vessels and uteroplacental arteries. Different indices mainly reflect the ratio between systolic and diastolic flow velocities.

Diastolic flow velocities in relation to systolic velocities increase with gestational age in the uteroplacental vessels (until 24 weeks) and in the umbilical artery (Fig. 3), while a small but significant increase in Pulsatility Index in the aorta suggests increased peripheral resistance within the fetus.[29] These data suggest an expansion of the placental circulation both on the fetal and placental side. In the fetal lamb, on the contrary, the cardiac

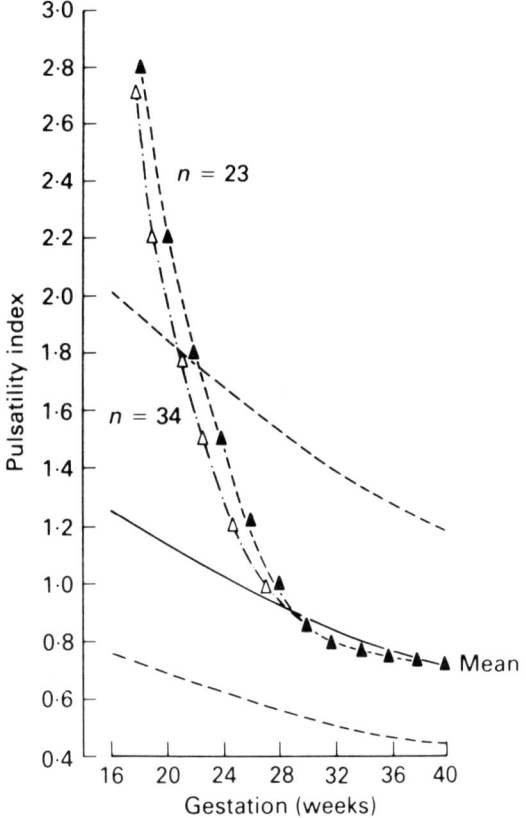

Fig. 3 The pulsatility index from the umbilical artery. The regression line from the present study before (△—·—△) and after (—) correction for fetal heart rate is demonstrated; △---△, the regression line derived from Reuwer et al (1984) and reference ranges (----) after correction for heart rate are also shown.[29] From: Pearce JM et al: British Journal of Obstetrics and Gynaecology 1988; 95:248. By kind permission of the authors and the publishers.

output has been described as being constant in relation to the fetal weight, and the placenta receives a larger fraction of the cardiac output at mid-gestation than at term.[30]

Blood pressure

Recordings of blood pressure in the mid-trimester human fetus are scanty. Castle & Mackenzie[31] recorded the pressure in the umbilical artery in 13 fetuses at 18–21 weeks before termination of pregnancy and found it to be on average 15.2 mmHg (∼2.0 kPa)—range = 6–26. We measured umbilical vein pressure in 15 fetuses undergoing direct intravascular transfusion (IVT) for Rh alloimmunization at 20–33 weeks (Fig. 4).[32] Mean umbilical vein pressure was 4.5 mmHg (0.6 kPa)—range = 1–9—and did not correlate with gestational age. The release of catecholamines following hypoxia has been shown to be positively related to gestational age in animals[33] and an increase in umbilical vein pressure during acute hypoxia has been recorded by us in a human fetus at 31 weeks; no observations have been made in the second trimester fetus. The increase in umbilical vein pressure after an intravascular transfusion is directly correlated with the change in fetal haematocrit (Fig. 5) and is inversely correlated with gestational age;[32] this may reflect maturational asynchrony of sympathetic

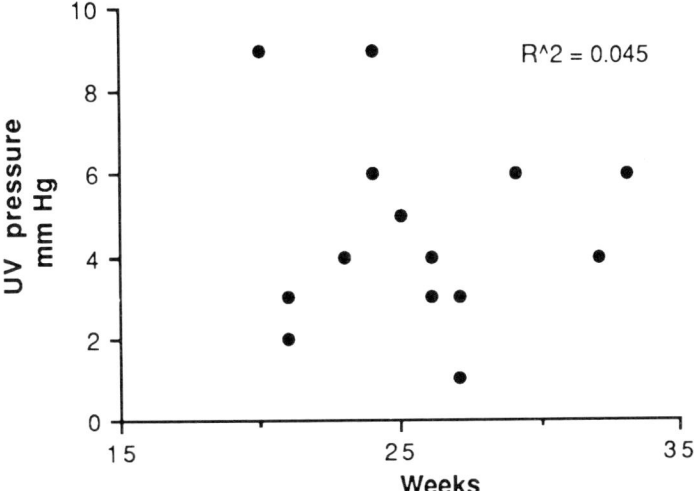

Fig. 4 Umbilical vein (UV) pressure vs gestational age (P = n.s.). (Nicolini et al, unpublished observations.)

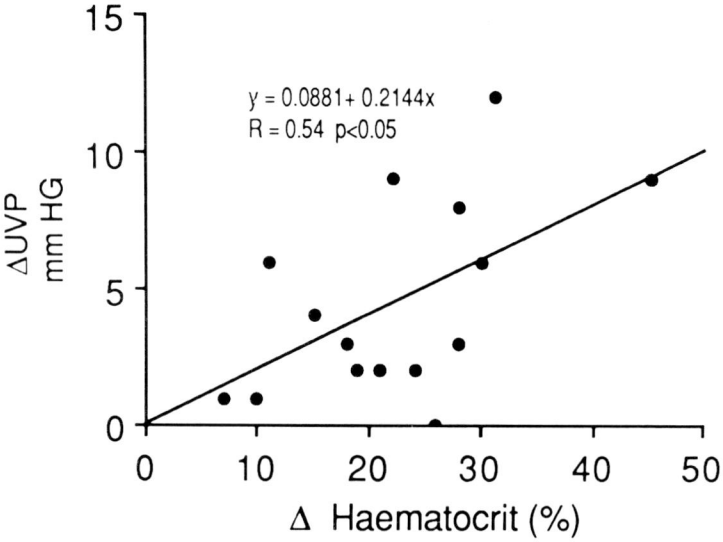

Fig. 5 Change in umbilical vein pressure (ΔUVP) vs increase in fetal haematocrit following intravascular transfusion for Rh alloimmunization. (Nicolini et al, unpublished observations.)

and parasympathetic tone or the reduction in the vascular sensitivity to catecholamines which occurs with advancing gestation.

Blood volume

Fetuses with Rh alloimmunization have also been studied to provide in vivo measurements of the feto-placental blood volume in the second trimester.[34] The feto-placental blood volume rises from 25 ml at 18 weeks to 150 ml at 31 weeks (Fig. 6), but during the same time interval it decreases from 117 ml per kg of fetal weight to 93 ml per kg.

ACID-BASE BALANCE

The maintenance of a normal fetal acid-base balance depends on the efficiency of the utero-placental blood flow, placental transfer of oxygen and carbon dioxide and the fetal cardiovascular system. In normal pregnancies, pH does not change with gestational age, but Po_2 shows a significant negative correlation with gestational age both in the umbilical vein and artery (Fig. 7).[35] On the contrary, there is a positive correlation with gestational age for Pco_2 both in the umbilical vein and artery and for bicarbonate,

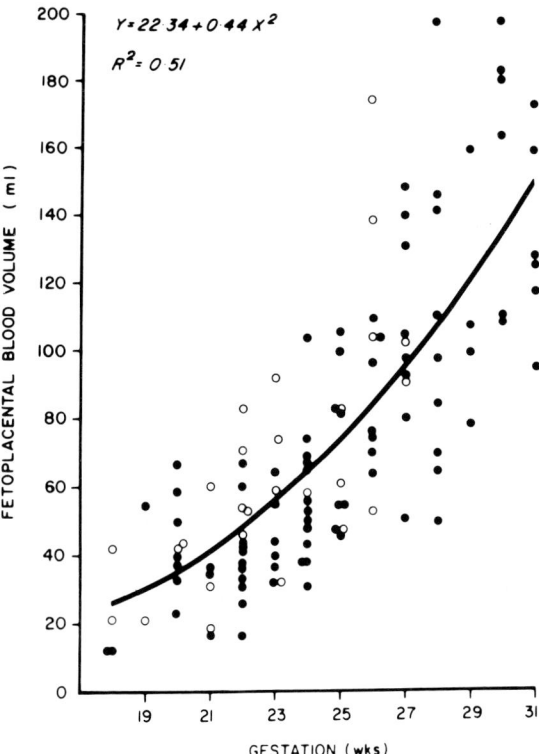

Fig. 6 Estimated fetoplacental blood volume. Open symbols represent hydropic fetuses.[34] From: Nicolaides KH et al: American Journal of Obstetrics and Gynecology 1987; 157:50. By kind permission of the authors and the publishers.

base excess, and lactate in the umbilical vein only.[35] The decrease in fetal Po_2 is compensated by the rise in fetal haemoglobin; the total oxygen content is therefore not modified by gestation (Fig. 8). Normal ranges for the mid-trimester fetus have been established. The fall in fetal Po_2 may be interpreted as proof of impairment of feto-maternal exchange with advancing pregnancy or of increased oxygen consumption by the feto-placental unit. The latter seems more likely, in view of a parallel decrease of Po_2 in the intervillous space and the increase in fetal base excess and bicarbonate which would be otherwise unexplained. The increase in lactate in the umbilical vein and not in the artery also supports this hypothesis and suggests that a larger amount of lactate is produced by the placenta in late pregnancy as a major substrate for the fetus.

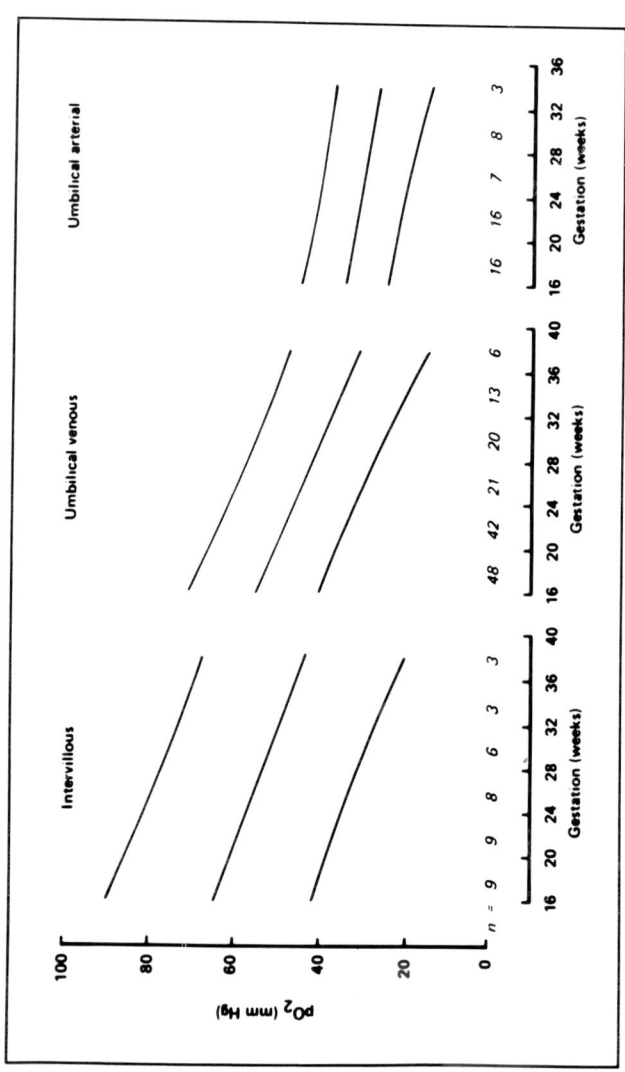

Fig. 7 Change of Po_2, with gestational age (mean and 95% confidence intervals) in intervillous, umbilical venous and arterial blood.[35] From: Soothill PW et al: Fetal Therapy 1986; 1:168. By kind permission of the publishers.

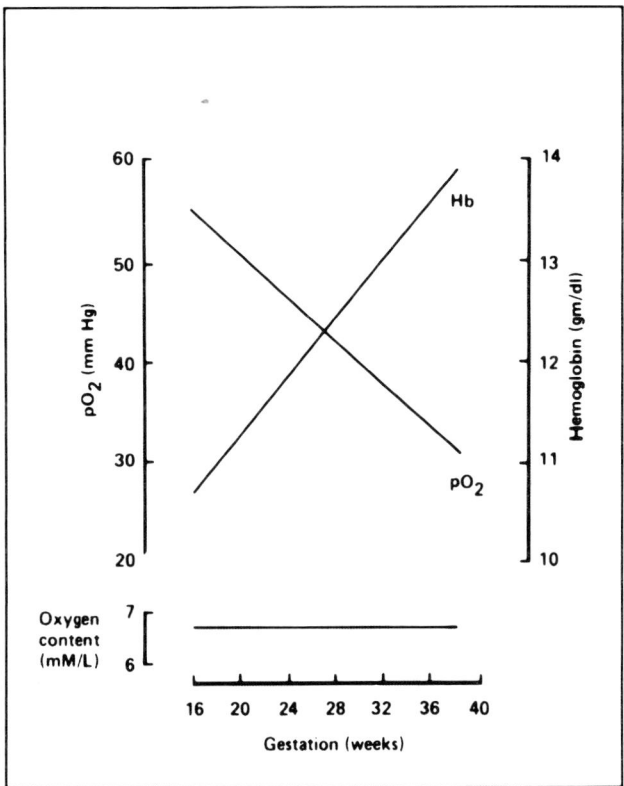

Fig. 8 The relationship between umbilical venous Po_2, Hb and oxygen content to gestation. The rise in Hb (r + 0.42, n = 117, $P < 0.0001$) and fall in umbilical venous Po_2 (Fig. 2) maintained a constant blood oxygen content (r = -0.02, n = 90, NS).[35] From: Soothill PW et al: Fetal Therapy 1986; 1:168. By kind permission of the publishers.

LUNGS

In the fetus, the lungs receive only 10% of total cardiac output. They secrete fluid which in the fetal lamb has been shown to have similar osmolality to fetal plasma, having however a higher concentration of Cl^- and a lower content of HCO_3^- and proteins.[36] The lung dimensions are difficult to evaluate precisely in vivo and are mainly studied indirectly by ultrasound. The ratio of fetal thoracic to abdominal circumference is the parameter mostly used. Linear growth has been demonstrated in this way, as a ratio of 0.89 remains constant throughout pregnancy.[5] Fetal breathing movements appear to be necessary to allow normal lung development as their inhibition by bilateral phrenectomy in lambs[37] and section of the cervical cord in fetal rabbits[38] cause severe hypoplastic changes. Fetal breathing movements have been extensively studied in the human by different techniques (Fig. 9). An increase in the percentage of time during which the fetus is breathing occurs with advancing gestational age. During apnoea there is a positive pressure inside the lungs compared with amniotic fluid, causing a net outflow of lung fluid. Amniotic fluid thus contains substances secreted by the lung tissue which can be studied to predict lung maturity. Normal ranges of different biochemical indices have been established. Figure 10 illustrates the changes in concentration of phosphatidylinositol and phosphatidylglycerol in the amniotic fluid after 20 weeks' gestation.[40]

KIDNEYS

The ratio of renal to abdominal circumference remains constant at 0.27–0.30 throughout pregnancy.[8] The functional maturation of the fetal kidney shows, however, a non-linear trend. The number of nephrons is in fact close to the final number at mid-gestation and nephrogenesis is complete at 34 weeks.[41] We (unpublished) have found major changes in the fetal urine with gestational age. Osmolality and the concentration of Na^+ and PO_4^{2-} decrease with advancing gestation. Na^+ decreases from a mean value of 100 mmol/l at 15 weeks to values below 60 after 25 weeks (Fig. 11); at this stage, PO_4^{2-} is always less than 0.5 mmol/l, while values up to 1.5 can be observed between 16 and 25 weeks. The urinary concentration of creatinine shows a positive correlation with gestational age. Values between 60 and 150 µmol/l are found in the mid-trimester and between 100 and 230 during the third trimester. No changes occur with gestation in the urinary concentration of urea (range = 4–14 µmol/l), K (range = 1–8 mmol/l) and Ca^{2+} (range = 0.05–1.4 mmol/l). These results suggest a progressive increase both in tubular reabsorption and in glomerular filtration rate. The latter is in contrast with observations in preterm newborns, in whom few changes occur in the glomerular filtration rate until the 34th week post-conception.[42]

As already mentioned, fetal urine production, as estimated by serial changes in bladder volume measured by ultrasound, increases with gestational age and so does the maximal bladder volume.[16]

In our studies of fetal bladder pressure, this was recorded in one

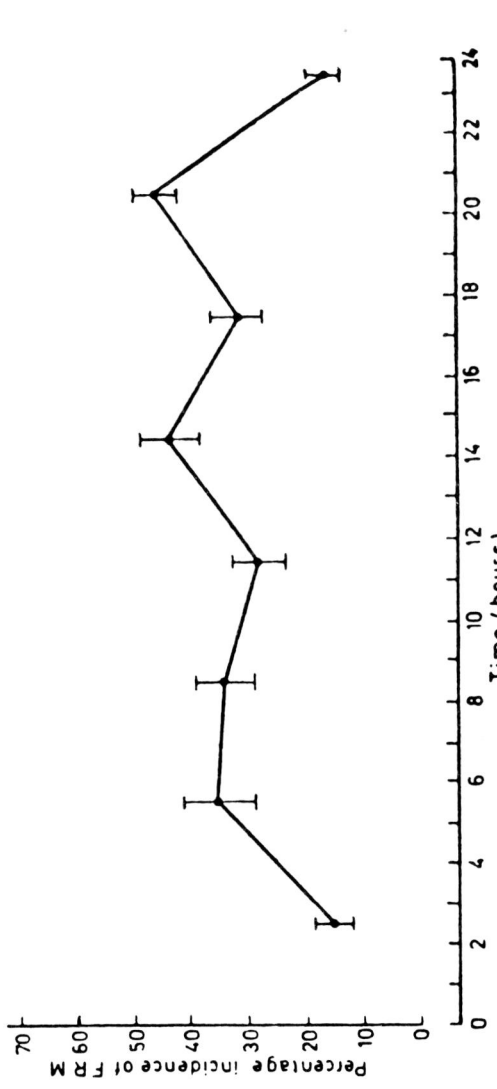

Fig. 9 The mean ± standard error of percentage incidence of fetal respiratory movements (FRM) in 21 normal fetuses over a 24 hour period.[39] From: Roberts A et al: British Journal of Obstetrics and Gynaecology 1979; 86:4. By kind permission of the authors and publishers.

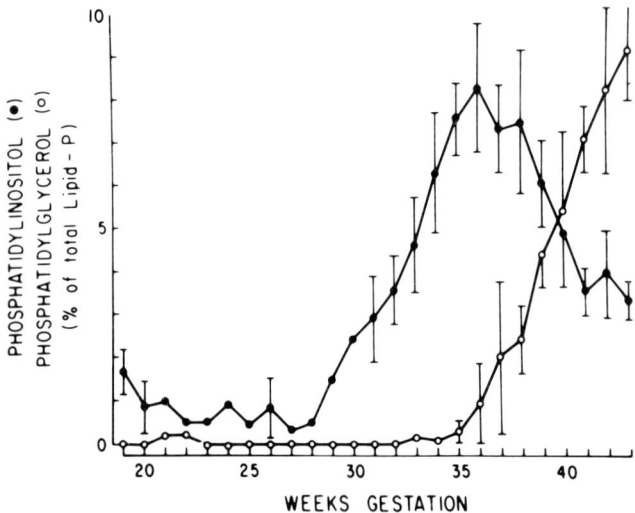

Fig. 10 Changes of phosphatidylglycerol and phosphatidylinositol in the amniotic fluid with gestation.[40] From: Hallman et al: American Journal of Obstetrics and Gynaecology 1976; 125:613. By kind permission of the authors and the publishers.

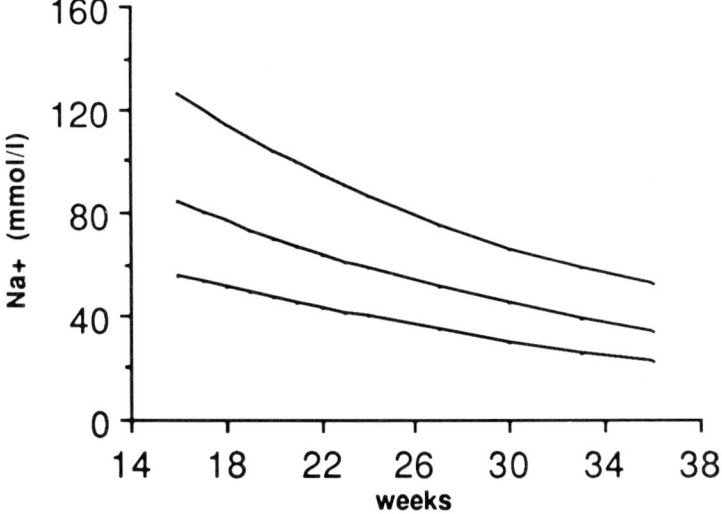

Fig. 11 Changes in concentration of Na^+ in fetal urine during gestation. (Nicolini and Rodeck, unpublished observations.)

patient at 26 weeks before an intraperitoneal transfusion. The pressure was 5 mmHg (~ 665 Pa), (3 mmHg (~ 400 Pa) above the intraabdominal pressure) and micturition was observed when the bladder pressure rose to 8 mmHg (~ 1 kPa). It is noteworthy that bladder pressure in cases of posterior urethral valves was comparable. Thus, renal dysplasia associated with obstructive uropathy is probably related to a relatively low, but continuous pressure in the bladder.

FETAL BLOOD

Normal ranges for haematological, biochemical, enzymatic and hormonal indices have been established in the fetus since a relatively easy approach to the fetal circulation has become available, initially by fetoscopy[43] and subsequently by transabdominal needling under ultrasonic guidance from the cord[44] or the intrahepatic tract of the umbilical vein.[45]

Haematology

Table 2 and Figure 12 illustrate changes in different haematological indices during the trimester. There is a positive correlation with gestational age for haemoglobin, haematocrit and red cell number. On the contrary, mean corpuscular volume, reticulocytes and nucleated red cells decrease significantly with gestational age. The myeloid series does not show any significant change apart from eosinophils and basophils which increase. The platelet count remains constant.

Table 2 Mean blood cell values in the mid-trimester fetus. From Daffos et al.[46] and Millar et al.[47]

Weeks	Red cells $\times 10^{12} \, l^{-1}$	White cells $\times 10^9 \, l^{-1}$	Platelets $\times 10^9 \, l^{-1}$	Haemoglobin g dl^{-1}	Haematocrit %
18	2.44	4.3	204	11.1	34.1
20	2.77	4.3	244	11.7	36.9
22	2.98	4.2	260	12.4	38.4
24	3.17	4.3	275	12.6	39.1
26	3.35	4.4	269	12.9	40.5
28	3.60	4.6	290	13.4	41.6

Weeks	Mean cell haemoglobin pg	Reticulocytes $\times 10^9 \, l^{-1}$	Nucleated red cells $\times 10^9 \, l^{-1}$
15	45.4	0.63	2.1
17	45.4	0.43	2.5
19	42.5	0.36	1.7
21	40.6	0.23	0.8

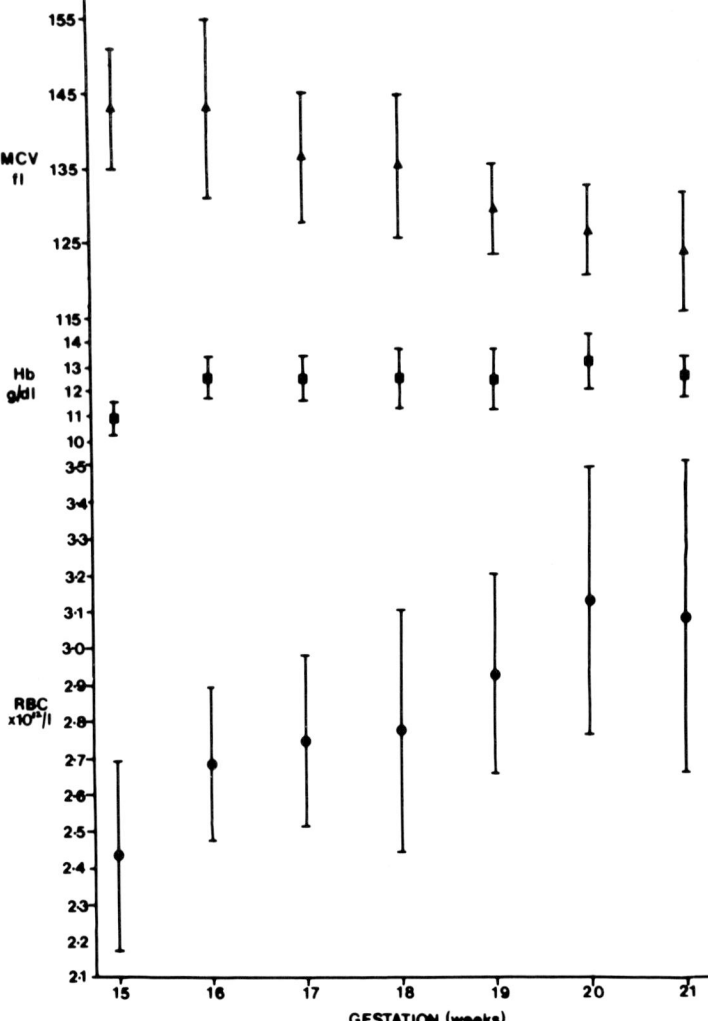

Fig. 12 The distribution (mean and S.D.) of mean cell volume (fl), haemoglobin concentration (g/dl) and red blood cell count ($\times 10^{12}/l$) in human fetal blood at 15–21 weeks gestation.[47] From: Millar DS et al: Prenatal Diagnosis 1985; 5:367. By kind permission of the publishers.

Coagulation

In Table 3 normal values for coagulation factors are reported.[48] Gestational age ranged between 18 and 22 weeks and no significant changes were found.

Table 3 Coagulation factors in the fetus between 18 and 22 weeks.[48] By courtesy of R S Mibashan and D S Millar

Assay	Unit	Mean	SD	Range
I	mg/dl	60	8.5	43–70
I:Ag	mg/dl	63	9.3	45–78
V:C	% of Norm.	56	9.4	45–76
VIII:C	u/dl	39	6.5	25–57
vWF:Ag	u/dl	58	10.3	51–79
II:C	% of Norm.	17	2.0	15–20
II:Ag	% of Norm.	17	1.5	15–20
VII:C	% of Norm.	20	2.8	14–24
IX:C	u/dl	9.1	1.5	5.9–11.8
IX:Ag	u/dl	4.3	1.7	1.7–8.2
X:C	% of Norm.	20	4.2	14–26
Protein C:Ag	% of Norm.	11	2.6	6–15
XI:C	% of Norm.	13	2.2	10–18
XII:C	% of Norm.	21	3.6	13–25
AT III	% of Norm.	29	5.3	20–41
AT III:Ag	% of Norm.	29	4.6	20–38
Plasminogen	% of Norm.	24	1.5	22–26

All haemostatic factors are reduced compared with adult normal values; as for the vitamin K-dependent factors, similar coagulant and antigen values support the hypothesis that these low values are due to a defect in the synthesis related to liver immaturity and not to a deficit of vitamin K.

Biochemistry

Most of the present knowledge of normal fetal biochemistry has been achieved through the research of two groups, one in London (Rodeck et al.), the other in Paris (Daffos et al.).

Table 4 summarizes normal values in fetal blood at different gestational ages and the relation to maternal values for several biochemical indices is also provided.[49,50] Maternal-fetal gradients may be used as an index of transplacental passage and have been reported to be altered in pathological conditions. The major differences between maternal and fetal values concern total protein content and albumin in particular; fetal levels of albumin reach maternal levels only around the 30th week (Fig. 13) and this increase parallels the fall in fetal alphafetoprotein (Fig. 14). On the contrary, phosphorus and bilirubin are found in higher concentration in the fetus than in the mother. Simultaneous measurements of venous and arterial umbilical blood could provide information

Table 4 Mean values for different biochemical indices. Derived from Moniz et al.[49] and Forrestier et al.[50]★

	Unit	Maternal blood	Fetal blood	Gestational age weeks
Sodium	mmol/l	135	136	15–22
		136	135.5	26–30
		136.5	135.5	31–38
Potassium	mmol/l	3.35	3.6	15–22
		3.45	3.55	26–30
		3.55	3.55	31–38
Urea	mmol/l	4.3	2.6	20–26★
		3.1	3.0	15–22
		2.95	3.2	26–30
		2.7	3.3	31–38
Creatinine	µmol/l	67	64	20–26★
		45	38.5	15–22
		43.5	42	26–30
		38.5	45	31–38
Calcium	mmol/l	2.27	2.25	20–26★
		2.38	2.18	15–22
		2.31	2.18	26–30
		2.24	2.35	31–38
Phosphate	mmol/l	1.09	1.13	15–22
		1.01	1.14	26–30
		1.00	1.10	31–38
Uric acid	µmol/l	215	167	20–26★
Bilirubin (total)	µmol/l	8.6	26.8	20–26★
		<10	11	15–22
		<10	14	26–30
		<10	23	31–38
Glucose	mmol/l	4.4	2.8	20–26★
Triglycerides	mmol/l	1.4	0.89	20–26★
Cholesterol	mmol/l	6.6	1.5	20–26★
Albumin	g/l	34.9	21.4	20–26★
		34	17	15–22
		33	26	23–30
		33	32	31–38
Total protein	g/l	69.6	30.4	20–26★
		63.5	28.5	15–22
		62.5	39.5	23–30
		60	51	31–38
Alkaline phosphatase	iu/l	60	197	20–26★
		83.5	144	15–22
		113	191	23–30
		125	263	31–38
Aspartate transaminase	iu/l	12.9	21.1	20–26★
		<10	15.5	15–22
		<10	20	23–30
		<10	22	31–38
Creatine kinase	iu/l	48	62	20–26★
Lactic dehydrogenase	iu/l	132	261	20–26★
Gamma-glutamyl transferase	iu/l	19	24.4	20–26★

PHYSIOLOGY OF THE MID-TRIMESTER FETUS 845

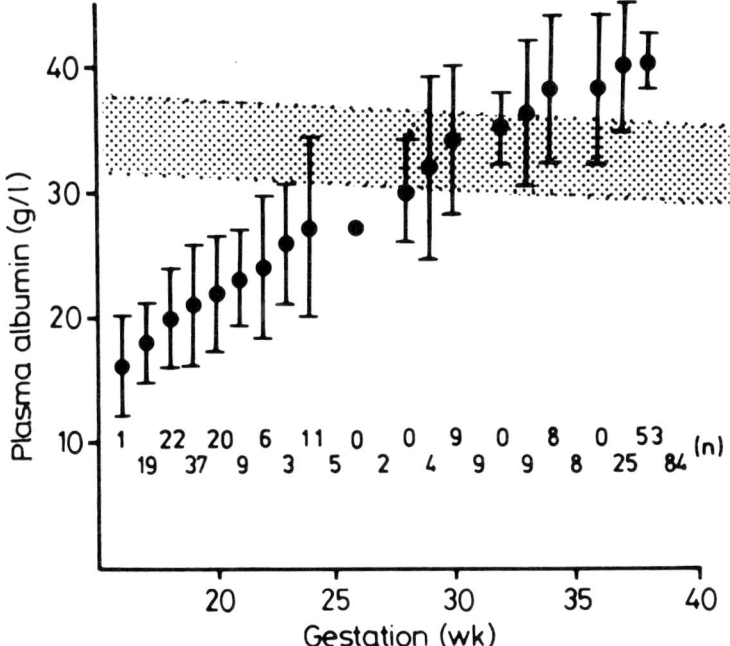

Fig. 13 Fetal plasma albumin concentration (mean 2 SD). Maternal range in shaded area.[49] From: Moniz CF et al: Journal of Clinical Pathology 38: 1985; 38:468.

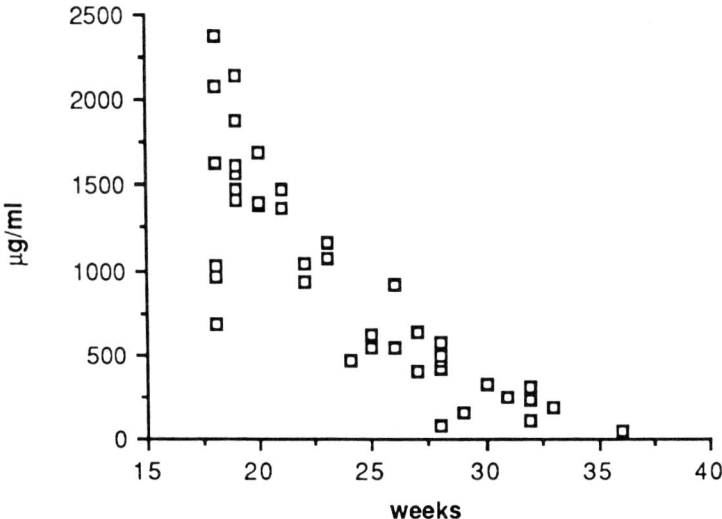

Fig. 14 Changes in fetal serum alphafetoprotein (AFP) with gestation. (Nicolini and Rodeck, unpublished observations.)

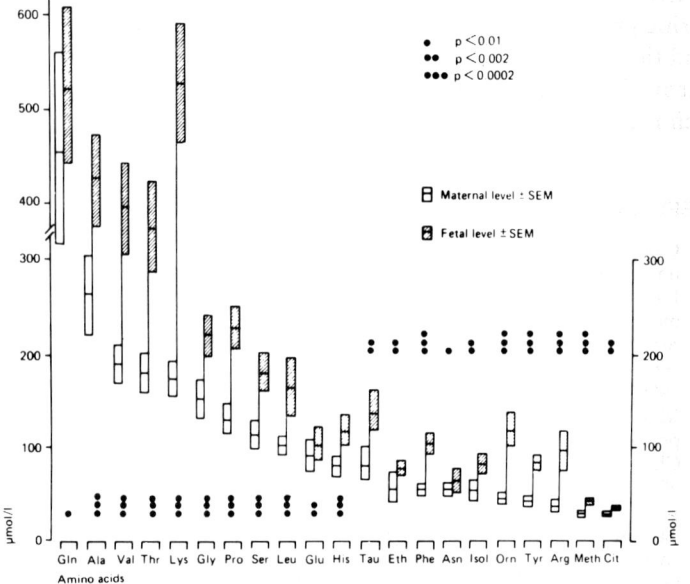

Fig. 15 Comparison of maternal venous plasma amino acids in descending order with fetal umbilical venous amino acids. Bars show mean ± SEM.[51] From: McIntosh N et al: Biology of the Neonate 1984; 45:218. By kind permission of the publishers.

on fetal uptake and synthesis. Unfortunately, this is not possible in the human except in rare circumstances. Data provided here refer to venous blood and reflect therefore mainly the efficiency of placental transfer. A typical example is the amino acids, which are higher in fetal than in maternal blood (Fig. 15)[51], but a positive umbilical venous-arterial gradient can be demonstrated at term.[52] Thus, higher fetal values are explained in this instance mainly by an active mechanism of transplacental passage.

CONCLUSION

Fetal medicine has grown out of its infancy. Continuous recording of fetal heart rate and blood sampling from the scalp in labour were the first techniques for evaluating fetal wellbeing in utero. The body of knowledge acquired in the last ten years now covers several aspects of fetal physiology throughout the whole of gestation. This has been the basis for the diagnosis of congenital diseases, for more effective treatment of pathologies such as feto-maternal alloimmunization,[53] for better management of intrauterine growth retardation[54] and is the prelude to other diagnostic and therapeutic approaches to the fetus from early development to birth. The continuum between obstetrics and neonatology is being defined and perinatal medicine is therefore a reality.

REFERENCES

1 Campbell S, Newman GB. Growth of the fetal biparietal diameter during normal pregnancy. Br J Obstet Gynaecol 1971; 78: 513
2 Hadlock FP, Deter RL, Harrist RB. Fetal head circumference: Relation to menstrual age. Am J Roentgenol 1982; 136: 649
3 Smith PA, Johansson D, Tzannatos C et al. Prenatal measurement of the fetal cerebellum and cysterna cerebello-medullaris by ultrasound. Prenat Diagn 1986; 6: 133
4 Mayden K, Tortora M, Berkowitz RL. Orbital diameters: A new parameter for prenatal diagnosis and dating. Am J Obstet Gynecol 1982; 144: 289
5 Chitkara U, Rosenberg J, Chervenak FA et al. Prenatal sonographic assessment of the fetal thorax: normal values. Am J Obstet Gynecol 1987; 156: 1069
6 Jeanty P, Romero R. Obstetrical Ultrasound. New York: McGraw-Hill, 1984
7 Campbell S, Wilkin D. Ultrasonic measurement of fetal abdomen circumference in the evaluation of fetal weight. Br J Obstet Gynaecol 1975; 82: 689
8 Grannum PAT, Bracken M, Silverman R, Hobbins JC. Assessment of fetal kidney size in normal gestation by comparison of kidney circumference to abdominal circumference ratio. Am J Obstet Gynecol 1980; 136: 294
9 Hohler CW, Quetel TA. Femur length: Equations for computer calculation of gestational age from ultrasound measurements. Am J Obstet Gynecol 1982; 143: 479
10 Queenan JT, O'Brien GB, Campbell S. Ultrasonic measurement of the fetal limb bones. Am J Obstet Gynecol 1980; 138: 287
11 Deter RL, Harrist LB, Hadlock FP et al. Longitudinal studies of fetal growth with the use of dynamic image ultrasonography. Am J Obstet Gynecol 1982; 143: 545
12 Deter RL, Rossavik IK, Harrist RB et al. Mathematical modelling of fetal growth: Development of individual growth curve standards. Obstet Gynecol 1986; 66: 156
13 Rossavik IK, Deter RL, Hadlock FP. Mathematical modelling of fetal growth. IV. Evaluation of trunk growth using the abdominal profile area. J Clin Ultrasound 1987; 15: 31
14 Todros T, Ferrazzi E, Groli C et al. Fitting growth curves to head and abdomen measurements of the fetus: A multicentric study. J Clin Ultrasound 1987; 15: 95
15 Abramovich DR. Fetal factors influencing the volume and composition of liquor amnii. J Obstet Gynaecol Br Commonw 1970; 77: 865
16 Campbell S, Wladimiroff JW, Dewhurst CJ. The antenatal measurement of fetal urine production. J Obstet Gynaecol Br Commonw 1973; 80: 686
17 Abramovich DR, Garden A, Jandial L et al. Fetal swallowing and voiding in relation to hydramnios. Obstet Gynecol 1979; 54: 15
18 Queenan JT, Thompson W, Whitfield CR, Shah SI. Amniotic fluid volumes in normal pregnancies. Am J Obstet Gynecol 1972; 114: 34
19 Hutchinson DL, Hunter CB, Neslen ED et al. The exchange of water and electrolytes in the mechanism of amniotic fluid formation and the relationship to hydramnios. Surg Gynecol Obstet 1955; 100: 391

20 Seeds AE. Current concepts of amniotic fluid dynamics. Am J Obstet Gynecol 1980; 138: 575
21 Seeds AE, Koch HC, Myers RE, Stolte LAM, Hellegers AE. Changes in rhesus monkey amniotic fluid pH, $P\text{co}_2$ and bicarbonate concentration following maternal and fetal hypercarbia and fetal death in utero. Am J Obstet Gynecol 1967; 97: 67
22 Abramovich DR, Page KR. Pathways of water transfer between liquor amnii and the feto-placental unit at term. Eur J Obstet Gynecol 1973; 3: 155
23 Dallaire L, Potier M. Amniotic fluid. In: Milunsky A, ed. Genetic disorders and the fetus. New York: Plenum Press, 1986: p. 53
24 Druzin ML, Hutson JM, Edersheim TG. Relationship of baseline fetal heart rate to gestational age and fetal sex. Am J Obstet Gynecol 1986; 154: 1102
25 Patrick J, Campbell K, Carmichael L, Natale R, Richardson B. Daily relationships between fetal and maternal heart rates at 38 to 40 weeks of pregnancy. Can Med Assoc J 1981; 124: 1177
26 Smith CV, Phelan JP, Paul RH. A prospective analysis of the influence of gestational age on the baseline fetal heart rate and reactivity in a low risk population. Am J Obstet Gynecol 1985; 153: 780
27 Natale R, Nasello-Paterson C, Turliuk R. Longitudinal measurements of fetal breathing, body movements, heart rate, and heart rate accelerations and decelerations at 24 to 32 weeks gestation. Am J Obstet Gynecol 1985; 151: 256
28 Dierker LJ, Pillay SK, Sorokin Y, Rosen MG. Active and quiet periods in the preterm and term fetus. Obstet Gynecol 1982; 60: 65
29 Pearce JM, Campbell S, Cohen-Overbeek T, Hackett G, Hernandez J, Royston JP. References ranges and sources of variation for indices of pulsed Doppler flow velocity waveforms from the utero-placental and fetal circulation. Br J Obstet Gynaecol 1988; 95: 248
30 Rudolph AM, Heymann MA. Circulatory changes during growth in the fetal lamb. Circ Res 1970; 26: 289
31 Castle BM, MacKenzie IZ. In vivo observations on intravascular blood pressure in the fetus during mid-pregnancy. In: Rolfe P, ed. Fetal physiological measurements. London: Butterworths, 1986: p. 65
32 Nicolini U, Talbert GB, Fisk NM, Rodeck CH. Pathophysiology of pressure changes during intrauterine transfusion. 1988 (submitted for publication)
33 Weismann DN, Robillard JE. Renal haemodynamic responses to hypoxemia during development: Relationships to circulating vasoactive substances. Pediatr Res 1988; 23: 155
34 Nicolaides KH, Clewell WH, Rodeck CH. Measurement of human fetoplacental blood volume in erythroblastosis fetalis. Am J Obstet Gynecol 1987; 157: 50
35 Soothill PW, Nicolaides KH, Rodeck CH, Campbell S. Effect of gestational age on fetal and intervillous blood gas and acid-base values in human pregnancy. Fetal Therapy 1986; 1: 168
36 Strang LB. Neonatal respiration—Physiological and clinical studies. Oxford: Blackwell, 1977
37 Fewell JE, Lee CC, Kitterman JA. Effects of phrenic nerve section on the respiratory function of fetal lambs. J Appl Physiol 1981; 51: 293
38 Wigglesworth JS, Desai R. Effects on lung growth of cervical cord section in the rabbit fetus. Early Hum Dev 1980; 3: 51
39 Roberts AB, Little D, Cooper D, Campbell S. Normal patterns of fetal activity in the third trimester. Br J Obstet Gynaecol 1979; 86: 4
40 Hallman M, Kulovich M, Kirkpatrick E, Sugarman RG, Gluck L. Phosphatidylinositol and phosphatidylglycerol in amniotic fluid: Indices of lung maturity. Am J Obstet Gynecol 1976; 125: 613
41 Potter EL, Thierstein ST. Glomerular development in the kidney as an index of fetal maturity. J Pediatr 1943; 22: 695

42 Arant BS. Developmental patterns of renal functional maturation compared in the neonate. J Pediatr 1978; 92: 705
43 Rodeck CH, Campbell S. Sampling pure fetal blood by fetoscopy in second trimester of pregnancy. Br Med J 1978; 2: 728
44 Daffos F, Capella-Pavlovsky M, Forestier F. Fetal blood sampling during pregnancy with use of a needle guided by ultrasound: A study of 606 consecutive cases. Am J Obstet Gynecol 1985; 153: 655
45 Bang J, Bock TE, Trolle D. Ultrasound-guided fetal intravenous transfusion for severe rhesus haemolytic disease. Br Med J 1982; 284: 373
46 Daffos F, Forestier F. Medicine et biologie du foetus humaine. Paris: Maloine, 1988
47 Millar DS, Davis LR, Rodeck CH, Nicolaides KH, Mibashan RS. Normal blood cell values in the early mid-trimester fetus. Prenat Diagn 1985; 5: 367
48 Millar DS, Mibashan RS, Rodeck CH, Nicolaides KH. Coagulation in the normal human mid-trimester fetus. Prenat Diagn 1988 (In press)
49 Moniz CF, Nicolaides KH, Bamforth FJ, Rodeck CH. Normal reference ranges for biochemical substances relating to renal, hepatic, and bone function in fetal and maternal plasma throughout pregnancy. J Clin Pathol 1985; 38: 468
50 Forestier F, Daffos F, Rainout M, Bruneau M, Trivin F. Blood chemistry of normal human fetuses at mid-trimester of pregnancy. Pediatr Res 1987; 21: 579
51 McIntosh N, Rodeck CH, Heath R. Plasma amino acids of the mid-trimester human fetus. Biol Neonate 1984; 45: 218
52 Hayashi S, Sanada K, Sagawa N, Yamada N, Kido K. Umbilical vein-artery differences of plasma amino acids in the last trimester of human pregnancy. Biol Neonate 1978; 34: 8
53 Rodeck CH, Nicolaides KH, Warsof SL, Fysh WJ, Gamsu HR, Kemp JR. The management of severe rhesus isoimmunization by fetoscopic intravascular transfusions. Am J Obstet Gynecol 1984; 150: 769
54 Nicolaides KH, Soothill PW, Rodeck KH, Campbell S. Ultrasound-guided sampling of the umbilical cord and placental blood sampling to assess fetal wellbeing. Lancet 1986; i: 283

Extreme prematurity: The aetiology of preterm delivery

Philip R Bennett
Queen Charlotte's Maternity Hospital, London

Murdoch G Elder
Institute of Obstetrics and Gynaecology, Hammersmith Hospital, London

> Preterm delivery will follow either a decision to terminate the pregnancy before term for fetal or maternal reasons, or spontaneous preterm labour. A number of previously more important causes of prematurity have declined in incidence due either to improvements in prevention or treatment of the problem. Rhesus haemolytic disease of the newborn is now relatively rare and all severe cases should be managed in specialist centres. The introduction of prophylactic measures, such as the administration of anti-D globulin, and the success of intraperitoneal or intravascular fetal transfusion techniques has greatly reduced the frequency of the disease as a cause of extreme prematurity. Severe pre-existing maternal diseases—for example hypertension, chronic renal disease or systemic lupus—still account for a small number of preterm deliveries. With improvements in the management of pregnancy in diabetics and those with gestational diabetes, including the introduction of specialist clinics and home monitoring of blood glucose concentrations, there is rarely a need for very preterm delivery in this group. Most infants in neonatal units today will have been delivered following: severe pre-eclampsia; intrauterine growth retardation; antepartum haemorrhage; or spontaneous preterm labour.

PRE-ECLAMPSIA AND INTRAUTERINE FETAL GROWTH RETARDATION

It is probable that severe intrauterine growth retardation and pre-eclampsia share some common aetiological factors. Severe growth retardation is uncommon without pre-eclampsia and severe pre-eclampsia is rarely associated with a normally grown fetus. Pre-eclampsia occurs more frequently in primigravid women or in those who have a new sexual partner. It is also more common in those with pre-existing hypertension, multiple pregnancy, immunological disease, or a hydatidiform mole. The syndrome is of hypertension, oedema and proteinuria. As its severity increases placental and renal function become further impaired and cerebral oedema causes hyper-reflexia. The condition may go on to become eclampsia, characterised by generalised grand-mal type fits, and severe hypertension may cause placental and cerebral vascular accidents.

Termination of the pregnancy brings pre-eclampsia to an end. This gave rise to the old concept that the condition results from circulating toxins originating in the placenta and to the old name of pre-eclamptic toxaemia. No toxin was ever identified and the name is now falling into disuse.

There appears to be a significant familial factor in the aetiology of pre-eclampsia. Chesley et al.[1] have observed an incidence of recurrence of the disease in the daughters and grand-daughters of women with severe pre-eclampsia which is consistent with it having autosomal recessive inheritance. The increased incidence in primigravid women, those with new sexual partners and those whose partners express similar major histocompatibility antigens, suggests a role for the immune system in the aetiology of pre-eclampsia. Many major issues concerning the interactions between trophoblast and the maternal immune system remain unsolved. It appears that villous trophoblast does not express antigens of the major histocompatibility complex although extravillous trophoblast expresses a number of immunologically distinguishable surface antigens including histocompatibility and ABO antigens. Pre-eclampsia may result from development of hostile antitrophoblast maternal antibodies but several studies have failed to demonstrate a rise in antiHLA antibodies.[2,3] Similarly studies of maternal lymphocyte function or circulating immune complex levels have not demonstrated differences between normal and pre-eclamptic pregnancies.[4,5] There is evidence, however, for the deposition of IgG, IgM and fibrin in the kidneys of pre-eclamptic women.[6] An attractive theory is that the basic immunological defect in pre-eclampsia is a failure in the development of protective antibodies. This would explain the increased incidence in couples who share histocompatibility antigens, a group who also experience a high rate of early pregnancy loss, and also the improvement in pregnancy outcome following maternal sensitisation by injection of paternal leucocytes.[7] It would also explain the apparent protective effect of prior blood transfusion.

Histological studies of the placenta and placental bed have demonstrated that pre-eclampsia is associated with abnormal placentation. During normal early placentation extravillous trophoblast invades the lumen of the decidual portion of the spiral arteries replacing the maternal endothelial cells, destroying musculoelastic tissue and reducing resistance to blood flow. A second wave of trophoblast invasion occurs at between 14 and 20 weeks into the myometrial portions of the arteries causing similar changes and a further reduction in vascular resistance. In women who develop pre-eclampsia this second wave of trophoblast invasion does not seem to occur, the spiral arteries do not dilate as pregnancy advances, blood flow to the uterus is inadequate and fetal growth is impaired.[8] The histological appearances of the spiral arteries in pre-eclampsia are similar to those seen in association with rejected renal transplants suggesting that there may be an immunological mechanism.[9] Similar abnormalities have been described in women who bear severely growth retarded infants but who do not exhibit signs of pre-eclampsia. The use of Doppler ultrasound studies which assess patterns of blood flow in the uteroplacental vessels during the second trimester may prove to be useful in predicting pregnancies at risk.

Abnormal platelet behaviour may be another aetiological factor in pre-eclampsia, initiating occlusion of the spiral arteries supplying the placental bed. Excessive platelet aggregates precede fibrin deposition and reduction in the lumen of the vessel. Thrombocytopaenia occurs in severe pre-eclampsia and even if there is only a slight reduction in platelet count there is an increase in the proportion of immature platelets indicating an increased turnover. Platelet function, as determined by their ability to respond to aggregatory stimuli in vitro, is diminished in pre-eclampsia.[10,11] This process appears to precede the appearance of the clinical signs of moderate to severe pre-eclampsia.[12] This could be due to platelets that have already been involved in an aggregatory process, disaggregating and recirculating. At present this is speculation rather than fact.

In normal pregnancy there is an increase in cardiac output but a decrease in total peripheral vascular resistance. Despite an increase in angiotensin II levels there is a reduction in blood pressure especially during the second trimester. Gant et al.[13]

demonstrated a loss of the refractoriness to angiotensin II in women who develop pre-eclampsia before the condition becomes clinically manifest. This has led to the development of the angiotensin sensitivity test, in which the need to infuse significantly reduced amounts of angiotensin to cause a 20 mmHg rise in blood pressure in early pregnancy accurately predicts the onset of pre-eclampsia in up to 50% of subjects, whereas in those destined for a normal pregnancy, much larger concentrations of angiotensin are needed to cause a similar rise.

There is evidence that the refractoriness of the vasopressor effects of angiotensin II seen in normal pregnancy is mediated by prostaglandins. Ingestion of prostaglandin synthesis inhibitors abolishes this refractoriness[14] and a similar effect can be seen in animals taking a diet deficient in prostaglandin precursors.[15] Infusion of prostaglandin E_2 into pregnant women further blunts their vasopressor response to angiotensin II.[16]

It is becoming apparent that prostaglandin synthesis is abnormal in women with pre-eclampsia. Urinary prostaglandin E_2 levels rise during pregnancy but in pre-eclampsia the rise is less marked.[17] More importantly, pre-eclampsia appears to be associated with a relative deficiency of prostacyclin (prostaglandin I_2) production. This compound is a potent vasodilator and inhibits platelet aggregation. It counteracts the effects of thromboxane A_2 which is a powerful vasopressor and platelet aggregatory substance. Several studies have demonstrated reduced production of prostacyclin by placental, fetal and maternal tissues in pre-eclampsia and fetal intrauterine growth retardation, with reduced circulating levels and urinary excretion.[18,19] Many of the signs of pre-eclampsia can be explained by alteration in prostaglandin synthesis and in particular, the balance between prostacyclin and thromboxane. Hypertension may be due to failure to protect against the effects of normally elevated angiotensin II. The already poor uteroplacental circulation may be further compromised by an increase in vascular tone and the formation of thrombi within it. If severe placental infarction occurs release of thromboxane could lead to further thrombus formation, further infarction, disseminated intravascular coagulation and acute episodes of more severe hypertension. In addition to changes on the maternal side of the placenta Remuzzi et al.[20] have found that prostacyclin production by fetal umbilical vessels is impaired in pre-eclampsia. Glance et al[21] have shown that vasodilator prostaglandins antagonise the vasopressor effect of angiotensin II in the fetoplacental circulation in vitro. It is possible that the increase in placental resistance to fetal blood flow in severe growth retardation, seen in Doppler ultrasound studies as increased pulsatility or reversal of flow in diastole, may be mediated by a reduction in local prostacyclin synthesis.

Reduced prostacyclin production may be associated with redirection of metabolism of its precursor arachidonic acid via the cyclo-oxygenase enzyme to other compounds possibly leading to an increase in thromboxane synthesis. There may also be increased metabolism via the lipoxygenase enzyme to leukotrienes and other hydroxy-eicosanoids. These compounds have been found to be circulating in elevated levels in women with pre-eclampsia.[22] Their actions include the ability to modulate capillary permiability and to cause oedema, a fundamental sign of pre-eclampsia. 15-hydroxyeicosatetraenoic acid is known to be an inhibitor of prostacyclin formation. Interestingly systemic lupus, strongly associated with pregnancy loss including that from pre-eclampsia, is known to cause inhibition of prostacyclin synthesis, and its associated microangiopathy is similar to that of pre-eclampsia.[23] There is growing evidence that the therapeutic use of compounds which modulate the prostacyclin:thromboxane ratio—such as low dose aspirin, or dipyridamole—may improve the outcome in pregnancies complicated by pre-eclampsia.[24,25]

ANTEPARTUM HAEMORRHAGE

The two major causes of antepartum haemorrhage are placental abruption and placenta praevia. Placental abruption is the premature separation of the placenta before or during labour. Its consequences will depend upon the degree of separation. Whilst a small abruption may go almost unnoticed, a major abruption will result in massive intrauterine maternal blood loss and places the lives of both mother and fetus at risk. The aetiology of placental abruption remains essentially unknown. There appears to be a relationship between abruption and maternal age, parity and socioeconomic status. There are isolated reports of placental abruption in association with severe abdominal injury following assault or a road traffic accident.[26] Placental separation following sudden decompression of polyhydramnios has been described, as has abruption associated with attempts at external cephalic version.[27]

Maternal folate deficiency was once thought to be an important aetiological factor in placental abruption,[27] but later work has failed to support this theory.[28] It has been suggested that preconception folate deficiency may be of importance.[29] This may explain the decreasing incidence of the condition in the Western World as general maternal health improves.

There is an association between maternal hypertensive diseases and placental abruption. There remains controversy as to cause and effect. Naeye et al.[30] suggest that abruption occurs before hypertension and that the hypertension is a consequence and not a cause of abruption. However, the initiating event in abruption appears to be uterine vasospasm and subsequent relaxation causing vascular engorgement, arteriolar rupture and placental infarction.[29] These events are similar to those seen in the pathology of pre-eclampsia and the consequent hypertension may be due to the release of vasoactive substances from the infarcted placenta. Furthermore there appears to be an association between placental abruption and elevated maternal alpha feto protein levels.[29] This suggests that the primary event is abnormal placentation and that the stage is set for abruption earlier than might otherwise be thought.

Placenta praevia is the attachment of the placenta to the uterus within the lower uterine segment. As the lower segment enlarges and the cervix effaces towards the end of pregnancy there is a tendency for the placenta to shear off. The more centrally it is placed over the cervical os the earlier the bleeding and the greater is the blood loss. Placenta praevia is presumed to be a consequence of implantation of the blastocyst into the lower part of the uterus. It is more likely therefore to occur in cases of multiple pregnancy and when the placenta is unusually large as in placenta membranacea.

PRETERM LABOUR

Preterm labour remains a significant problem in obstetric practice. It accounts for up to 10% of all births but 85% of perinatal deaths in otherwise normal babies.[31] There are associations between preterm labour and maternal age, weight, small stature, high parity, low social and poor nutritional status. Previous recurrent abortion, whether spontaneous or induced and previous preterm labour are indicators that a subsequent pregnancy may end with preterm delivery. Complications of pregnancy, including antepartum haemorrhage, hypertension, multiple pregnancy and congenital malformations are all associated with the onset of labour before term. None of these factors is, however, directly implicated as a cause of preterm labour. Despite the presence of more than one of these factors the prediction of preterm labour in a subsequent pregnancy is unreliable.

It has recently become apparent that infection or abnormal colonisation of the maternal genital tract may be an important factor in the aetiology of preterm labour. Most of the evidence implicating infection as a cause of preterm labour is based on two observations. Firstly all types of infection consequent to ascending genital bacterial invasion namely chorioamnionitis, neonatal sepsis and maternal endometritis are more commonly found after preterm birth. Secondly certain organisms in the vaginal flora are more often found in women with preterm premature rupture of membranes.[32]

A full understanding of the mechanisms by which preterm labour may be initiated will only be gained when the mechanism of the onset of labour at term is fully understood. Although it is clear that fetal signals control the onset of parturition in certain animals through changes in the activity of the pituitary-adrenal axis evidence for this in man is lacking. There is good evidence that prostaglandins play a central role in the process of human parturition. Prostaglandins are used in the induction of labour or abortion, and inhibitors of prostaglandin synthesis, such as indomethacin, will delay or stop labour. Prostaglandin and prostaglandin metabolite levels rise significantly in amniotic fluid before labour and in serum during labour and certain prostaglandins are known to be powerful oxytocic substances. There is now a large body of evidence to support the theory that labour at term is initiated by an increase in the synthesis of prostaglandins, in particular prostaglandin E_2 by either the fetal membranes or the decidua—although the stimulus to this increase has not yet been established.

Although bacteria do not themselves synthesise prostaglandins genital tract infection is associated with an inflammatory response. Leukocytes are highly active in the synthesis of prostaglandins and of other arachidonic acid metabolites, such as the leukotrienes.[33] This alone may be sufficient to initiate labour. Leukocytes have also been found to release substances which stimulate prostaglandin synthesis in other tissues. Polymorphonuclear leukocytes from patients with rheumatoid arthritis cause an increase in synthesis of prostaglandins by synovial cells in culture[34] and monocytes activated by addition of bacterial endotoxins release interleukin 1 which stimulates prostaglandin synthesis in amnion cells in culture.[35]

Common bacterial pathogens have been shown to release substances which stimulate arachidonic acid metabolism in amnion cells. If amnion cells are collected at elective caesarean section at term, before labour, and established in culture they metabolise endogenous arachidonic acid to a range of lopoxygenase enzyme products and synthesize little if any prostaglandins. The roles of these lipoxgenase enzyme products have not been established clearly although 5-hydroxyeicosatetraenioc is weakly oxytocic[36] and may be the mediator of Braxton-Hicks contractions. If amnion cells are established in culture following spontaneous vaginal delivery arachidonic acid metabolism is markedly increased and there is a change in the ratio of cyclo-oxygenase to lipoxygenase enzyme activity, such that prostaglandin E_2 synthesis is greatly increased. Addition of bacterial products to amnion cell cultures established before labour causes an increase in arachidonic acid metabolism similar to that seen in association with spontaneous labour.[37] Phospholipase A_2 is the enzyme which releases the prostaglandin precursor arachidonic acid from esterification in cell membrane phospholipids and makes it available for metabolism. Addition of phospholipase A_2 to these amnion cell cultures produces an effect similar to those seen prior to labour. Bacteria are known to possess phospholipase activity.[38] Therefore it is possible that it is by release of that enzyme that genital tract pathogens may stimulate prostaglandin synthesis in the fetal membranes and thereby initiate preterm labour.

Dilation of the cervix for curettage or to procure abortion may damage the cervix sufficiently to cause incompetence. Some studies[39] have shown an increase in the risk of preterm delivery following induced abortion. The World Health Organization collaborative study (1979) found an association between abortion and subsequent preterm delivery in some European cities but not in others. It is probable that the greatest risk is following excessive dilatation of the cervix at late termination of pregnancy and that gentle moderate dilatation and vacuum evacuation confers little risk. It appears that there is an increase in the incidence of preterm labour following cone biopsy of the cervix.[40] Cervical incompetence classically results in midtrimester abortion in which the pregancy is lost with minimal uterine activity. It is possible, however, that a minor degree of incompetence of the internal os might result in funneling and distortion of the fetal membranes within the cervical canal, and the release of prostaglandins from the membranes and the cervix itself. This might then initiate the cascade of prostaglandin synthesis associated with early labour and lead to the onset of uterine contractions and preterm delivery.

Multiple pregnancy and polyhydramnios are associated with preterm delivery. This may be simply a consequence of overdistention of the uterus stimulating prostaglandin synthesis in the fetal membranes, decidua or myometrium. Although the factor responsible for the initiation of labour at term is yet undiscovered it is highly likely to be fetal in origin. It is possible that such a factor would come into play earlier in the case of a multiple pregnancy.

Once the mechanism of the onset of parturition in man has become more fully understood it may be possible to reliably predict and prevent preterm labour. Multiple pregnancy can never be completely eradicated. Although a twin pregnancy is usually associated with a good outcome, fetal numbers in excess of two are often associated with extreme prematurity. With improved monitoring during ovulation induction regimens iatrogenic multiple pregnancies should become less common. Whether cervical cerclage confers any benefit where cervical incompetence is suspected is currently being examined by a major multicentre trial. Routine bacteriological examination of the genital tract in pregnancy may allow prediction of early parturition in some cases. An important factor in protection of the vagina from infection is the maintenance of an acidic environment hostile to most microorganisms. It is possible that the simple measurement of vaginal pH which increases in the presence of abnormal bacterial colonisation may have a predictive value. These organisms can release phospholipase A_z and could alter membrane arachidonic acid metabolism significantly whilst the lactobacillus, thought to be important in maintaining vaginal acidity has no effect on prostaglandin production within the uterus (Bennett et al. 1988—unpublished observations.[41])

REFERENCES

1 Chesley LC, Annito JE, Cosgrove RA. The familial factor in toxaemia of pregnancy. Obstet Gynecol 1963; 32: 303
2 Scott JS, Jenkins DM. Immunogenic factors in the aetiology of pre-eclampsia. J Med Genetics 1976; 13: 200
3 Jenkins DM, Need JA, Rajah SM. Deficiency of specific HLA antibodies in severe pregnancy toxaemia. Clin Exp Immunol 1977; 27: 485

4 Petrucco OM, Thompson NM, Lawrence JR, Weldon MW. Immunofluorescent studies in renal biopsies in pre-eclampsia. Br Med J 1978; 1: 473
5 Knox FG, Stagno S, Volanakis JE, Huddleston JF. A search for antigen antibody complexes in pre-eclampsia; further evidence against immunological pathogenesis. Am J obstet Gynecol 1978; 132: 87
6 Petrucco OM. Aetiology of pre-eclampsia. In: Studd J, ed. Progress in Obstetrics and Gynaecology, Vol 1, London: Churchill Livingstone, 1981
7 Taylor C, Faulk WP. Prevention of recurrent abortion with paternal leukocyte transfusions. Lancet 1981; ii: 68
8 Robertson WB, Brosens I, Dixon HG. Maternal blood supply and fetal growth retardation. In: van Assche FA, Robinson WB, eds. Fetal growth retardation. Edinburgh: Churchill Livingstone, 1981
9 Robertson WB, Brosens I and Dixon HG (1975) Uteroplacental vascular pathology. Eur J Obstet Gynecol Reprod Biol 1975; 5: 47
10 Howie PW, Prentice CRM, McNicol GT. Co-agulation fibrynolysis and platelet function in pre-eclampsia essential hypertension and plancental insufficiency. Journal Obstet Gynecol Brit Com 1971; 78: 992–1003
11 Whigham KA, Howie PW, Drummond AH, Prentice CRM. Abnormal platelet function in pre-eclampsia. B.J. Obstet Gynecol 1978; 85: 1 28–32
12 Lennon A, Sullivan M, Elder MG. Platelet function in pre-eclampsia. 1988 (Unpublished observations)
13 Gant NF, Daley GL, Chad S, Whalley PJ, McDonald PC. A study of angiotensin II pressor response throughout primigravid pregnancy. J Clinic Invest 1973; 52: 2682
14 Everett RB, Worley RJ, McDonald PC, Gant NF. Effects of prostaglandin synthetase inhibitors on the pressor response to angiotensin II in human pregnancy. J Clin Endocrinol Metab 1978; 46: 1007
15 O'Brian PMS, Broughton Pipkin F. The effects of deprivation of prostaglandin precursors on vascular sensitivity to angiotensin II and on the kidney in the pregnant rabbit. Br J Pharmacol 1979; 65: 29
16 Broughton Pipkin F, Hunter JC, Turner SR, O'Brian PMS. Prostaglandin E_2 attenuates the pressor response to angiotensin in pregnant subjects but not in non pregnant subjects. Am J Obstet Gynecol 1982; 142: 168
17 Pedersen EB, Christiensen NJ, Christiensen P. Pre-eclampsia- a state of prostaglandin deficiency? Hypertension 1983; 5(1): 105
18 Stuart MJ, Sunderji SG, Yamba T. Decreased prostacyclin production; a characteristic of chronic placental insufficiency syndromes. Lancet 1981; i: 1126
19 Jogee M, Myatt L, Elder MG. Prostacyclin production by placental cells in culture in pregnancy complicated by growth retardation. Br J Obstet gynaecol 1983; 90: 247
20 Remuzzi G, Marchesi D, Schieppati A, Mecca G. Plasmatic regulation of vascular prostacyclin in pregnancy. Br Med J 1981; 282: 512
21 Glance DG, Elder MG, Myatt L. Prostaglandin production and stimulation by angiotensin II in the isolated perfused human placental cotyledon. Am J Obstet Gynecol 1985; 151: 387
22 Maseki M, Nishigaki I, Hagihara M, Tomoda Y, Yaki KL. Lipid peroxidase levels and lipid content of serum lipoprotein fragments of pregnant subjects with or without pre-eclampsia. Clin Chim Acta 1981; 115(2): 155
23 Carreras LO, Muchin SJ, Deman R. Arterial thrombus, intrauterine death and lupus anticoagulant; detection of immunoglobulins which interfere with prostacyclin formation. Lancet 1981; i: 244
24 Beaufils M, Uzan S, Dunismuni R, Colan JC. Prevention of pre-eclampsia by early anti-platelet therapy. Lancet 1985; (i): 840
25 Wallenburg HCS, Makovitz JW, Dekker GA, Rotmans P. Low dose aspirin prevents pregnancy induced hypertension and pre-eclampsia in angiotensin sensitive primigravida. Lancet 1986; i: 1

26 Crosby WM, Costiloe JP. Safety of lap belts restraint for pregnant victims of automobile collisions. New Eng J Med 1971; 284: 632
27 Hibbard BM, Hibbard ED. Aetiological factors in abruptio placentae. Br Med J 1963; 2: 1430
28 Naeye RL. Abruptio placentae and placenta praevia: Frequency, perinatal mortality and cigarette smoking. Obstet Gynecol 1980; 55: 707
29 Egley C, Cefalo RC. Abruptio placenta. In: Studd J, ed. Progress in Obsetrics and Gynaecology, Vol 5. London: Churchill Livingstone, 1985
30 Naeye RL, Harkness WL, Utts J. Abruptio placentae and perinatal death; a prospective study. Am J Obstet Gynecol 1977; 128: 740
31 Rush RW, Keirse MJNC, Howat P. The contribution of preterm delivery to perinatal mortality Br Med J 1976; 2: 9653
32 Minkoff H. Prematurity; Infection as an aetiological fator. Obstet Gynecol 1983; 62: 137
33 Gemsa D, Leser HG, Seitz M, Dieman W, Barlin E. Membrane pertubation and stimulation of arachidonic acid metabolism. Mol Immunol 1982; 19: 1287
34 Hamilton JA, Clarris BJ, Fraser JRE, Niall MC. Peripheral blood mononuclear cells stimulate prostacyclin levels in human synovial fibroblast-like cells. Rhumatol Int 1985; 5: 121
35 Romero R, Mitchell M, Duras S. A possible mechanism for premature labor in gram negative maternal infection: A monocyte product stimulates prostaglandin release by the amnion. Abstr 219, 32nd Ann Meeting Soc Gynecol Invest 1985
36 Bennett PR, Myatt L, Elder MG. Effects of lipoxygenase products of arachidonic acid upon contractility of human pregnant myometrium in vitro. Prostaglandins 1987; 33: 837
37 Bennett PR, Rose MP, Myatt L, Elder MG. Preterm labour: Stimulation of arachidonic acid metabolism in human amnion cells in culture by bacterial products. Am J Obstet Gynecol 1987; 156(3): 649
38 Bejar R, Curbello V, Davis C, Gluck L. Premature labor and bactrial sources of phospholipase. Obstet Gynecol 1981; 57: 473
39 Wright CSW, Campbell S, Bragley S. Second trimester abortion after vaginal termination of pregnancy. Lancet 1972; i: 1278
40 Jones JM, Sweetnam P, Hibbard BM. The outcome of pregnancy after cone biopsy, a case control study. B.J. Obstet Gynecol 1979; 86: 913–916.
41 Bennett PR, Myatt L, Elder MG. Production of phospholipase A_2 by potential vaginal pathogens. 1988 (Unpublished observations)

Epidemiology of birth before 28 weeks of gestation

Alison Macfarlane
National Perinatal Epidemiology Unit, Radcliffe Infirmary, Oxford

Susan Cole
Information and Statistics Division, Common Services Agency for the Scottish Health Service, Edinburgh

Ann Johnson
Oxford Region Child Development Project, John Radcliffe Hospital, Oxford

Beverley Botting
Medical Statistics Division, Office of Population Censuses and Surveys, London

> Information about the incidence of birth before 28 weeks of gestation is very scanty in the United Kingdom as gestational age is not recorded when live births are registered. Data from the Scottish Morbidity Records SMR2 system and the Scottish Stillbirth and Neonatal Mortality Survey show an apparent rise in incidence between the mid 1970's and mid 1980's. This probably reflects increased reporting. There is a raised incidence of births before 28 weeks of gestation among women under 20 and aged 40 and over, and there are marked social class differences.
>
> While mortality among very small babies has fallen dramatically over the past 20 years, it is difficult to assess trends and variations in morbidity among the surviving children. There have been few population based studies and those which have been done have not measured outcome in comparable ways. Suggestions are therefore made about the steps which need be taken to make better use of the data which are being collected through routine systems and special studies.

Despite the growing professional and public interest in the care given to babies born before 28 weeks of gestation, very little is known about their epidemiology. Even the data which do exist about the incidence and outcome of pregnancy before 28 weeks tend to be incomplete and subject to biases of various kinds. This chapter explores reasons for this and tries to interpret the available data about the incidence of births before 28 weeks of gestational age, their birthweights and the mortality and morbidity associated with these births. It also suggests ways in which data collection could be improved.

DATA FROM ROUTINE SOURCES

Gestational age is not among the items recorded when live births are registered in the four countries of the United Kingdom. While it is recorded on stillbirth certificates, late fetal deaths are only registrable as stillbirths if they have reached 28 or more completed weeks of gestation. In Scotland, if parents wish it, a late fetal death of less than 28 weeks gestation may be registered as a still birth. This occasionally occurs, with between 0 and 12 such registrations taking place each year.

In Scotland, information about gestational age is collected through the SMR2 maternity discharge system.[1] As well as being used to monitor the patterns of maternity care given and the backgrounds of the women receiving it, this system also acts as a framework for the Scottish Stillbirth and Neonatal Mortality Survey.[2] In this ongoing survey, the Information and Statistics Division in Edinburgh asks health boards for information about stillbirths and neonatal deaths registered in Scotland. In addition, since 1984, health boards have been requested to supply information about fetal deaths from 20 to 27 weeks of gestation, or weighing 500g or more. At present, these still appear to be under-reported in the Surveys.[2] compared with the fuller information collected routinely through the SMR2 system.

So far, there is no comparable source of data in England, Wales or Northern Ireland. Some English regions run perinatal mortality surveys[3] and Wales did an extensive 'one-off' survey,[4] following a rise in its perinatal mortality rate in 1981.

Up to 1980 for England and Wales, and from 1981 to 1985 for England only, data about in-patient stays in maternity departments, including gestational age, were collected through the Maternity Hospital In-patient Enquiry (HIPE). This was a 10% sample of all discharges from NHS maternity departments. It was hoped that, despite a number of known problems,[5] data from this source could be used to look at associations between low gestational age and other factors. When gestational age was tabulated by birthweight, however, it was found that a considerable proportion of babies with gestational ages coded as being between 20 and 28 weeks, had recorded birthweights in excess of 2.5 kg (Macfarlane A J, unpublished observations). As it is not known whether there is a systematic source of error in these data, the analyses had to be abandoned.

The Hospital In-patient Enquiry was superceded by the Hospital Episode System which brings together national information about all stays in NHS hospitals. The Maternity Hospital Episode System came into operation on 1 April 1988 and gestational age is among the items recorded in its minimum dataset. At the time of writing, it is too early to comment on the quality of the data collected.

For the present, however, Scotland is the only UK country with usable national data about gestational age at birth.

SPECIAL STUDIES

Although there have been many studies of very small babies, most have been hospital-based and have analysed the data in terms of birthweight. Very few studies have either been population-based or have used gestational age as a criterion. The discussion which follows is restricted to studies which satisfied one of these criteria and makes no claims to be a comprehensive review of studies done since the mid 1970's. Instead the aim is to highlight major themes and methodological problems. There has been a marked tendency for studies based on geographically defined populations to use birthweight as a criterion while studies focusing on gestational age have tended to use hospital populations.

A study of 149 infants born between 20 and 28 weeks gestation over the five year period 1980–1984 in Ninewells Hospital, Dundee, Scotland was not strictly population-based but described itself as such, on the grounds that all women in the city deliver in this hospital.[6] In the Netherlands, a survey of 1338 infants born alive in 1983 after less than 32 weeks gestation, or weighing less than 1.5 kg represented a response rate of 94% of such infants born in the country as a whole.[7,8] A smaller survey in the Northern Region of England covered pregnancies of at least 24 but less than 32 completed weeks of gestation to residents of the Region in 1983 (Wariyar UK, Richmond S, unpublished observations).

More recently, two further studies were done in the Oxford Region. The ongoing Oxford Region Low Birthweight Study covers registered deaths to residents of the Oxford Region and babies admitted to special care after being born alive to residents of the Region at 28 or fewer weeks of gestation in the years 1984–86 (Johnson MA, unpublished observations). A second study covered a much shorter time span, September 1986 to February 1987. As it was done by searching labour ward registers and records of gynaecology wards it is likely to have a more complete coverage. It included all live births and fetal deaths before 30 weeks of gestation in the Oxford Region to residents of the region but did not cover births occurring to them outside the region. Other population based studies covered 139,[9] 255[10] and 351[11] births respectively and used birthweight as a cut-off point. One of these implied it was population-based but was not as it included all births in a geographically defined area of Australia.[10]

The other studies which used gestational age as a criterion were all hospital-based and tended to be relatively small, apart from a study of 730 babies born between 23 and 32 weeks of gestation in the Regional Perinatal Unit in Toronto, Canada.[12] Five other hospital-based studies covered from 62 to 307 babies of very low gestational age.[13-17]

The information collected in these studies and the question of whether they can be used to make comparisons between births at different places and times is discussed in what follows.

INCIDENCE OF BIRTH BEFORE 28 WEEKS

Most studies have focused on the survival of and prevalence of impairment among babies born before 28 weeks of gestation rather than on their incidence, or the incidence of fetal death. This may be a reflection of the fact that, particularly at the lower end of the gestational age range, many babies who are born alive die very shortly after birth.

Table 1 shows that live births, at 20–23 weeks of gestation accounted for 0.029% of live births in Scotland over the years 1980–84 and that live births at 24–25 and 26–27 weeks accounted for 0.073 and 0.15% respectively.[18]

In the Netherlands, the incidence was much lower with births at 24–25 weeks of gestation accounting for 0.039% of the 170 246 live births in 1983 and births at 26–27 weeks accounting for 0.106%.[8]

Not surprisingly, compared with live births, a much higher percentage of fetal deaths occurred before 28 weeks of gestation. In Scotland, fetal deaths at 20–23, 24–25 and 26–27 weeks accounted for 33.1, 10.3 and 6.4% respectively of all stillbirths plus fetal deaths at 20 or more completed weeks of gestation.[18]

Table 1 Births with very low gestational age, Scotland 1980–84

a) *Live births*

Year	\multicolumn{8}{c}{Gestational age, weeks}							All live births	
	20–23		24–25		26–27		28 or more			
	Number	Percentage	Number	Percentage	Number	Percentage	Number	Percentage	Number	Percentage
1980	30	0.044	48	0.071	105	0.16	67523	99.73	67706	100.0
1981	17	0.025	34	0.050	92	0.13	68349	99.79	68492	100.0
1982	18	0.027	55	0.084	99	0.15	65409	99.74	67781	100.0
1983	18	0.028	47	0.073	89	0.14	64461	99.76	64615	100.0
1984	27	0.042	67	0.103	128	0.20	64676	99.66	64521	100.0
1980–84	110	0.033	251	0.076	513	0.15	330418	99.74	331292	100.0

b) *Stillbirths and late abortions*

Year	\multicolumn{8}{c}{Gestational age, weeks}							All still births and late abortions	
	20–23		24–25		26–27		28 or more			
	Number	Percentage	Number	Percentage	Number	Percentage	Number	Percentage	Number	Percentage
1980	279	31.7	101	11.5	64	7.3	436	49.5	880	100.0
1981	295	34.2	92	10.7	56	6.5	419	48.6	862	100.0
1982	271	34.5	81	10.3	46	5.9	386	49.4	786	100.0
1983	236	32.4	71	9.8	48	6.6	373	51.2	728	100.0
1984	234	32.8	63	8.8	39	5.5	377	52.9	713	100.0
1980–84	1315	33.1	408	10.3	253	6.4	1993	50.2	3969	100.0

Source: Information and Statistics Division

Some studies did not relate the numbers of very pre-term births to total births, but did compare numbers of live births and fetal deaths. In Ninewells Hospital, Dundee, 50 of the 149 pregnancies ending between 20 and 28 weeks of gestation resulted in a live birth. In the Northern Region of England in 1983, the percentages born alive ranged from 36% at 24 weeks of gestation to 68% at 27 weeks of gestation as Table 2 shows. Thus, these were similar to the 38% born alive in Scotland at 24–25 weeks and 69% at 26–27 weeks.

The data for Scotland come from national statistics and the Netherlands data from a survey with many participants. In both cases therefore, many different people will have been involved in the assessment of gestational age. It is unlikely, therefore to be estimated as consistently as can be possible in studies from a single hospital[6] or small geographical area.

Estimates of gestational age based on last menstrual period (LMP) are likely to be unreliable if the woman has an irregular cycle or has recently been using oral contraceptives. Although current practice is to use ultrasound scans to reduce uncertainty, a study in Aberdeen found that women with an uncertain LMP were less likely than women with certain dates to book for antenatal care before 20 weeks.[19] Estimates of gestational age based on ultrasound scans after 20 weeks are likely to be less accurate than those based on scans earlier in pregnancy.

Scottish routine statistics record both gestational age calculated from LMP and clinicians' 'best estimate', without specifying how this should be derived. The extent to which discrepancies can arise is illustrated in Table 3. All other data from Scotland in this article use gestational age based on the 'best estimate'. Close examination of the data collected in 1980–84 has revealed some apparent errors in cases with incongruous birthweights for gestational age. Use of these data has led to the introduction of more rigorous checks in subsequent years.

Table 2 Births before 28 weeks of gestation, Northern Region, 1983

	\multicolumn{4}{c}{Completed weeks of gestation}
	24	25	26	27
Antepartum deaths	28	23	19	12
Intrapartum deaths	5	6	6	2
Live births	19	22	27	30
Total	52	51	52	44
Percentage born alive	36	43	52	68

Source: Wariyar and Richmond, unpublished observations

Table 3 Discrepancies between gestational age derived by 'best estimate' and gestational age calculated from date of last menstrual period, Scotland, 1984

Estimated gestational age, weeks	Numbers of live births for which estimated and calculated gestational ages:			Total live births
	are the same	differ by one week	differ by more than one week	
21	1	0	1	2
22	4	0	2	6
23	10	2	3	15
24	12	4	8	24
25	19	3	13	35
26	30	17	22	69
27	29	7	24	60
Total	105	33	73	211

Source: Information and Statistics Division, Scotland

Table 4 Distribution of live births before 28 weeks of gestation by mother's age, Scotland 1980–84

Mother's age	Percentage of babies with mothers in each age group			
	Singletons 20–27 weeks gestation	All live births	Multiples 20–27 weeks gestation	All live births
Under 20	18.4	10.1	18.5	6.6
20–24	32.4	32.9	30.2	27.8
25–29	27.0	33.9	32.3	34.7
30–34	16.7	17.2	10.6	22.2
35–39	4.1	5.0	6.3	7.5
40+	1.4	0.8	2.1	1.2
All ages	100.0	100.0	100.0	100.0
Number	636	321521	189	6156

Source: Information and Statistics Division, Scotland

VARIATIONS IN INCIDENCE

The distribution of very pre-term live births in Scotland according to their mother's age is shown in Table 4 and compared with that for all live births. For both singletons and multiples there is an excess of live births before 28 weeks among women under 20 and, for multiple births, a slight excess in the 20–24 age group. There also appear to be very slight excesses among women aged 40 or over.

The Netherlands survey covered a broader range of gestational ages including births before 32 weeks or under 1.5 kg and thus had a higher proportion of live births. As a result, less marked difference between the study group and the general population would be expected. Also, compared with Scotland, births in general are more highly concentrated among women aged 25–29. Despite this, Table 5 shows that the study group also showed excesses of women under 20 or aged 40 or over, compared with births in the Netherlands as a whole.

The distribution of live births in Scotland before 28 weeks of gestation by mother's height is given in Table 6. This shows an

Table 5 Distribution of preterm and small for gestational age infants by mother's age, Netherlands, 1983

Mother's age	Percentage of babies with mothers in each group	
	Study population*	General population
Under 20	4.5	2.7
20–24	25.7	23.7
25–29	39.7	44.0
30–34	22.3	23.1
35–39	6.0	5.7
40+	1.7	0.9
All mothers with stated age	100.0	100.0
Percentage unstated	2.9	—
Total births	1338	170246

*Infants born alive after 32 weeks or less of gestation or weighing less than 1500g
Source: POPS study[8]

Table 6 Distribution of live births before 28 weeks of gestation by mother's height, Scotland 1980–84

Mother's height cm	Percentage of babies with mothers in each height group			
	Singletons		Multiples	
	20–27 weeks gestation	All live births	20–27 weeks gestation	All live births
<150	5.6	3.4	0.6	2.0
150–154	14.9	13.5	12.6	11.6
155–159	28.4	26.9	24.6	24.1
160–164	26.5	30.6	41.7	32.5
165–169	17.2	18.0	13.1	21.1
170–174	6.7	6.2	5.7	6.8
175+	0.7	1.4	2.3	1.9
All mothers with stated height	100.0	100.0	100.0	100.0
Percent unstated	15.9	5.0	7.4	5.4
Numbers of births	636	321531	189	6156

Source: Information and Statistics Division, Scotland

excess of short and tall women amongst mothers of very pre-term singleton babies compared with all singleton births in Scotland. These differences were not seen among mothers of multiple births.

Given the known inter-relationship between social class and both mothers' ages and heights,[20] it is not surprising to find social class differences in the incidence of birth before 28 weeks in Table 7. This contrasts with earlier analyses by birthweight which have not found social class differences in the very lowest weight groups.[20] The social classes shown are based on the fathers' occupation of babies born within marriage. The 'not stated' category includes instances where the parents are not married as well as those where the parents are married but the father is unemployed. Overall, this group has a particularly high incidence of short gestational age for both multiple and singleton births.

In the Netherlands study the mother's social class was recorded for parents of 841 of the 1338 births studied. Both parents' occupations were recorded and the highest social class was tabulated. Unfortunately, however, because of the high non-response and the absence of comparable data for all births, incidence rates within social class could not be calculated. This was also true of

Table 7 Incidence of pre-term birth by social class of father, Scotland 1980–84

Social class of father	Percentage of live births with gestational age			
	20–27 weeks	28–31 weeks	32–36 weeks	Under 37 weeks
Singletons				
I Professional	0.12	0.31	2.8	3.3
II Intermediate	0.14	0.44	3.6	4.2
III Skilled	0.19	0.52	4.1	4.8
IV Partly skilled	0.20	0.61	4.4	5.2
V Unskilled	0.22	0.71	4.8	5.7
Not stated	0.27	0.82	5.6	6.7
All	0.20	0.60	4.4	5.2
Numbers of births	636	1902	14043	16581
Multiples				
I Professional	1.4	4.5	31.3	37.2
II Intermediate	1.4	5.5	25.7	32.6
III Skilled	3.0	6.2	31.6	40.9
IV Partly skilled	2.5	6.0	31.8	40.6
V Unskilled	2.1	7.4	36.2	45.7
Not stated	5.2	7.1	33.9	46.2
All	3.1	6.3	32.4	41.8
Numbers of births	189	383	1983	2555

Source: Information and Statistics Division, Scotland

the data about ethnic origin recorded for 1214 of the mothers in the study.

Apart from these two sources there seems to be little information about the background of women having very pre-term babies. Some other studies collected information, but did not report incidence by social class. The available data suggest, however, that there is an excess of very pre-term births among women under 20 and that there is a marked social class gradient.

BIRTHWEIGHT AND ITS RELATIONSHIP TO GESTATIONAL AGE

As birthweight is so much more easily measurable than gestational age, most of the population-based studies of very small babies use it as a criterion, so it is important to consider the relationship between them. Tables 8 and 9 give data for Scotland and the Netherlands respectively.

In Scotland 3.5% (2 out of 57) of singleton and 13.3% (4 out of 30) of multiple live births at 20–23 weeks were recorded as having

Table 8 Percentage distribution of birthweight of live births by gestational age, Scotland 1980–84

Birthweight (g)		Gestational age, weeks		
		20–23	24–25	26–27
Singletons				
Under 500		15.8	1.7	0.5
500–999		77.2	83.8	52.6
1000–1499		3.5	14.5	44.4
1500 and over		3.5	—	2.5
All with stated	Percent	100.0	100.0	100.0
birthweight	Number	57	173	365
Number with unstated birthweight		8	14	20
Multiples				
Under 500		34.6	14.0	—
500–999		65.4	82.0	64.5
1000–1499		—	4.0	35.5
1500 and over		—	—	—
All with stated	Percent	100.0	100.0	100.0
birthweight	Number	26	50	93
Number with unstated birthweight		3	5	12

Source: Information and Statistics Division, Scotland

Table 9 Percentage distribution of birthweights of live birth before 28 weeks of gestational age, Netherlands, 1983

Birthweight (g)	Gestational age, weeks		
	Under 24	24–25	26–27
Under 500	25	0	0
500–999	75	93	49
1000–1499	0	7	49
1500 and over	0	0	1
All live births before 28 weeks	100	100	100
Number of births	8	69	180

Source: POPS study[8]

birthweights of 1.5 kg or over. This seems unlikely and could arise from inaccuracies in either estimating or recording gestational age or birthweight although some apparently incongruous birthweights for gestational age are known to have been associated with hydropic infants, twin-to-twin transfusion syndrome or congenital anomalies. In addition, just over 14% of babies in this gestational age group did not have recorded birthweights. Taken as a whole, therefore, the data for this gestational age range may be somewhat unreliable.

In the 24–25 and 26–27 week groups there were fewer missing values. For singletons at least, there was broad similarity between the data for Scotland and the Netherlands, apart from an absence of babies with birthweights under 500g in the 24–25 week group in the Netherlands.

Most of the standard birthweight for gestational age charts were compiled in the 1960's or early 1970's, since which time new techniques have become available for assessing gestational age. Most of the standard charts start at 28 weeks of gestation, and those which contain data relating to earlier gestational ages are based on very small numbers of births in this time period.

More recently, an analysis based on terminations, births and babies admitted for neonatal care in three Sheffield hospitals, derived birthweight distributions for terminations, spontaneous abortions and live births from 14 to 42 weeks of gestation.[21] It concluded that the birthweight distributions for live births and spontaneous abortions between 20 and 28 weeks of gestation differed very little from each other, although this was based on very small numbers of events.

Two studies have pointed to the way the statistical relationship between birthweight and gestational age has been modified by the increasing tendency to do Caesarean sections at low gestational ages for babies whose fetal growth is abnormal. In one English hospital, 35% of births at 25 to 31 weeks of gestation in 1982–84 were by elective Caesarean section and a further 13% were emergency Caesarean sections. The corresponding rates for the same hospital for the years 1968–72 were 3% and 2% respectively.[22] In the John Radcliffe Hospital, Oxford, 226 of the 803 live births at gestational ages of 34 weeks or less followed induction of labour or an elective Caesarean section.[22]

In both cases, average birthweights and in the second, average head circumferences of babies born following elective delivery were significantly lower than those following spontaneous delivery at the same gestational age.[22,23] Because of this, births following elective delivery were excluded from the new birthweight for gestational age tables which were derived.[22,24] Although elective delivery is relatively uncommon among births before 28 weeks of gestation compared with those between 28 and 34 weeks,[8,22,23] the parts of these tables which relate to births before 28 weeks are set out in Table 10.

The first set of centiles are derived from births in five hospitals over a three year time span and the second from births in one hospital over a seven year period. Both are based on relatively

Table 10 Smoothed birthweight centiles for live births before 28 weeks of gestation, following spontaneous onset of labour
a) *Based on data from five hospitals 1982–84*[21]

Gestational age, weeks	Number of births	Standard deviation, g	Smoothed birthweight centiles, g				
			3rd	10th	50th	90th	97th
25	16	90	550	615	760	905	970
26	38	154	630	715	890	1065	1150
27	35	166	720	820	1020	1220	1320

b) *Based on data from births in the John Radcliffe Hospital, Oxford 1978–84*[23]

Gestational age, weeks	Number of births	Standard deviation, g	Smoothed birthweight centiles, g				
			3rd	10th	50th	90th	97th
24	9	136	510	600	740	880	970
25	17	114	550	630	790	950	1030
26	25	124	600	700	870	1050	1140
27	29	191	680	790	980	1180	1280

small numbers of observations. Despite these problems they are remarkably consistent with each other.

TRENDS IN THE INCIDENCE OF BIRTHS BEFORE 28 WEEKS OF GESTATION

Although there have been year to year fluctuations, the percentage of live births in Scotland at gestational ages 20–27 weeks increased over the period 1975–85, as can be seen in Table 11. These births accounted for 0.26% of live births reported in the SMR2 system in the years 1981–85 combined compared with 0.20% in 1976–80. Table 1 shows that over the period 1980–84 there was an increase in the incidence of births at 24 to 27 weeks of gestation but no clear trend in births between 20 and 23 weeks.

The period 1975–85 also saw an increase in the reported incidence of live births with birthweights under 750g. These accounted for 0.08% of live births in 1981–85 compared with 0.06% in 1976–80. The corresponding figures for births from 20–27 weeks of gestation of babies born weighing less than 750g were 0.07% and 0.05% respectively.

There is no information about gestational age at birth in England, but trends in the incidence of extremely low birthweight were broadly parallel to those seen in Scotland. Data from DHSS' LHS 27/1 low birthweight returns showed that the percentages of live born babies weighing 1 kg or less increased from 0.23 of live births in 1976 to 0.30 in 1986.[25] They also accounted for an increasing percentage of live births weighing 2.5 kg or less, 3.6% in 1976 rising to 4.4% in 1986. Similar trends were seen in birth registration data for England and Wales, where the recording of birthweight has been relatively complete since 1983.

Does this represent an increase in the incidence of births before 28 weeks or a change in recording? A common explanation is that reporting could well have become more complete as a consequence of the rise of intensive care. Babies who might, in the past, have been regarded as miscarriages are now admitted to intensive care and, as a result, are notified and registered.

There are, however, other changes which may have influenced decisions about the distinction between live births and miscarriages or fetal deaths before 28 weeks of gestation. In Scotland, where information about late abortions or miscarriages before 28 weeks of gestation is collected through the SMR2 system, there appears to have been a shift in reporting over the years 1975 to

Table 11 Trends in the incidence of very short gestation and very low birthweight among live births in Scotland, 1975–85

Year	Births at 20–27 weeks of gestation — Number	Percentage of live births	Births with birthweights under 750g — Number	Percentage of live births	Births at 20–27 weeks of gestation with birthweights under 750g — Number	Percentage of live births	Live births reported to SMR2
1975	123	0.19	40	0.06	31	0.05	65112
1976	102	0.16	28	0.04	21	0.03	64082
1977	121	0.20	40	0.06	30	0.05	61810
1978	122	0.19	31	0.05	25	0.04	63960
1979	139	0.21	37	0.06	32	0.05	67038
1980	170	0.25	59	0.09	43	0.06	67247
1981	139	0.20	46	0.07	34	0.05	68063
1982	166	0.25	54	0.08	47	0.07	65193
1983	146	0.22	51	0.08	43	0.07	64242
1984	209	0.32	58	0.09	47	0.07	64521
1985	189	0.29	60	0.09	54	0.08	64634

Source: Information and Statistics Division, Scotland

1985, as Table 12 shows. In 1975, 19.9% of births at 20–27 weeks of gestation were recorded as live, compared with 36.5 ten years later. There were also marked increases in 1979 and in 1984 in the percentages of live births. The second of these increases coincided with the addition in 1984 of late fetal deaths to the Scottish Stillbirth and Neonatal Death Survey. In addition, from 1984 onwards, the survey report has contained exhortations to clinicians to report live births as such.[2]

Similarly, an exercise in the Mersey Region of England highlighted the failure to weigh all infants at birth and to report all neonatal deaths and consequent inaccuracies in the LHS 27/1 low birthweight returns.[26] Once this became known, data accuracy improved considerably and this led to major shifts in reported birth and mortality rates.

These are probably not the only instances where a conscious desire to improve statistics have led to fuller reporting of live births. Another factor which may have contributed to this is changes in attitudes to parents who experience the loss of a baby born alive before 28 weeks of gestation. Although there are no statistics on the subject, anecdotal evidence suggests that parents are becoming more likely to have the opportunity to see and hold the baby and view its fate as a death rather than a miscarriage.[27]

Taken together, the data suggest an apparent increase in the incidence of live births at very low gestations, but it is likely that this is a consequence of fuller reporting.

Table 12 Late abortions and live births at 20–27 weeks of gestation, Scotland 1975–85

Year	Late abortions	Live births	Live births as percentage of total
1975	476	123	20.5
1976	403	102	20.2
1977	452	121	21.1
1978	489	122	20.0
1979	360	139	27.9
1980	421	170	28.8
1981	433	139	24.3
1982	398	166	29.4
1983	355	146	29.1
1984	336	209	38.3
1985	296	189	39.0

Source: Information and Statistics Division, Scotland, SMR2 returns

MORTALITY OF BABIES BORN BEFORE 28 WEEKS

Mortality rates from various studies which used gestational age as a criterion are brought together in Table 13. While many reported death rates at single weeks of gestational age, the data have, as far as possible, been grouped for gestational ages of 20-23, 24-25 and 26-27 weeks.

Another feature is the difference in mortality rates used. In the past neonatal mortality was the accepted criterion, but it had already been recognized by the beginning of the 1980's that deaths attributable to causes originating in the perinatal or neonatal period were actually occurring in the postneonatal period.[28-31] As a result a number of studies used survival to hospital discharge as a criterion, whereas in others it was not quite clear what cut-off point was used to describe the babies as 'surviving'. Table 13 is annotated to indicate studies in which this is unclear.

Comparisons between studies done in different countries, at different time periods and using differently defined mortality rates are fraught with problems.[20] Even despite these, there is a tendency for the mortality rates reported in population-based studies to be higher than those from hospital-based studies. Exceptions to this are the two studies done in Vermont and New Hampshire[16] and in Boston,[13] USA. In Scotland there appeared to be little or no difference between the mortality rates of babies from singleton and multiple births, but it may be that the numbers involved were too small to reveal any such differences.

Even among babies of similar gestational ages, mortality can vary according to birthweight as Table 14 shows. Among singletons born at 24-25 and 26-27 weeks of gestation and multiple births at 26-27 weeks in Scotland mortality decreased with increasing birthweight.

The study comparing the two nurseries in Vermont and New Hampshire stressed the importance of using both birthweight and gestational age groupings to compare neonatal units.[16] This found a similar trend in birthweight specific mortality at gestational ages below 28 weeks in the Hanover, New Hampshire nursery. In the Burlington, Vermont nursery the numbers of babies were too small to detect any trend. This study analysed birthweight in 250g groupings.

In the Netherlands study the data were analysed in greater detail

Table 13 Mortality rates reported in studies of birth before 28 weeks of gestation

Population studied	Years	Gestational ages	Number of live births	Deaths before							
				One week		One month		One year		Hospital discharge	
				No	%	No	%	No	%	No	%
Netherlands[7,8]	1983	Under 24	8	8	100	8	100			8	100
		24–25	67	55	82	58	87			60	90
		26–27	180	76	42	90	50			95	53
Scotland, singletons	1980–84	20–23	65			62	95	62	95		
		24–25	187			135	72	150	80		
		26–27	385			196	51	236	61		
Scotland, multiple births	1980–84	20–23	29			28	97	28	97		
		24–25	55			46	84	46	84		
		26–27	105			63	60	74	70		
Northern Region, England	1983	24–25	41	29	71	32	78				
		26–27	57	26	46	29	51				
Oxford Region, England	Sep 1986–Feb 1987	24–25	26	21	81	21	81	21	81	21	81
		26–27	24	11	46	13	54	14	58	14	58
Oxford Region, England	1984–86	Under 24	14			14	100	14	100	14	100
		24–25	83			64	77	68	82	68	82
		26–27	144			62	43	71	49	69	48
Ninewells Hospital, Dundee Scotland[6]	1980–84	20–28	50	21	42	24	48				
Liverpool Maternity Hospital, England[17]	1980–85	Under 28	307							181*	59
Women's College Hospital, Toronto,	1979–82	23	7	6	86					6	86
		24–25	67	23	34					25	37

Table 13 (*Continued*)

Population studied	Years	Gestational ages	Number of live births	Deaths before One week No	%	Deaths before One month No	%	Deaths before One year No	%	Hospital discharge No	%
Canada[12]		26–27	105	24	23					26	25
Queen Victoria Medical Centre, Melbourne, Australia[14]	Jan 1977– Jun 1981	24–25 26–27	45 84							30 31	67 37
Children' Hospital, Buffalo, USA[15]	Jul 1977– Jun 1980	24–25 26–27	27 35							17* 11*	63 31
Two intensive care nurseries in Burlington, Vermont and Hanover, New Hampshire, USA[16]	1976–79	Under 25 26–27	38 64							34 37	89 58
St Margaret's Hospital for Women, Boston, USA[13]	1977–80	24–25 26–27	35 76							30* 40*	86 53

*Definition of survival not clearly specified in paper

Table 14 Infant mortality by birthweight and gestational age, Scotland 1980–84

Birth weight g	Gestational age, weeks					
	20–23		24–25		26–27	
	Live births	Infant mortality[+]	Live births	Infant mortality[+]	Live births	Infant mortality[+]
Singletons						
Under 500	9	1000	3	1000	2	1000
500–999	44	954	145	800	192	667
1000–1499	2	1000	25	680	162	518
1500 and over	2	500	—	—	9	667
Not known	8	1000	14	1000	19	790
Total	65	954	187	802	385	623
Multiple births						
Under 500	9	1000	7	857		
500–999	17	1000	41	829	60	800
1000–1499	—	—	2	1000	33	455
1500 and over	—	—	—	—	—	—
Not known	3	667	5	800	12	917
Total	33	848	55	836	105	705

[+] Rate per 1000 live births
Source: Information and Statistics Division, Scotland

using 100g birthweight groups.[7,8] There was no clear inverse relationship between neonatal mortality and birthweight among babies born at gestational ages below 28 weeks. Such a relationship was, however apparent when all gestational ages were combined and mortality decreased markedly as birthweights increased from 0.5 to 1.5 kg.

In England and Wales, where it is not possible to analyse data by gestational age, very marked differences between birthweight groups were apparent when stillbirth, neonatal, postneonatal and infant mortality rates among very low birthweight babies were analysed in 100g groups. Some of these data are shown in Table 15 and plotted in Figure 1.

Both of these show wide differences in mortality within the conventional 500g groupings and also differences in the age at death. Thus, for example among singletons the infant mortality rate was 870.3 deaths per thousand live births in the 500–599g group compared with 395.2 among babies weighing from 900–999g. In the 500–599g group, 92.2% of infant deaths oc-

Table 15 Infant mortality rates and percentages of deaths occurring at different ages, England and Wales 1982–86

Birthweight g	Singletons						Multiples				
	Live births	Infant mortality rate	\multicolumn{3}{c	}{Percentages of deaths which were}		Live births	Infant mortality rate*	\multicolumn{3}{c	}{Percentages of deaths which were}
			early neonatal	late neonatal	post neonatal				early neonatal	late neonatal	post neonatal
Under 1500	22399	315.0	75.7	11.8	12.5	5214	318.8	76.6	12.5	10.8
Under 500	529	527.4	96.4	1.8	1.8	132	916.7	99.2	0.8	0.0
500–599	563	870.3	92.2	4.5	3.3	176	926.1	92.6	4.3	3.1
600–699	1048	792.0	86.6	7.5	5.5	274	861.3	89.4	7.6	4.2
700–799	1384	648.8	78.7	10.0	11.2	259	691.1	83.2	9.5	7.3
800–899	1735	522.8	74.4	13.2	13.4	367	580.4	80.3	7.5	6.1
900–999	2095	395.2	72.6	14.2	13.2	457	420.1	68.2	17.7	14.1
1000–1099	2454	284.4	70.6	13.3	16.0	503	324.1	65.6	18.4	16.0
1100–1199	2627	223.8	69.0	17.0	14.0	587	224.9	59.1	22.0	18.9
1200–1299	2868	193.9	69.4	14.4	16.2	656	163.1	61.8	27.4	15.7
1300–1399	3345	143.2	66.0	13.6	20.5	793	97.1	63.6	7.8	28.6
1400–1499	3751	134.1	64.6	15.3	20.1	1010	78.2	55.7	15.2	29.1

*per 1000 live births
Source: Office of Population Censuses and Surveys

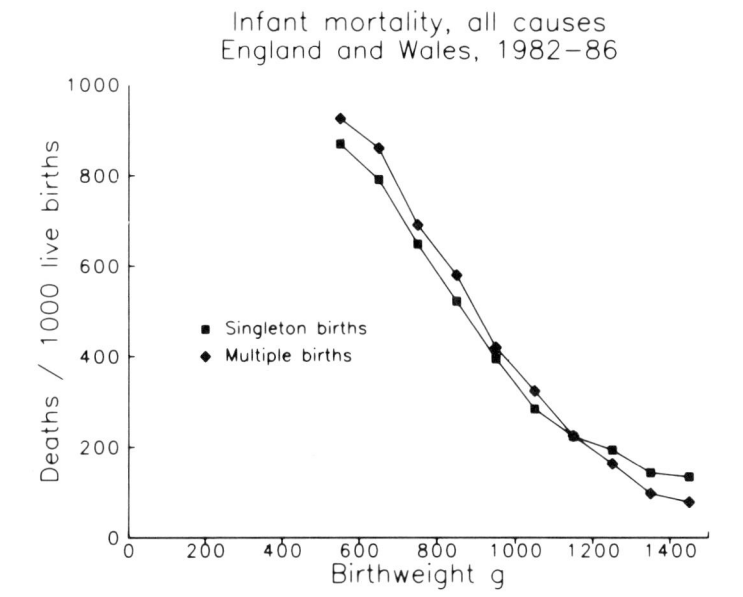

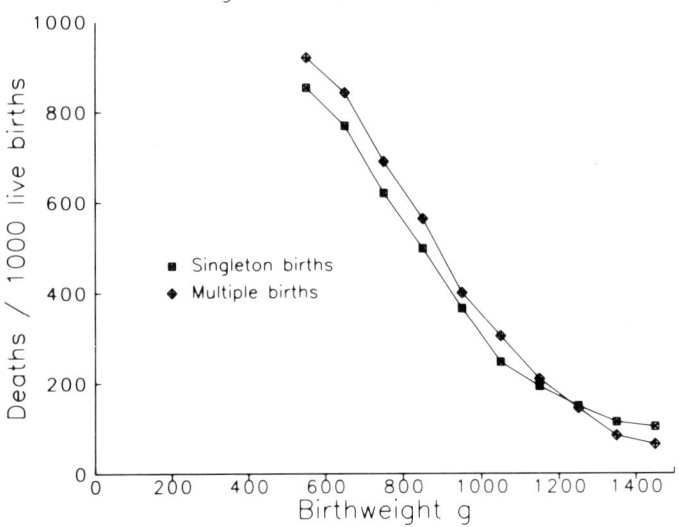

Fig. 1 Infant mortality among babies with birthweights under 1500g, England and Wales, 1982–1986: a) All causes of death; b) All causes except congenital malformations. (Source: Office of Population Censuses and Surveys.)

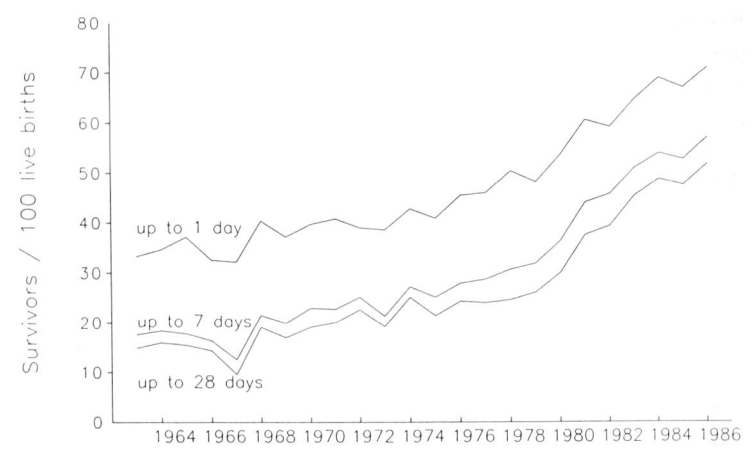

Fig. 2 Survival rates at birthweights 1000g and under England and Wales, 1963–86 (Source: DHSS LHS 27/1 low birthweight returns).

curred in the early neonatal period compared with 72.6% in the 900–999g group.

Figure 1 illustrates the differences in mortality between singleton and multiple births. Under 1100g infant mortality is higher for multiple births, while above this weight the reverse is the case. Deaths attributed to congenital malformations are excluded from the second graph in Figure 1. Because of the higher death rate from congenital malformations among singleton births, the death rate from all other causes does not exceed that for multiple births until the 1200–1299g group.

It is not possible to extend this analysis back to earlier years. Birthweight data were not collected at birth registration until 1975 and reporting was incomplete before 1983. It is, however, possible to derive less detailed data for neonatal deaths over a longer timespan from DHSS' low birthweight notifications. These are plotted, in terms of survival rates, in Figure 2, and show dramatic changes in survival rates since the mid 1960s. In 1986 the neonatal mortality rate for babies weighing up to 1 kg was 48.1 per 1000 live births compared to 85.1 per 1000 live births in 1963.

MORBIDITY

This marked increase in survival rates makes the question about morbidity among the survivors increasingly important. Many of the studies of births before 28 weeks included a follow-up of the survivors, but it is difficult to compare morbidity rates from study to study or over time, because different measures were used and data were collected at different ages.

The study from Toronto counted what it described as 'major developmental handicaps' of mental retardation, spastic diplegia, quadriplegia, hemiplegia, blindness, hydrocephalus, hypotonia and periventricular leukomalacia. It is commented that 'In this series, since the incidence of major developmental handicap was almost the same at 6 months after discharge as at 18 months, this former time frame was accepted and minor degrees of handicap were excluded'.[12]

In the study at Ninewells Hospital, Dundee, each of the 24 surviving infants' progress was recorded for a minimum of 18 months following delivery;[6] of these 8 had a 'handicap'. These were either right or left hemiplegia, spastic diplegia, blindness, microcephaly, or osteogenesis imperfecta.

Other studies report more systematic and specific assessments of morbidity in considerable detail. In both hospital[14] and population[11] based studies in Melbourne, Australia, children were assessed at the age of two years, corrected for gestational age at delivery, by staff who had not been involved in their care during their stay in intensive care units. The assessments were detailed and included cerebral palsy, sensorineural deafness, visual impairment, development as measured by the Bayley Scales[32] and other developmental and psychological assessments.

This information was used to classify children as having severe, moderate, mild or no functional handicap using criteria based on 'current findings on psychometric tests, unequivocal neurologic signs and confirmed sensory deficits'.[11] If this is compared with the World Health Organization's (WHO's) definitions[33] set out in Table 16, it would appear that the authors were attempting to assess impairment rather than handicap.

In the McMaster Health Region infants were assessed at their 'due date', and at 3, 6, 12 and 24 months corrected age and 3 years chronological age.[10] They had detailed physical examinations and developmental status was assessed using selected items from the Bayley Scales of Infant Development[32] and the Stanford-Binet Test.[34] The children were tested for visual impairments including retrolental fibroplasia and for hearing impairments.

The information collected was classified in both neurologic and

Table 16 WHO recommended definitions of impairments, disabilities and handicaps

Impairments
Concerned with abnormalities of body structure and appearance and with organ or system function, resulting from any cause; in principle, impairments represent disturbances at the organ level.

Disabilities
Reflecting the consequences of impairment in terms of functional performance and activity by the individual; disabilities thus represent disturbances at the level of the person.

Handicaps
Concerned with the disadvantages experienced by the individual as a result of impairment and disabilities; handicaps thus reflect interaction with adaptation to the individual's surroundings.

Source: International Classification of Impairments, Disabilities and Handicaps[33]

functional terms. In contrast with the classification used in the Melbourne studies, 'The functional classification scheme was developed to provide a summary judgement of the quality of each child's ordinary activities and skills of daily living. Assignment to one of four categories (normal, or mild, moderate or major dysfunction) was based on a combination of the child's everyday function and the degree of additional caretaking burden for children with developmental abnormalities'.[10] This falls somewhere between the definitions of disability and handicap in the WHO classification.

Neurologic handicaps, on the other hand, 'consisted of definitive problems such as cerebral palsy, hydrocephalus, microcephaly, mental retardation and blindness'.[35] This approximates more to the definition of 'functional handicap' in the Melbourne studies and is consistent with the WHO definition of impairment. In the McMaster study the classifications were based on assessments at three years except for children born in 1980, the last year in the cohort studied. In this case they were based on data collected at the two year follow-up. As a consequence of all these differences it was found to be almost impossible to compare the findings of the Melbourne and McMaster studies.[11]

There were further differences again in the studies done in Wolverhampton[9] and in the Northern Region. In Wolverhampton children were seen between the ages of three and seven and given a physical examination and tests of motor skill, hearing, vision and development. They were also rated by teachers. Handicap was classified as follows:

> Children were classified as having a major handicap if their condition precluded education at a normal school. Partial sightedness or hemiplegia did not prevent normal schooling. Children with lesser disabilities including squint, clumsiness and epilepsy were classified as having a minor handicap, as were dull children and those over age 5 with very indistinct speech.[9]

This was one of the few studies which attempted to have a control group. It used normal birthweight siblings as controls, but 29 of the 67 surviving children had no such sibling.

Comparisons were also made with eight earlier studies. The author felt that the rates of major or moderate handicap were 'broadly comparable' with the 14% found at Wolverhampton, but went on to comment that 'The wide range of minor handicap rates (6–40% of survivors) reflects differences in definition, age at follow-up and tests performed.[9]

The Northern Region survey set out to measure the prevalence of severe disability among all survivors who reached the age of two years. Pointing to the absence of an agreed definition of severe disability it used 'cerebral palsy severe enough to hamper the normal physical activities that are appropriate for the child's age or a Griffiths General Quotient more than three standard deviations below the mean. Hearing loss severe enough to require bilateral hearing aids or likely to need special educational provision or visual loss of similar severity were also included' (Wariyar UK and Richmond S, unpublished observations).

In this study all the surviving children were traced, but this was not always the case to the same extent in all other studies. To explore the importance of this, the Northern Region identified children who had been difficult to trace. This included those who had been adopted or fostered, those whose parents initially refused the interview or repeatedly failed to attend, those who moved more than twice within the Region and those who left the Region or emigrated. Twenty six of the 230 survivors fell into one or more of these categories. When the children were ranked in groups by their General Quotient derived from the Griffiths assessment, it was found that the lower scoring groups contained higher proportions of children who were difficult to trace.

This calls into question the findings of studies in which follow-up has been incomplete. When compounded with differences in definition, this makes it difficult to draw any firm conclusions about long term morbidity in children born before 28 weeks of gestation.

DISCUSSION

In the early 1950s when programmes of care were being set up for what were then described as 'premature babies', the importance of collecting statistics to monitor and evaluate them was strongly emphasized.[36-39] Since then, while the care provided has changed out of all recognition, the standards of data collection have not progressed greatly, despite the revolution in computing technology.

It is clear that very preterm and very small babies born in recent years have better chances of surviving than those born in the 1950s and 1960s. The magnitude of these changes and the extent to which they reflect changes in incidence, changes in reporting, changes in the effectiveness and accessibility of intensive care or changes in other factors is far less clear. Furthermore there are no reliable estimates of changes in morbidity rates among survivors.

There are also, no long term series of data which could be used to assess changes in the incidence of birth before 28 weeks. The data for Scotland suggest increases over time in the reporting of live births at this gestation, but it is not clear to what extent this arises from increased rates of referral to intensive care, changes in policies towards bereaved parents or simply improvements in data collection. Longer term series of data about the incidence of low and very low birthweight show an apparent disproportionate increase in the incidence of birthweights below 1000 or 1001g compared with other low weight births. This suggests that the trends reflect increases in reporting rather than in incidence.

The question arises as to whether birthweight or gestational age is a better criterion to use for analysis. It is true that birthweight can be measured much more accurately and consistently than gestational age. Statistically, two studies have concluded that birthweight is a better predictor of mortality than is gestational age.[40,41]

From a practical point of view, however, it has been pointed out that obstetricians faced with decisions about whether to intervene at very short gestations have no knowledge of the baby's birthweight.[13-15] They can only, therefore, base their decisions on the very scanty data about survival by gestational age. In addition, if through an oversight the baby is not weighed at birth, then the birth weight will never be known, but gestational age can be estimated retrospectively from information in casenotes. Paediatricians who know both birthweight and gestational age should be on firmer ground, or at least would be if fuller and more reliable data were available.

In England, gestational age should now be being collected on a national scale through the Maternity Hospital Episode System (HES). Unfortunately, however, this system does not contain information about deaths outside hospital or in hospitals outside the district of birth. As very small and immature babies are the ones most likely to be referred outside their district of birth for intensive care, this is a major problem. In addition the baby's record in Maternity HES is closed at 28 days after birth, even though, increasingly, deaths in intensive care occur after this.[28-31] In this case, the death would be recorded elsewhere in HES, but not in the record containing information about the birth.

If, however, Maternity HES files were linked to the Office of Population Censuses and Survey's infant mortality linked files, it would be possible to calculate birthweight and gestational age specific mortality rates for babies at ages up to one year. Attention also needs to be given to validity checks on birthweight and gestational age data to ensure that the errors which occurred in Maternity HIPE and in the SMR2 system in the early 1980s are not carried over into the new system.

Even if mortality data which can now be produced only in Scotland become available on a national scale in the other countries of the United Kingdom, there will still be a need for follow-up studies to assess morbidity. There is clearly a lot of work under way in this area, but unfortunately the majority of studies are hospital based and do not collect data in a comparable way. While it is only natural for clinicians to want to follow up children for whom they have cared, restricting data collection in this way will end up with biased data which may be misleading for monitoring care. It is possible to identify births to residents of NHS districts through birth notification forms and through draft entries of birth registrations both of which are forwarded to the mother's district of residence. The findings from Newcastle underline the importance of following up even the children who are most difficult to find.

It is also important to agree criteria for measuring morbidity. Although studies which measure handicap attempt to tackle questions about the implications of disability and impairment for the lives of the children concerned, these still beg questions about the extent to which these subjectively reflect the circumstances in which they live and the support available to them. Measuring impairment avoids these important questions but leads to measurements which can be more validly compared from study to study. Whatever else is measured, there is clearly a need for agreement on a minimum set of comparable data.

The same applies to follow-up intervals. Admittedly, it is difficult to balance the need for a long enough follow-up period against the need to monitor and evaluate rapidly changing patterns of care. In theory, it should be possible to set up follow-up studies which draw on data from child health computer systems. At the present time there are differences in the systems available and the extent to which districts may or may not have implemented them. This means that some time is likely to elapse before it might be feasible to use them in this way. It is intended to try to explore this possibility through the Oxford Region Child Development Project.

Even if better data become available, there will still be problems in interpreting them. How far, for example, do differences in outcome in centres providing varying levels of care and changes over time reflect differences in the quality of care, how far selective referral and how far other factors such as socio-economic differences in the circumstances to which children are discharged?[42-45] To some extent it may be possible to tackle some of these questions by incorporating a control group, but there are undoubted problems in selecting controls.[9] Other questions may be unanswerable without doing randomized trials.

One of the most difficult questions is the extent to which death is to be considered a necessarily adverse outcome, in cases where the alternative may be the survival of a severely impaired child.[12,46-50] There are many different ethical and cultural considerations which may shape the views of parents and staff and affect their views. Added to this is the problem of taking decisions in a climate where there is much popular support for neonatal care coupled with high expectations, but constraints on resources for providing this expensive form of care. At the same time debates about this often overlook the infinitely greater constraints on resources to allow people with disabilities to reach their full potential in their lives.

Studies in the 1950s placed considerable emphasis on ethnic and gender differences in mortality among 'premature' births,[39,51] and suggested the need for socio-economic analyses.[39] Although the need for collecting socio-economic data has been stressed again much more recently,[52] the studies quoted here do not seem able to do so in analysable way. Given the social class differences observed in Scotland in the incidence of birth before 28 weeks of gestation, this is an important deficiency. It may also be a reflection of the fact that the need for finding ways to prevent 'prematurity' was mentioned more prominently in the 1950s,[36] than in recent studies.

A new study, which seems to be moving on from most of those described here has recently started in the Avon district in England. Each baby born before 33 weeks of gestation has two controls, one born on the same day and one born on the baby's estimated date of delivery. These controls are being matched for sex, ethnic group, marital status, size of sibship and social class. The study will look at the babies' environmental conditions and use of health services during their first year of life (Baum D, Emond A, personal communication). Although there may be problems arising from matching out social factors, it will be interesting to see whether, as well as adopting this broader approach, the study manages to avoid some of the pitfalls discussed here and provide further insights into the context of very preterm births.

CONCLUSIONS

Live births before 28 weeks of gestational age accounted for 0.26% of live births in Scotland over the years 1980–84. There are no data for other countries of the United Kingdom. Much higher proportions of both multiple and singleton births at this gestation occurred to women under 20 than was the case for births as a whole. As with all preterm births, births before 28 weeks of gestation were almost twice as likely to occur to women married to men in unskilled occupations than to those with husbands in professional occupations.

The apparent increase over the past ten years in the incidence of live births before 28 weeks in Scotland and of live births with birthweights under 1 kg is likely to reflect more complete reporting.

Both routinely collected statistics and special studies done over the last 30 years point to increased survival rates of babies weighing under 1 kg or born before 28 weeks, although the chances of survival are virtually zero for babies born before 24 weeks or with birthweights under 500g. Mortality rates decrease from 24 to 27 weeks and with increasing birthweight at each gestational age. When mortality rates are tabulated by birthweight alone there are marked differences between 100g groupings from 500g to 1.5kg.

Neonatal mortality rates have for some time been an inadequate measure of outcome of care in neonatal units and deaths later in infancy should be included. Survival to hospital discharge may perhaps be a more appropriate measure than neonatal mortality, but is not sufficiently precise as discharge criteria are not uniform. The time of discharge may depend on other factors as well as the conditions of babies, and it is unclear to what extent rates of survival to hospital discharge allow for readmissions. The cut off point for any survival rates quoted should be stated clearly.

In any case neonatal and either postneonatal or infant mortality rates should be quoted as well, even though the latter will inevitably include deaths which may occur long after discharge from neonatal care or among babies to whom no long-term specialist care was given. Mortality rates should be based on resident rather than hospital populations and should allow for socio-economic differences between populations, as well as differences in the care they receive and the way this can depend on hospital of birth and whether babies were transferred after birth to specialist centres.

Much of this is already possible in Scotland. It may be some time before the other countries of the United Kingdom are able to provide mortality rates by gestational age on a national scale. It would appear that the most suitable approach is through linking data from the NHS data collection systems with civil registration data. Meanwhile there is a potential for local studies and a need to give attention to the quality of gestational age data.

The longer term outcome for surviving babies born before 28 weeks of gestation is far from clear. Although many follow-up studies are done, too many are hospital-based, contain small numbers of children, or use only birthweight and not gestational age as a criterion. Few have information about the socio-economic background of the parents and control groups are extremely rare. Follow-up intervals, completeness of follow-up and outcome measures vary from study to study. It is often unclear whether impairment, disability or handicap are being measured. Few studies attempt to relate outcome to the child's circumstances on discharge from hospital. This is an important omission given the raised incidence of preterm birth in general and birth before 28 weeks in particular, at the lower end of the social scale.

Recommendations have already been made about the design, analysis and reporting of follow-up studies,[52,53] but it is not clear to what extent they have been heeded. It is important to take them further to develop and implement more specific guidelines for doing special studies and using routine data collection systems to monitor the outcome of pregnancy before 28 weeks and the care given to these babies. There will still be difficult ethical questions but at present these are even harder than they need be because of the shortage of reliable information.

As a consequence of this it is still necessary to echo the British Paediatric Association's recommendations, made as long ago as 1951:

> There is need for research into the causes and prevention of prematurity and into the value of various methods of treatment. Regular appraisal of results is of great importance and accurate statistics are required...[36]

ACKNOWLEDGEMENTS

We should like to thank Phillipa Claiden for typing this article, Lesley Mutch, Unni Wariyar and Sam Richmond for permission to use unpublished data and the Information and Statistics Division in Edinburgh and the Medical Statistics Unit, Office of Population Censuses and Surveys in London for providing additional tabulations. Alison Macfarlane and Ann Johnson are funded by the Department of Health and Social Security.

REFERENCES

1 Cole S. Scottish maternity and neonatal records. In: Chalmers I, McIlwaine G, eds. Perinatal audit and surveillance. London: Royal College of Obstetricians and Gynaecologists, 1980
2 Information and Statistics Division. Scottish stillbirth and neonatal death report 1986. Edinburgh: ISD, 1987
3 Mutch L. Archive of locally based perinatal surveys. Oxford: National Perinatal Epidemiology Unit, 1986
4 Welsh Office. Wales perinatal mortality initiative 1984–86. Cardiff: Welsh Office, 1986
5 Department of Health and Social Security, Office of Population and Censuses and Surveys, Welsh Office. Hospital In-patient Enquiry Maternity Tables 1977–1981. Series MB4 No. 19. London: HMSO, 1986
6 Walker EM, Patel NB. Mortality and morbidity in infants born between 20 and 28 weeks gestation. Br J Obstet Gynaecol 1987; 94: 670–674
7 Verloove-Vanhorick SP, Verwey RA, Brand R, Bennebroek Gravenhorst J, Keirse MJNC, Ruys JH. Neonatal mortality risk in relation to gestational age and birthweight. Lancet 1986; i: 55–57
8 Verloove-Vanhorick SP, Vervey RA. Project on preterm and small for gestational age infants in the Netherlands 1983. Doctoral thesis. Leiden, Netherlands 1987

9. Lloyd BW. Outcome of very low birthweight babies from Wolverhampton. Lancet 1984; ii: 739–741
10. Saigal S, Rosenbaum P, Stoskopf B, Sinclair JC. Outcome in infants 501 to 1000g birthweight delivered to residents of the McMaster Health Region. J Pediatr 1984; 105: 969–976
11. Kitchen W, Ford G, Orgill A et al. Outcome in infants with birthweight 500 to 999g. A regional study of 1979 and 1980 births. J Pediatr 1984; 92: 921–927
12. Milligan JE, Shennan AT, Hoskins EM. Perinatal intensive care: where and how to draw the line. Am J Obstet Gynecol 1984; 148: 499–503
13. Herschel M, Kennedy JL, Kayne HL, Henry M, Cetrulo CL. Survival of infants born at 24 to 28 weeks gestation. Obstet Gynecol 1982; 60: 154–158
14. Yu VYH, Orgill AA, Bajuk B, Astbury J. Survival and 2-year outcome of extremely preterm infants. Br J Obstet Gynaecol 1984; 91: 640–646
15. Dillon WP, Egan EA. Aggressive obstetric management in late second-trimester deliveries. Obstet Gynecol 1981; 58: 685–690
16. Philip AGS, Little GA, Polivy DR, Lucey JF. Neonatal mortality risk for the eighties: the importance of birth weight/gestational age groups. Pediatrics 1981; 68: 122–130
17. Weindling AM, Cook RWI. The outcome for infants of less than 28 weeks' gestation. Paper given at the Conference of the British Paediatric Association, York 15 April, 1988
18. Information and Statistics Division. Birthweight statistics 1980–84. Edinburgh: ISD, 1987
19. Hall MH, Carr-Hill RA, Fraser C, Campbell D, Samphier ML. The extent and antecedents of uncertain gestaton. Br J Obstet Gynaecol 1985; 92: 445–451
20. Macfarlane AJ, Mugford M. Birth counts: statistics of pregnancy and childbirth. London: HMSO, 1984
21. Keen DV, Pearse RG. Birthweight between 14 and 42 weeks gestation. Arch Dis Child 1985; 60: 440–446
22. Lucas A, Cole TJ, Gandy GM. Birthweight centiles in preterm infants reappraised. Early Hum Dev 1986; 13: 313–322
23. Yudkin PL, Aboualfa M, Eyre JA, Redman CWG, Wilkinson AR. Influence of elective preterm delivery on birthweight and head circumference standards. Arch Dis Child 1987; 62: 24–29
24. Yudkin PL, Aboualfa M, Eyre JA, Redman CWG, Wilkinson AR. New birthweight and head circumference centiles for gestational ages 24 to 42 weeks. Early Hum Dev 1987; 15: 45–52
25. DHSS. Birth notifications: 1976–1986. Low weight births and mortality. Summary information from form LHS 27/1, 1986, England. London: DHSS, 1987
26. Powell TG, Pharoah POD, Cooke RWI. How accurate are the perinatal statistics for your region? Community Med 1987; 9: 226–231
27. Walker I. Killing for kindness. New Society 1988; 83(1319): 13
28. Hack M, Merkatz IR, Jones PK, Fanaroff AA. Changing trends of neonatal and postneonatal deaths in very low birthweight infants. Am J Obstet Gynecol 1980; 87: 833–838
29. Arneil GC, Brooke H, Gibson AAM, Harvie A, McIntosh H, Patrick WJA. Post-perinatal mortality in Glasgow 1979–81. Lancet 1982; ii: 649–651
30. Harper R, Rosenstein R, Sia C, Kiernay C. Should we continue to define neonatal mortality as death within the first 28 days of life? Pediatr Res 1979; 13: 390 (Abstract)
31. Yu VYH, Watkins A, Bajuk B. Neonatal and postneonatal mortality in very low birthweight infants. Arch Dis Child 1984; 59: 987–999
32. Bayley N. Bayley scales of infant development. New York: Psychological Corporation, 1969

33 World Health Organization. International classification of impairments, disabilities and handicaps. Geneva: WHO, 1980
34 Terman IM, Merrill MA. The Stanford-Binet Intelligence Scale (rev 3). Stanford, USA: Stanford University Press, 1972
35 Saigal S, Rosenbaum P, Stoskopf B, Milner R. Follow-up of infants 501 to 1,500 gm birthweight delivered to residents of a geographically defined region with perinatal intensive care facilities. J Pediatr 1982; 100: 606–613
36 British Paediatric Association. Memorandum on the care of premature babies in urban and rural areas. Arch Dis Child 1951; 26: 276–278
37 Dunham EC. Premature birth as a world health problem. Pediatrics 1951; 7: 262–268
38 Wegman ME. Statistics for premature infants. Pediatrics 1951; 8: 570–572
39 Silverman WA, Fertig JW, Kraus A. A proposed method of computing standardised death rates for premature nurseries. Pediatrics 1955; 15: 467–477
40 Susser M, Marolla FA, Fleiss J. Birthweight, fetal age and perinatal mortality. Am J Epidemiol 1972; 62: 197–204
41 Helier JL, Goldstein H. The use of birthweight and gestation to assess perinatal mortality risk. J Epidemiol Community Health 1979; 33: 183–185
42 Cooke RWI. Referral to a regional centre improves outcome in extremely low birthweight infants. Arch Dis Child 1987; 82: 619–621
43 Roper HP, Chiswick ML, Sims DG. Referrals to a regional neonatal intensive care unit. Arch Dis Child 1988; 63: 403–407
44 Verloove-Vanhorick SP, Verwey RA, Ebeling CBA, Brand R, Ruys JH. Mortality in very preterm and very low birthweight infants according to place of birth and level of care: results of a national collaborative survey of preterm and very low birthweight infants in the Netherlands. Pediatrics 1988; 81: 404–411
45 Goldenberg RL, Nelson KG, Koski JF, Cutter G, Cassady GE. Neonatal mortality in infants born weighing 501 to 1000 grams. Am J Obstet Gynecol 1985; 151: 608–611
46 Whitelaw A. Death as an option in intensive care. Lancet 1986; ii: 329–331
47 Campbell AGM. Which infants should not receive intensive care? Arch Dis Child 1982; 52: 569–571
48 Stinson R, Stinson P. The long dying of baby Andrew. Boston/Toronto: Little Brown, 1979
49 Kirkley WH. Fetal survival — what price? Am J Obstet Gynecol 1980; 137: 873–875
50 Pomerance JJ, Ukrainski CT, Ukra T, Henderson DH, Nash AN, Meredith JL. Cost of living for infants weighing 1000 grams or less at birth. Pediatrics 1978; 61: 908–910
51 Erhardt CL, Joshi GV, Nelson FO, Kroll BH, Weiner L. Influence of weight and gestation on perinatal mortality by ethnic group. Am J Public Health 1964; 54: 1841–1855
52 Kiely JL, Paneth N. Follow-up studies of low-birthweight infants: suggestions for design, analysis and reporting. Dev Med Child Neurol 1981; 23: 96–99
53 Editorial. The fate of the baby under 1501g at birth. Lancet 1980; i: 461–463

Lung development in the second trimester

J S Wigglesworth
Department of Paediatrics and Neonatal Medicine, Royal Postgraduate Medical School, London

> In the second trimester the human lung develops from a near-solid glandular organ to a hollow one containing all the elements needed for extra-uterine gas exchange. Mesenchymal-epithelial interactions control the structural and biochemical maturation basic to this process, while the associated quantitative growth of the lung requires continued airway distension by fetal lung liquid and fetal breathing movements. Lung growth, during this rapid phase of development, is particularly vulnerable to impairment by interference with fetal breathing, space for lung expansion or lung liquid retention. Oligohydramnios may cause severe impairment both in lung growth and eipthelial maturation. Despite continued ignorance of the precise mechanism of this effect it appears to be prevented by obstruction to tracheal fluid outflow.

The second trimester is the critical period for development of the lung as it is for many other organs and tissues. A major part of the spectrum of development from a gland-like secretory organ to one that is capable of gaseous exchange occurs during the brief period from 16–24 weeks gestational age. Not only differentiation but quantitative growth is at its maximum during this period, and the lung achieves its largest size relative to the body at this time. The smallest hindrance to normal growth during this period may have a disproportionate effect on quantitative growth and maturation. Thus the second trimester is a focal point for both physiology and pathology of the developing lung.

STRUCTURAL DEVELOPMENT

At the start of the second trimester the lung is in the pseudoglandular stage of development. The future air spaces are represented by narrow tubules of endodermally derived columnar epithelium surrounded by condensations of mesenchymal tissue and separated by a loose mesenchymal stroma. The tubules have basal nuclei and their cytoplasm is rich in glycogen (Fig. 1). At this stage the epithelium is undifferentiated and the lung capillaries show no specific relationship to the tubules. During this phase of development there is dichotomous branching of the bronchi to reach some 15–26 generations along the axial pathways by about 16 weeks.[1] The branching of the primitive epithelial tubules is known to take place under the control of the adjacent mesenchyme.[2] Mesodermal cells appear to enhance epithelial cell proliferation at specific sites by acting on the organisation of intracellular microfilaments and by modifying the spatial distribution of basement membrane components.[3-5] Mesenchymal–epithelial reciprocal inductive processes may well control a major part of basic pulmonary development throughout intrauterine life.[6] The epithelial cell population of the major airways differentiates into ciliated, goblet and basal cells from the proximal end out to the periphery as does the formation of smooth muscle and cartilage.

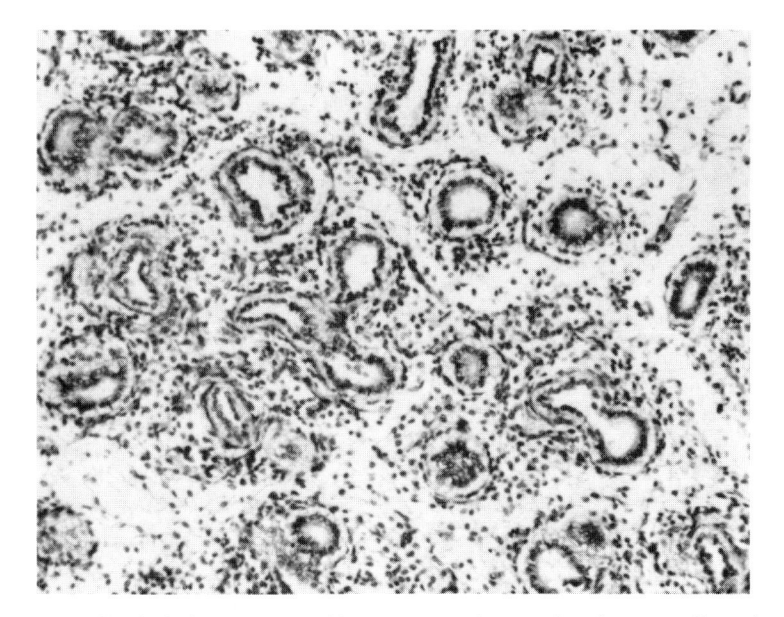

Fig. 1 Histological appearance of lung at 15 weeks gestation: haematoxylin and eosin (H & E) stain, magnification × 160. The gland-like tubules of the developing lung are surrounded by condensations of the mesenchymal stroma

At about 17 weeks gestational age the basic parenchymal structure changes to the canalicular form. This is characterised by flattening of the epithelium of the tubules to a low cuboidal form in association with dilatation of their lumina (Fig. 2). At some sites the capillaries within the adjacent mesenchyme become apposed to the epithelium which flattens further to form the first blood-air barriers. In effect this phase of lung development represents the transition of the lung to a hollow fluid-containing organ from its initial solid state. Individual neuroendocrine cells and neuro-epithelial bodies can be detected from early in the second trimester, and serotonin, calcitonin and bombesin can be detected by imunocytochemistry from 20 weeks of gestational age.[7-9]

At about 23–24 weeks of gestation the peripheral respiratory epithelium differentiates into the two characteristic cell types, the flattened Type 1 pneumonocytes and the Type 2 pneumonocytes with surface microvilli and cytoplasmic osmiophilic lamellar bodies, the site of surfactant formation. At the same time there is a progressive increase in blood air barriers and the dilating air spaces become recognised as saccules (Fig. 3). Small deposits of elastin appear within the saccular walls and delineate the site of

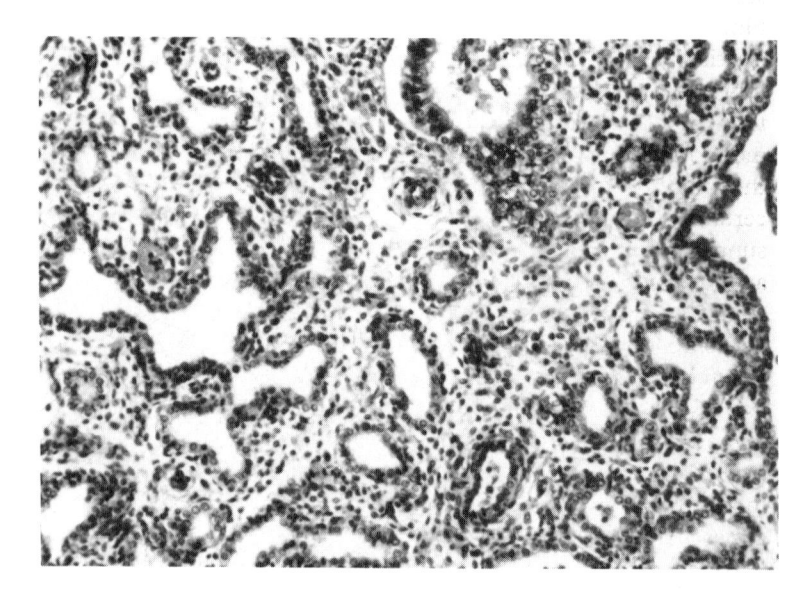

Fig. 2 Lung at 20 weeks gestation: (H&E × 160). Canalicular stage of development with fluid-filled peripheral airways lined by cuboidal epithelium

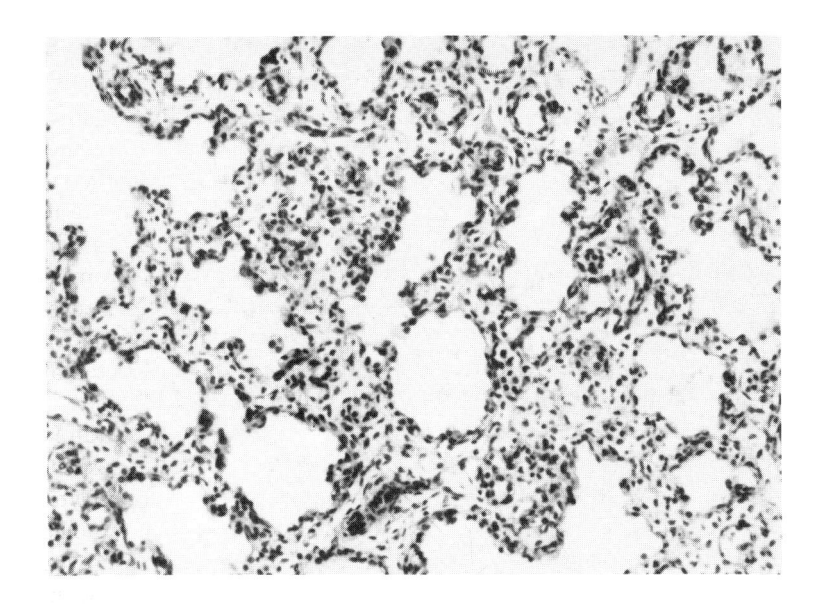

Fig. 3 Lung at 26 weeks gestation: (H&E × 160), showing saccular structure

future formation of alveolar septa. The earliest stage of alveolar septal formation seen at this stage consists in the development of blunt mesenchymal ridges with capillaries and small bundles of elastin fibres near the tips. In traditional descriptions of prenatal lung development this phase has been described as persisting to term,[10] but recent studies have been shown that alveolar formation commences by 32 weeks gestation or earlier.[11,12] However, the lung of the second trimester fetus delivered at up to 28 weeks is certainly in a saccular stage and only marginally capable of supporting extra-uterine life. Although Type 2 cells are differentiated and surfactant is present within osmiophilic lamellar bodies from 23–24 weeks, the concentration of surfactant is very low and its composition differs significantly from that at term.[13] Stimulation of surfactant production by the action of glucocorticoids, of extrinsic or intrinsic origin, is not due to a direct effect on the Type 2 cells but involves stimulation of the fibroblasts to secrete a small protein, fibroblast–pneumonocyte factor, which in turn induces surfactant synthesis.[14] This represents another example of a mesenchymal–epithelial interaction.

Apart from purely quantitative differences in the amounts of elastin and extent of elaboration of the respiratory portion of the lobule a major difference between the saccular and alveolar stages of development lies in the relation of the capillaries to the air spaces. During the saccular phase the capillaries project at one surface into the air spaces (Fig. 4), whereas the development of alveoli allows the septal capillaries to be exposed to air on two surfaces.

QUANTITATIVE GROWTH

Fetal lung growth is very rapid during the second trimester both in terms of weight and of cell population as measured by DNA. The weight of the lungs relative to that of the body rises to about 4% in the early second trimester and then gradually falls.[15] By 28 weeks the lung tissue represents about 2.5% of body weight, and is due to fall to about 1.5% by term.[16] The lung DNA increases slowly until about 16 weeks after which there is rapid increase with doubling of DNA content between 17 and 20 weeks, and again by 28 weeks.[17]

FUNCTIONAL ASPECTS OF LUNG GROWTH

Studies of experimental animals have revealed two functional activities of the fetal lung that appear to be of major importance for

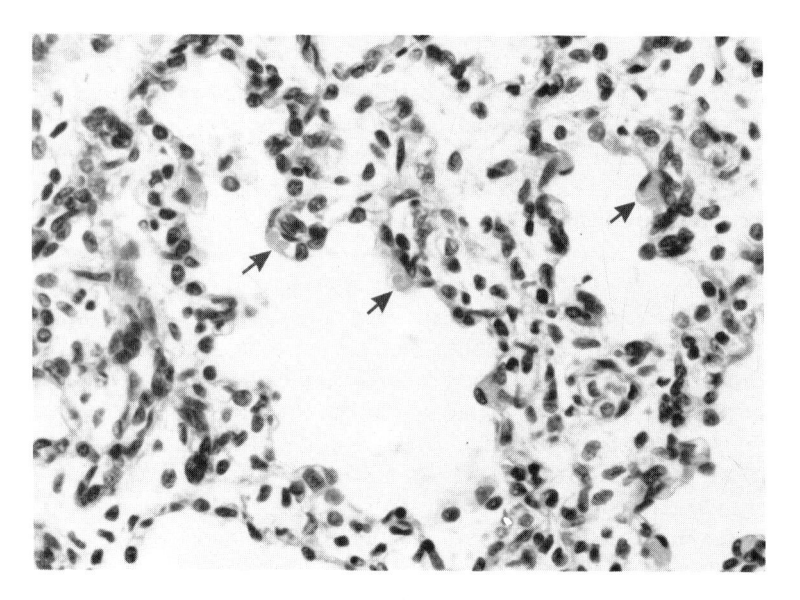

Fig. 4 Detail of lung shown in Fig. 3: (H&E × 450). Capillaries projecting into the air spaces are arrowed

lung growth. Studies on the fetal lamb have shown that the chloride rich fluid which fills the airspaces and airways *in utero* is secreted at rates of up to 15 ml per kg body weight per hour.[18] Continual drainage of this liquid through a tracheal tube in the chronic fetal lamb preparation results in lung hypoplasia.[19] Conversely the obstruction to drainage of the fluid into the amniotic cavity by tracheal ligation leads to massive expansion of the fetal lung with the retained liquid.[19]

The other form of fetal respiratory function which has been extensively studied in recent years in both animal and human fetuses is fetal breathing movements. These commence from early in the second trimester as episodic low amplitude high frequency activity in the diaphragm associated with paradoxical movement of the thoracic wall. There are bursts of this respiratory activity at a frequency of up to 4Hz separated by periods of quiescence.[20-22] Experimental studies on rabbit and lamb fetuses have shown that surgical procedures which prevent these movements, or their associated transpulmonary pressure changes, cause severe lung hypoplasia.[23-25] Thus abolition of fetal breathing by cervical cord transection in the fetal rabbit during the pseudoglandular stage of development causes a 70% reduction in lung growth as measured by the increment of DNA, although the operation does not interfere with development of the thoracic wall structures or the diaphragm.[24] The effects of high cord transection on fetal lung growth were confirmed by Liggins and colleagues using fetal lambs.[25] These workers caused equally severe lung hypoplasia by inserting a flexible silastic membrane into the chest wall to abolish the pressure swings from fetal breathing while allowing it to continue.[26] Other operations to abolish fetal breathing, such as phrenic nerve section,[27,28] cause diaphragmatic atrophy and may lead to lung compression by abdominal contents.

Although the importance of lung liquid as a moulding and stretching influence on the developing respiratory epithelium seems readily understandable it is unclear as to how fetal breathing movements may have any effect. Presumably the transpulmonary pressure swings, or the distortion of lung geometry, enhance the effects of liquid distension. There is little evidence that thyroid and pituitary hormones have any significant influence on quantitative lung growth although they may be of importance for maturation.[29] Similarly studies to date on growth factors such as EGF have demonstrated a role in maturation of surfactant but not in quantitative growth.[30]

OTHER FACTORS INVOLVED IN LUNG GROWTH

These include normal intrathoracic space to allow lung growth and a normal volume of amniotic fluid. Experimental reduction of intrathoracic space in the fetal lamb has been used as one model for production of lung hypoplasia.[31,32] The importance of amniotic fluid is discussed below. These factors seem to be linked to fetal breathing and to the volume of liquid retained in the fetal airways. The exact relationship between the various factors remain incompletely understood.

VULNERABILITY OF LUNG DEVELOPMENT

From the previous sections it can be seen that the fetal lung passes from an extremely immature state of proliferating epithelial tubules within a mass of mesenchyme to a relatively well differentiated saccular organ capable of sustaining extrauterine respiration within a brief period of some 8–10 weeks. It is now clear that this period of maximum growth and differentiation of the lung is also a period of considerable vulnerability. Any influence interfering with the factors mentioned above, liquid secretion and retention, fetal breathing movements, thoracic space and amniotic fluid volume, may have a disastrous effect on fetal lung growth.[33,34] Indeed the demonstration of lung hypoplasia as a consequence of interference with one or more of these factors constitutes the major evidence for their importance in control of normal fetal lung growth.

Effects of oligohydramnios

The syndrome of oligohydramnios presenting early in the second trimester, usually as a result of premature rupture of the membranes, has become widely recognised since the introduction of ultrasound for fetal monitoring. The infants are typically born in the late second or early third trimester, and frequently have severe respiratory distress syndrome associated with lung hypoplasia.[35-38] Hislop and colleagues[39] found a reduction in generations of bronchial branching in such cases, which suggested an onset before 17 weeks gestation.

A recent study found that oligohydramnios was most likely to be associated with impaired lung growth if membranes were ruptured before 26 weeks gestation and had been ruptured for over 5 weeks before birth.[37] It has also been claimed that a period of ruptured membranes as short as 5 days may impair lung growth.[38] Study of the effects of experimental oligohydramnios in the guinea pig fetus at varying time periods has shown that lung growth is most readily impaired in the canalicular phase.[40] Amniocentesis with minimal removal of amniotic fluid on a single occasion has been shown to result in lowered alveolar counts in the monkey fetus at term.[41] Although fetal breathing movements have been recorded in fetuses with renal agenesis,[42] a recent study has reported that occurrence of normal fetal breathing movements in cases of oligohydramnios is associated with preservation of lung development.[43] This work implies that the effect of oligohydramnios in impairing lung growth is due in part to inhibition of fetal breathing. A separate and larger study has failed to show such an effect,[44] although it has been argued that differences in the definition of effective fetal breathing movements may account for the discrepancy.[45] The combination of experimental oligohydramnios and cervical cord transection during the canalicular phase in the fetal rabbit has been shown to cause more severe lung hypoplasia than either operation alone,[46] which might indicate some protective effect of fetal breathing in this species. Other postulated mechanisms for lung hypoplasia in this condition are thoracic compression and disturbance of the normal fluid volume and pressure within the airways.

The effects of oligohydramnios on the lungs are quite distinctive. There is impairment both in quantitative lung growth in terms of DNA and elaboration of airspaces and an arrest of maturation of the respiratory epithelium with a lack of development of elastic tissue within the alveolar septa.[47] Undifferentiated epithelial tubules remain prominent at the periphery of the poorly developed acini into the third trimester (Fig. 6). These narrow peripheral airways suggest strongly that there has been reduction of airway fluid content over a period of time. The maturational defect may be more important than the decrease in lung size in determining the severity of respiratory distress in these infants. Indeed the increase in lung weight which occurs rapidly following commencement of mechanical ventilation,[48] may sometimes obscure the underlying lung hypoplasia if the infant survives for 24 hours or so. The original state of the lung can then only be established on histological criteria. Morphometric studies on the hypoplastic lungs of guinea-pig fetuses subject to oligohydramnios have shown a quantitative decrease in elastic tissue, similar to the effect observed in the human fetus.[49]

Other causes of lung hypoplasia

Other conditions associated with lung hypoplasia are listed in Table 1. Study of DNA content in normally grown and hypoplastic lungs indicated that cellular proliferation in the hypoplastic group had been impaired from before 20 weeks gestation irrespective of the type of lung hypoplasia.[17] Examination of the graph of lung DNA content against gestation suggested that impairment in lung cell proliferation had dated in most cases from about the time of transformation from the pseudoglandular to the canalicular stage of development (Fig. 5). This is in agreement with the experimental findings quoted above in the guinea pig fetus exposed to oligohydramnios. As described above the characteristic feature of this stage is the commencement of fluid retention by the airways. Oligohydramnios may prevent occurrence of this fluid accumulation. Such cases are now routinely recognised on ultrasound and may prompt initiation of measures to mitigate the cause or to perform termination if the hypoplasia (Fig. 6) is considered incompatible with extrauterine survival.

Table 1 Conditions associated with lung hypoplasia

Prolonged oligohydramnios	Renal agenesis Severe renal cystic dysplasia Obstruction of lower urinary tract, prune belly syndrome Prolonged rupture of membranes
Skeletal dysplasias affecting integrity of thoracic wall	Thanatophoric dwarfism Asphyxiating thoracic dysplasia Osteogenesis imperfecta (lethal variant)
Anomalies affecting development of diaphragm	Congenital diaphragmatic hernia Congenital muscular dystrophy Congenital amyoplasia of diaphragm
Anomalies or damage to CNS	Anencephaly Iniencephaly Anoxic-ischaemic lesions Meckel-Gruber syndrome
Miscellaneous conditions	Exomphalos Severe rhesus isoimmunisation Extralobar sequestration of lung with pleural effusion Other forms of non-immunologic hydrops

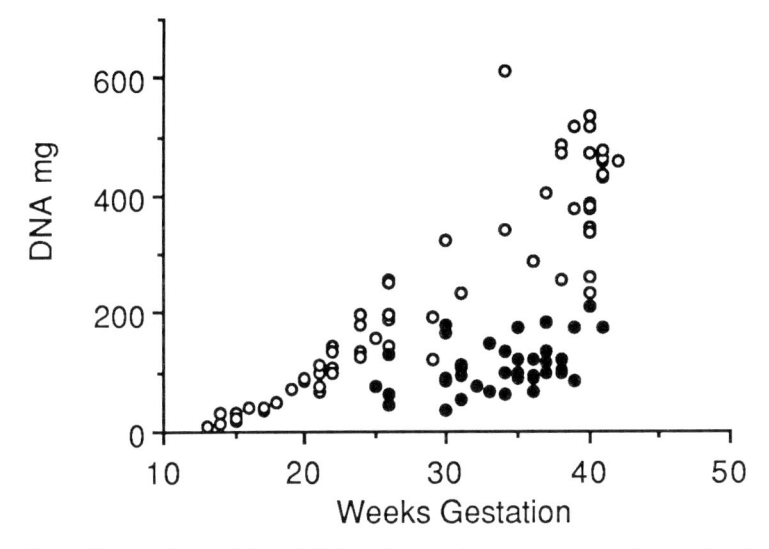

Fig. 5 Changes in total lung DNA with gestation: comparison of normal and hypoplastic lungs

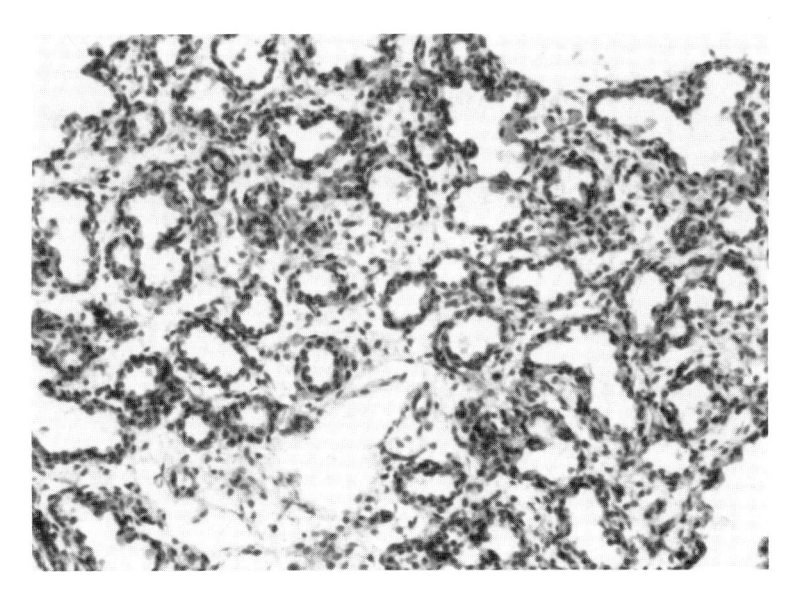

Fig. 6 Hypoplastic lung of an infant of 26 weeks gestation with lower urinary tract obstruction: (H&E × 160). Air spaces are mainly represented by tubules lined with cuboidal epithelium. Compare with Figures 3 and 4

Effects of laryngeal atresia

A form of pathology which sheds additional light on the mechanisms of lung growth control is laryngeal atresia. In those cases where laryngeal atresia occurs as an isolated defect without an associated tracheo-oesophageal fistula there is no route for escape of liquid from the airways apart from a pinhole sized pharyngotracheal duct.[50] The infants cannot usually be resuscitated at birth and present at autopsy with voluminous fluid-filled lungs. Although the wet weight of the lungs is about twice that expected on the basis of body weight this is mainly accounted for by the increased fluid volume and there is little increase in lung DNA.[51] Histological examination in such cases show a rather mature lung structure for gestation but without grossly distended air spaces (Fig. 7). Morphometric studies show an increase in lung surface area and alveolar number, and apparent advance in elastin maturation but no increase in disaturated phosphatidylcholine content.[51] The increase in alveolar number without increase in DNA implies that alveolar development in this condition is achieved by redistribution of cells rather than increase in cell number. A particularly interesting 'experiment of nature' is provided by cases

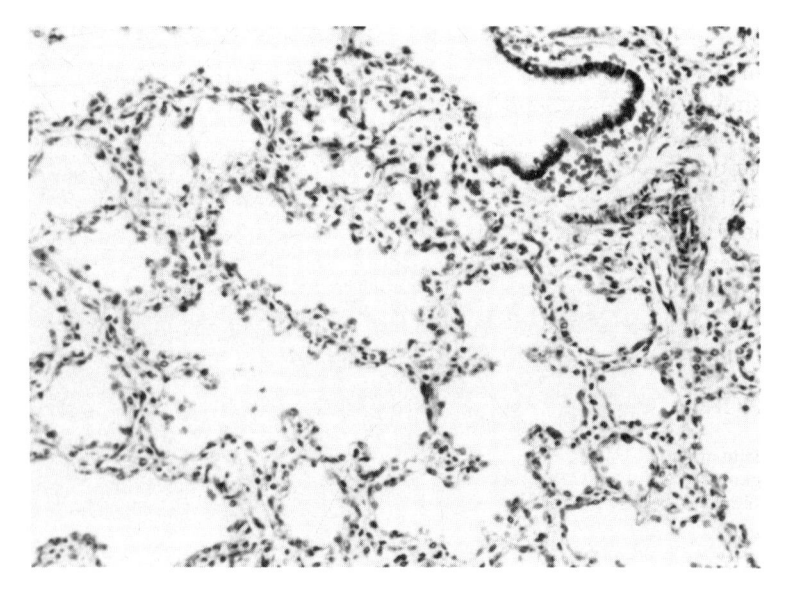

Fig. 7 Lung of an infant with congenital laryngeal atresia at 27 weeks gestation: (H&E × 160). Maturation appears more advanced than that of the normal lung shown in Figures 3 and 4

of cryptophthalmos-syndactyly (Fraser) syndrome where laryngeal atresia may be combined with renal agenesis and severe oligohydramnios. Biochemical and morphometric studies in one such case revealed voluminous lungs with mature alveolar structure in contrast to the hypoplasia and maturation arrest expected in renal agenesis.[51] Since the fixed lung distension resulting from laryngeal atresia might be expected to dampen fetal breathing movements, it appears that adequate maintenance of lung liquid volume and pressure is the most important single determinant of normal alveolar growth and maturation.

Other factors such as presence of normal amniotic fluid volume, adequate thoracic space and fetal breathing movements appear all to be contributory features which provide the appropriate milieu for fluid directed alveolar development in the normal anatomical condition in which the airways are in free communication with the amniotic cavity.

Effects of preterm birth and mechanical ventilation

The recognition of the importance of fluid distension for fetal lung growth and maturation raises the question as to the effects on lung growth of preterm birth and mechanical ventilation. Comparison of morphological and biochemical indices in such lungs with those of fresh stillbirths or very early neonatal deaths or cot death cases showed no abnormality in growth in the few instances when the infant had not been ventilated.[48] The effect of mechanical ventilation was to dilate the respiratory bronchioles and alveolar ducts and to impair development of alveoli, although there was an early increase in DNA and collagen content suggesting a stimulus to interstitial growth.[48] The long term effect in the most severely ill infants ventilated for hyaline membrane disease was to produce an emphysematous lung.[48,52]

ACKNOWLEDGEMENTS

I am grateful to W Hinkes of the RPMS Department of Medical Illustration for the photomicrographs. The work from the RPMS described in this chapter was supported by the MRC.

REFERENCES

1 Bucher U, Reid L. Development of the intrasegmental bronchial tree: the pattern of branching and development of cartilage at various stages of intrauterine life. Thorax 1961; 16: 207–218

2 Wessels, NK. Mammalian lung development: Interactions in formation and morphogenesis of tracheal buds. J Exp Zool 1970; 175: 455–466
3 Goldin GV, Hindman HM, Wessels NK. The role of cell proliferation and cellular shape change in branching morphogenesis of the embryonic mouse lung: analysis using aphidicolin and cytochalasins J Exp Zool 1984; 232: 287–296
4 Grant MM, Cutts NR, Brody JS. Alterations in lung basement membrane during fetal growth and type 2 cell development. Dev Biol 1983; 97: 173–183
5 Jascoll TF, Slavkin HC. Ultrastructural and immunofluoresence studies of basal-lamina alterations during mouse-lung morphogenesis. Differentiation 1984; 28: 36–48
6 Franzblau C, Hayes JA, Snider GL. Biochemical insights into the development of connective tissue. In: Hodson WA, ed. Development of the Lung. New York: Marcel Dekker, 1977: pp. 367–399
7 Cutz E, Chan W, Track NS. Bombesin, calcitonin and leu-enkephalin immunoreactivity in endocrine cells of human lung. Experientia 1981; 37: 765
8 Stahlman MT, Kasselberg AG, Orth DN, Gray ME. Ontogeny of neuroendocrine cells in human fetal lung. II. An immunohistochemical study. Lab Invest 1985; 52: 52
9 Stahlman MT, Jones M, Gray ME, Kasselberg AG, Vaughn WK. Ontogeny of neuroendocrine cells in human fetal lung. III. An electron microscopic immunohistochemical study. Lab Invest 1987; 56: 629–641
10 Hislop A, Reid L. Development of the acinus in the human lung. Thorax 1974; 29: 90–94
11 Langston C, Kida K, Reed M, Thurlbeck WM. Human lung growth in late gestation and in the neonate. Am Rev Respir Dis 1984; 129: 607–613
12 Hislop AA, Wigglesworth JS, Desai R. Alveolar development in the human fetus and infant. Early Hum Dev 1986; 13: 1–11
13 Bustos R, Kulovich MV, Gluck L, Gabber SG, Evertson L, Vargas C, Lowenberg E. Significance of phosphatidylglycerol in amniotic fluid in complicated pregnancies. Am J Obstet Gynecol 1979; 133: 899–903
14 Smith BT, Fletcher WA. Pulmonary epithelial-mesenchymal interactions: Beyond organogenesis. Hum Pathol 1979; 10: 248–250
15 Tanimura T, Nelson T, Hollingsworth RR, Shepard TH. Weight standards for organs from early human fetuses. Anat Rec 1971; 171: 227–236
16 Wigglesworth JS, Desai R, Aber V. Quantitative aspects of perinatal lung growth. Early Hum Dev 1987; 15: 203–212
17 Wigglesworth JS, Desai R. Use of DNA estimation for growth assessment in normal and hypoplastic fetal lungs. Arch Dis Child 1981; 56: 601–605
18 Mescher EJ, Platzker ACG, Ballard PL, Kitterman JA, Clements JA, Tooley WH. Ontogeny of tracheal fluid, pulmonary surfactant and plasma corticoids in the fetal lamb. J Appl Physiol 1975; 39: 1017–21
19 Alcorn D, Adamson TM, Brodecky V, Cranage S, Lambert TF, Ritchie BC. Effects of chronic tracheal ligation and drainage in the fetal lamb lung. J Anat 1977; 123: 649–660
20 Dawes GS, Knox HE, Leduc BM, Liggins CG, Richards JS. Respiratory movements and rapid eye movement sleep in the foetal lamb. J Physiol 1972; 220: 119–143
21 Boddy K, Dawes GS. Fetal breathing. Br Med Bull 1975; 31: 3–7
22 Fox HE, Inglis J, Steinbrecher M. Fetal breathing movements in complicated pregnancies. Am J Obstet Gynecol 1979; 134: 544–546
23 Wigglesworth JS, Winston RML, Bartlett K. Influence of the central nervous system on fetal lung development. Arch Dis Child 1977; 52: 965–967
24 Wigglesworth JS, Desai R. Effects on lung growth of cervical cord section in the rabbit fetus. Early Hum Dev 1979; 3: 51–65

25 Liggins GC, Vilos GA, Campos GA, Kitterman JA, Lee CH. The effect of spinal cord transection on lung development in fetal sheep. J Dev Physiol 1981; 3: 267–274
26 Liggins GC, Vilos GA, Campos GA, Kitterman JA, Lee CH. The effect of bilateral thoracoplasty on lung development in fetal sheep. J Dev Physiol 1981; 3: 275–282
27 Alcorn D, Adamson TM, Maloney JE, Robinson PM. Morphological effects of chronic bilateral phrenectomy or vagotomy in the fetal lamb lung. J Anat 1980; 130: 683–695
28 Fewell JE, Lee C, Kitterman JA. Effects of phrenic nerve section on the respiratory system of fetal lambs. J Appl Physiol 1981; 51: 293–297
29 Kitterman JA. Fetal lung development. J Dev Physiol 1984; 6: 67–82
30 Sundell HW, Gray ME, Serenius FS, Escobedo MB, Stahlman MT. Effects of epidermal growth factor on lung maturation in fetal lambs. Am J Pathol 1980; 100: 707–726
31 Harrison MF, Jester JA, Ross NA. Correction of congenital diaphragmatic hernia in utero. I. The model: intrathoracic balloon produces fetal pulmonary hypoplasia. Surgery 1980; 88: 174–182
32 Pringle KC. Human fetal lung development and related animal models. Clin Obstet Gynecol 1986; 29: 502–513
33 Lawrence S, Rosenfeld CR. Fetal pulmonary development and abnormalities of amniotic fluid volume. Semin Perinatol 1986; 10: 142–153
34 Wigglesworth JS. Factors affecting fetal lung growth. In: Walters DV, Strang LB, Geubelle F, eds. Physiology of the Fetal and Neonatal Lung. Lancaster: MTP, 1987; pp.25–36
35 Perlman M, Williams J, Hirsch M. Neonatal pulmonary hypoplasia after prolonged leakage of amniotic fluid. Arch Dis Child 1976; 51: 349–353
36 Fliegner JR, Fortune DW, Egger TR. Premature rupture of the membranes, oligohydramnios and pulmonary hypoplasia. Aust NZ J Obstet Gynaecol 1981; 21: 77–81
37 Nimrod C, Varela-Gittings F, Machin G, Campbell D, Wesenberg R. The effect of very prolonged membrane rupture on fetal development. Am J Obstet Gynecol 1984; 148: 540–543
38 Thibeault DW, Beatty EC, Hall RT, Bowen SK, O'Neill DH. Neonatal pulmonary hypoplasia with premature rupture of fetal membranes and oligohydramnios. J Pediatr 1985; 107: 273–277
39 Hislop A, Hey E, Reid L. The lungs in congenital bilateral renal agenesis and dysplasia. Arch Dis Child 1979; 54: 32–38
40 Moessinger AC, Collins MH, Blanc WA, Rey HR, James LS. Oligohydramnios-induced lung hypoplasia: the influence of timing and duration in gestation. Pediatr Res 1986; 20: 951–954
41 Hislop A, Fairweather DVI, Blackwell RJ, Howard S. The effect of amniocentesis and drainage of amniotic fluid on lung development in Macaca fascicularis. Br J Obstet Gynaecol 1984; 91: 835–842
42 Fox HE, Moessinger AC. Fetal breathing movements and lung hypoplasia: preliminary human observations. Am J Obstet Gynecol 1985; 151: 531–533
43 Blott M, Greenough A, Nicolaides KH, Moscoso G, Gibb D, Campbell S. Fetal Breathing movements as predictor of favourable pregnancy outcome after oligohydramnios due to membrane rupture in second trimester. Lancet 1987; ii: 129–131
44 Moessinger AC, Fox HE, Higgins A, Rey HR, Al Haideri M. Fetal breathing movements are not a reliable predictor of continued lung development in pregnancies complicated by oligohydramnios. Lancet 1987; ii: 1297–1300
45 Greenough A, Blott M, Nicolaides K, Campbell S. Interpretation of fetal breathing movements in oligohydramnios due to membrane rupture. Lancet 1988; i: 182–183

46 Adzick NS, Harrison MR, Glick PL, Villa RL, Finkbeiner W. Experimental pulmonary hypoplasia and oligohydramnios: relative contributions of lung fluid and fetal breathing movements. J Pediatr Surg 1984; 19: 658–663
47 Wigglesworth JS, Desai R, Guerrini P. Fetal lung hypoplasia: biochemical and structural variations. Arch Dis Child 1981; 56: 606–615
48 Hislop A, Wigglesworth JS, Desai R, Aber V. The effects of preterm delivery and mechanical ventilation on human lung growth. Early Hum Dev 1987; 15: 147–164
49 Collins MH, Moessinger Ac, Kleinerman J, James LS, Blanc WA. Morphometry of hypoplastic fetal guinea pig lungs following amniotic fluid leak. Pediatr Res 1986; 20: 955–960
50 Smith H, Bain D. Congential atresia of the larynx: a report of nine cases. Ann Otol Rhinol Laryngol 1965; 74: 338–349
51 Wigglesworth JS, Desai R, Hislop A. Fetal lung growth in congenital laryngeal atresia. Pediatr Pathol 1987; 7: 515–525
52 Sobonya RE, Loquinoff MM, Taussig LM, Thericault A. Morphometric analysis of the lung in prolonged bronchopulmonary dysplasia. Pediatr Res 1982; 16: 969–972

Adaptation of the respiratory system

A D Milner
Department of Child Health, University Hospital, Nottingham
A Greenough
Department of Child Health, King's College Hospital, London

> Apart from those examining the preterm babies reflex response to intermittent positive pressure ventilation, studies referred to in this paper have included only one or two babies of less than 28 weeks gestation. It is therefore not possible at the moment to state whether extreme immaturity is associated with changes which are just quantitatively or perhaps also qualitatively different from more mature pre-term babies, who are more stable and so easier to study. In particular, we need more information on the mechanical characteristics of these babies' lungs so that we can plan effective and safe forms of resuscitation. We also need to find ways of providing respiratory support without inducing broncho-pulmonary dysplasia and to learn more about respiratory control so that we can prevent apnoea.

The last 40 years has seen an impressive expansion in our knowledge of the growth, control and development of the respiratory system in the neonatal period. The majority of these studies have been on healthy, full-term babies who are reasonably easy to investigate. Although there are an increasing number of reports of lung function on pre-term babies, those under the age of 28 weeks have generally been considered to be too fragile and technically more difficult to study, so that most of our information is on babies who are more mature. We still do not know to what extent our current concepts can be applied to those who are extremely immature.

ANATOMICAL DEVELOPMENT

Although most stress has been placed on the importance of surfactant deficiency in the aetiology of the respiratory distress syndrome of preterm babies, those under the age of 28 weeks also have a major problem with anatomical immaturity. Indeed it is this which consistently sets the lower limit of viability to 23–24 weeks gestation.

At this stage (pre-acinar), the main airway branching system has been laid down and the adult pattern of cartilage distribution has already occurred. Other aspects of airway differentiation are also relatively complete. Mucus and globlet cells are present, although in reduced numbers and cilia are present on the lung epithelial cells down to the 15th/16th airway division[2] in similar distribution to that seen in older children and adults. Airways, however, do not terminate in a potential gas exchange system until 19/20 weeks when the primitive respiratory bronchiole develops as an extension of the respiratory airway.[3] This is initially lined by undifferentiated cuboidal epithelial cells. By 24 weeks the respiratory bronchioles have subdivided followed in 4 weeks by the appearance of transitional ducts and primitive sacules. Even at 24 weeks gestation it is possible to differentiate some of the lining cells into Type I and Type II pneumocytes[4] and the pulmonary capillaries then grow into close apposition with the epithelium. As close contact is reached, the epithelium thins so that there is a rippling effect with variable thickness. True alveoli do not appear until after 40 weeks gestation.

Surfactant is often detected in Type II pneumocytes as early as 22–23 weeks gestation,[5] closely followed by its appearance in the terminal air spaces. By 28 weeks gestation the terminal air spaces are well developed as out-pouches of the bronchioles. Type I and II pneumocytes are well differentiated and the Type I pneumocytes flattened to cover the extended respiratory exchange surface.[6] The capillaries by this time are close to the epithelium and allow easy gaseous exchange across the alveolar air/blood barrier.

LUNG EXPANSION AT BIRTH

Our information on the changes occurring at delivery and during the onset of respiration is based almost entirely upon the extrapolation of data obtained from babies born at, or close to term.[7] There is a small amount of data obtained from measurements carried out during resuscitation, showing that babies less than 28 weeks have relatively stiff lungs, even when allowance is made for their body size[8] (Table 1). There is no doubt that some babies with gestation as low as 24 weeks do have the ability to both expand their lungs and establish a functional residual capacity spontaneously, although currently we have no information on the pressures these babies generate in order to achieve this. In recent years, however, there has been a trend towards more active intervention at birth so that in many units all babies less than 28 weeks are electively ventilated and intubated at birth. There is some evidence that the prevention of asphyxia can reduce the incidence of the respiratory distress syndrome.[9] A controlled study from Australia also demonstrated that elective intubation is associated with lower mortality.[10] However, only 3% of the preterm babies in the control group received intubation, a very different pattern to that adopted in even the most conservative of units today. A smaller study (unpublished data), based in Nottingham, failed to show any difference in mortality or morbidity when elective intubation was compared to a policy of intervening if the baby showed any signs of respiratory distress or was not breathing within 30 seconds of delivery. This led to an overall intubation rate of 60% in the 'selective' group. However, all the nine 'selective' babies with a gestation of less than 28 weeks had received intubation.

There is also some debate on the inflation pressures which should be selected for resuscitating babies of less than 28 weeks gestation. The compliance measurements that we have available would suggest that pressures greater than those routinely used for full-term babies should be selected (Table 1). Certainly what measurements we have, indicate that the pressure of 30 cmH$_2$O (2.94 kPa) will not necessarily produce adequate gas exchange in these very immature babies.[8] There are, however, anxieties that

Table 1 Measurements of static respiratory compliance in babies less than 28 weeks gestation[8]

Gestation (weeks)	Birthweight (kg)	Compliance (ml/cmH$_2$O)*
25	0.78	0.49
25	0.84	0.07
27	1.07	0.32

*1 cmH$_2$O ≈ 98 Pa

the use of high pressures at birth may lead to pulmonary intestitial emphysema, a condition which at its most severe may prevent adequate gaseous exchange, even with very high inflation pressures and is associated with the development of broncho-pulmonary dysplasia.[11] It is obviously advisable to use as low an inflation as possible during resuscitation. Unfortunately, the babies going on to develop pulmonary intestitial emphysema are likely to be those with relatively stiff lungs at birth, who require relatively high pressures in order to achieve satisfactory lung expansion. There is obviously a very considerable need to collect more information on the changes occurring at birth. Meanwhile, it would seem reasonable to adopt a policy of providing respiratory support with a face mask[12] and progressing to intubation if the baby does not show an immediate response, with regular respiratory efforts, good skin perfusion and oxygenation within 30–60 seconds of delivery.

LUNG VOLUMES AND LUNG MECHANICS IN THE IMMEDIATE NEONATAL PERIOD

The mechanism by which the lung volume is maintained in the immediate neonatal period has been under some dispute. Some data suggests that even entirely healthy babies at term have relatively hyperinflated lungs. It is claimed that this is due to air-trapping, and persists for 1–2 days while lung fluid is reabsorbed.[12] Other studies have been unable to substantiate this[13] and evidence now indicates that lung volume in the hours after birth is maintained predominantly by a balance between the inward elastic recoil of the lungs and the outward recoil of the chest wall and respiratory muscles. There remains a striking difference between the measurement of the resting lung volume (functional residual capacity) using plethysmography and closed circuit helium techniques in the first few hours of life, suggesting that there is some trapped air, probably behind fluid within the airway.[14] In the healthy preterm baby there is more evidence to suggest that the lung volume is artificially elevated as a result of air-trapping and that this may persist for several weeks.[15,16] There is also evidence that the lung volume of preterm babies is dynamically elevated by relatively high respiratory rates and that inspiration commences before expiration is complete.[17] So far, these data have been limited to babies of 28 weeks gestation or older, due to technical problems, and we can only surmise that babies less mature than this are likely to show this tendency to hyperinflation, perhaps as a result of relatively compliant airways. This tendency to hyperinflation could explain the susceptibility of these very immature babies to broncho-pulmonary dysplasia and the Wilson–Mikity Syndrome.[16]

RESPIRATORY REFLEXES

Our data on neonatal respiratory reflexes has been provided by inspiratory pressure and tidal volume measurements during resuscitation and to a greater extent during intermittent positive pressure ventilation.

Respiratory activity during resuscitation

Studies on full-term babies requiring resuscitation have shown that most often the infant responds to the inflation pressure with a prolonged expiratory effort lasting for up to 2 seconds (47%).[18] On 11% of inflations there is an augmented inspiratory response (Head's paradoxical reflex) in which the baby's respiratory efforts augment the inflation pressure to provide a considerably larger tidal volume. On 28% of the measurements the babies made no respiratory effort whatsoever and on the remaining 14% there was a combined rejection and augmented inspiratory response in a single breath. Data on preterm babies (less than 36 weeks) showed that they more often responded with an augmented inspiratory response (23%) but only 8% of inflations showed the rejection response and a further 9% had a combined rejection and augmented inspiratory response.[8] Of the 3 babies less than 28 weeks, none showed the rejection response and one had an augmented inspiratory response—the only one producing an adequate tidal exchange.

Respiratory activity during intermittent positive pressure ventilation

We now have considerable information on the manner in which babies with gestation less than 28 weeks interact with the ventilator.[19-21] In a further study,[19,20] (Greenough, unpublished observations) 33 babies of less than 28 weeks gestation were investigated in the first 6 hours of life. All received intermittent positive pressure ventilation from birth for the idiopathic respiratory distress syndrome. Typically, the ventilator rate was 30/min with an inspiratory time of at least one second. Inspection of the inflation pressure, tidal volume and oesophageal pressure traces showed that 9 were making no respiratory effort whatsoever, 12 exhibited a Hering Breuer response with suppression of spontaneous respiratory efforts in response to inflation and the remaining 12 active expiratory efforts, i.e. the baby was actively expiring during the period of ventilator inflation (fighting the ventilator) (Table 2). Active expiratory reflex (AER) tended to occur in those with the lowest lung compliance ($P<0.01$). Infants who were hypoxic ($P_aO_2 < 40$ mmHg) or hypercarbic ($P_aCO_2 > 60$ mmHg) did not show any reflex activity but did make intermittent gasping efforts which were independent of the ventilator inflation pattern. The Head's paradoxical reflexes which occur so often during the resuscitation of full-term babies, occurred only when the ventilator rate was less than 20/min, i.e. the babies were well on the way to recovery. The frequency of this reflex was not related to gestational age, but did tend to occur more often in those babies who had relatively stiff lungs ($P<0.001$). Data after the first week of life are limited, but the Head's Paradoxical Reflex has not been seen in any infant of more than 5 days of age.

Two previous studies have shown that pneumothoraces occur almost exclusively in babies exhibiting AER and that the incidence of pneumothorax can be greatly reduced by selective paralysis of this group of babies.[21,22] Data are now available on 78 babies with a gestation of less than 28 weeks from the same author. Of these 37 had AER in response to ventilator settings of 30/min. Twenty-two were paralysed and 5 developed pneumothoraces, compared to all 15 of those who were not paralysed (Table 3). Only 2 of the remaining 41 babies who did not show AER went on to develop pneumothoraces, confirming that in severely immature babies AER was an unwelcome form of interaction and that selective use

Table 2 Patterns of respiratory interaction in 33 babies less than 28 weeks gestation[19,20] (Greenough, unpublished observation). All were less than 6 hours of age and receiving ventilator support at a rate of 30/minute

Gestation (weeks)	24	25	26	27
Number	3	6	10	14
Apnoea	1	3	2	3
Hering Breuer	1	3	5	3
Active Expiratory Reflex	1	0	3	8
Heads Paradoxical Reflex	0	0	0	0

Table 3 Effects of paralysis on the incidence of pneumothoraces in babies with a gestation of less than 28 weeks (Greenough, unpublished observations)

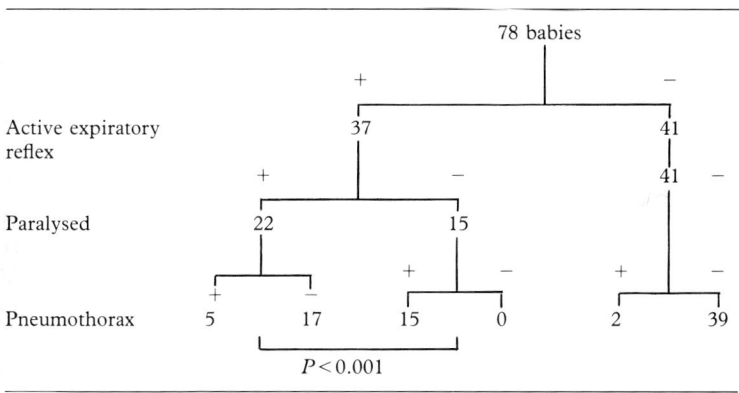

```
                              78 babies
                    ┌─────────────┴─────────────┐
                    +                           −
Active expiratory   37                          41
reflex              │                           │
               ┌────┴────┐                      41   −
               +         −
Paralysed      22        15
               │         │
            ┌──┴──┐   ┌──┴──┐              ┌────┴────┐
            +     −   +     −              +         −
Pneumothorax 5   17   15    0              2         39
            └─────────┬───────┘
                  P<0.001
```

of agents such as pancuronium could reduce the incidence of pneumothoraces.

An alternative approach has been to increase the ventilator rate in an attempt to synchronize this with the babies' own respiratory efforts,[23-25] in the hope that this might lead to improved gaseous exchange, while at the same time reducing the incidence of pneumothorax. Data has now been analysed on 21 babies[24,25] with a gestation less than 28 weeks who all had AER at a ventilator rate of 30/min. When the rate was increased to 60/min, 6 were breathing synchronously and at 100–120/min this had risen to 18 with only 2 showing AER and one with an irregular pattern of response (Table 4). Temporary disconnection of 8 babies, all less than 28 weeks gestation, from their ventilator, revealed that their own spontaneous rate ranged from 81–112/min with a mean of 94, slightly lower than the rate adopted in the ventilator study above, indicating that selection of rates a little above the babies' own spontaneous pattern will most easily lead to synchrony.[25]

Table 4 Effects of different ventilator frequencies on pattern of respiratory interaction in infants of less than 28 weeks gestation[24,25]

Rate/min	30	60	100–120
Active expiratory reflex	21	7	2
Mixed pattern	0	3	1
Synchronous breathing	0	6	18

APNOEA AND RESPIRATORY CONTROL

Over 80% of babies born less than 28 weeks gestation have apnoeic attacks, lasting at least 10 seconds and usually commencing on the 2nd or 3rd day of life in those not requiring ventilatory support. Recent studies measuring air flow and respiratory effort have shown that in preterm babies, including those less than 28 weeks, there are 3 separate patterns of apnoea.[26,27] Less than 50% of all apnoea is central in origin, i.e. due primarily to a cessation of respiratory drive. Although sometimes prolonged, most central apnoea is short in duration.[27] The mechanism for central apnoea remains controversial. There is evidence that central and peripheral chemosensitivity is reduced in those having apnoea.[28,29] In severely preterm babies hypoxia has a suppressive, rather than stimulatory effect on respiratory drive.[29,30] Henderson-Smart et al.[31] studied brain stem conduction times, using auditory evoked responses and found that babies having apnoea with gestations down to 28 weeks, had prolonged conduction times, compared to gestationally matched controls, suggesting a maturation delay. There is also now considerable interest in the role of neurotransmitters and neuromodifying secretions, including endorphin, substance P and adenosine—which all have a suppressant effect on the respiratory centre.[32]

Obstructive apnoea, i.e. regular and continuing respiratory efforts against a closed airway, is also occasionally seen, although relatively rarely in severely preterm babies and then usually only in those with brain damage.[27] Over 50% of the apnoeic episodes has been designated as 'mixed', as there is airway obstruction, usually at pharyngeal level,[37] but either only infrequent or intermittent respiratory efforts. In some preterm babies, including those less than 28 weeks, airway obstruction is present, as determined by an absence of cardiac artefact on the face mask pneumotachograph and yet they make no respiratory effort whatsoever.[26] The mechanism for this form of apnoea remains unclear, although there is now a well-recognized intercostal phrenic inhibitory reflex in which distortion of the chest wall, such as that which will occur if respiratory efforts are made against a closed airway, can lead to apnoea.[34] There is currently little information on this reflex in babies less than 28 weeks but Gerhardt and Bancalari[35] found that preterm babies not having apnoea had a greater prolongation of inspiratory effort when obstructed at end expiration compared to those having apnoea. In an earlier study Milner et al.[36] found that end expiratory obstruction during the measurement of thoracic gas volume in the total body plethysmograph frequently led to cessation of respiratory efforts while the obstruction was maintained. This occurred only in preterm babies with intermittent apnoea. The credence of the intercostal phrenic inhibitory reflex as a cause of mixed apnoea, has been increased by the study of Miller et al.[37] into the role of continuous positive airway ventilation in the prevention of apnoea. They found that this form of therapy had no influence whatsoever on the incidence of central apnoea, but effectively abolished both obstructive and mixed apnoea. They concluded that the continuous positive airway pressure acted by maintaining upper airway patency and so prevented chest wall distortion and thus the stimulation of the intercostal phrenic inhibitory reflex.

REFERENCES

1 Bucher U, Reid L. Development of the Intrasegmental bronchial tree: The pattern of branching and development of cartilage at various stages of intrauterine lung. Thorax 1961; 16: 207–218
2 Bucher U, Reid L. Development of the mucus secretive elements in human lung. Thorax 1961; 16: 219
3 Inselman LS, Mellins RR. Growth and development of the lung. J Pediatr 1981; 98: 1–15
4 Campieche M, Gautier A, Hermandez EI, Reymond A. An electron microscope study of the fetal development of human lung. Pediatrics 1963; 32: 976–994
5 Meyrick B, Reid L. The alveolar wall. Br J Dis Child 1970; 64: 121
6 Hislop A, Reid L. Growth and development of the respiratory system: Anatomical development, Ch. 20. In: Davis JA, Robbins J, eds. Scientific foundations of paediatrics, 2nd edn. William Heinemann; London, 1981
7 Milner AD, Vyas H. Lung expansion at birth. J Pediatr 1982; 101: 879–886
8 Hoskyns EW, Milner AD, Boon AW, Vyas H, Hopkin IE. Endotracheal resuscitation of preterm infants at birth. Arch Dis Child 1987; 62: 663–666
9 Robson E, Hey E. Resuscitation of preterm babies at birth reduces the risk of death from hyaline membrane disease. Arch Dis Child 1982; 57: 184–186
10 Drew JH. Immediate intubation at birth of very low birthweight infants: effect on survival. Am J Dis Child 1982; 136: 207–210
11 Watts JL, Ariagno RL, Brady JP. Chronic pulmonary disease in neonates after artificial ventilation: distribution of ventilation and pulmonary intestitial emphysema. Pediatrics 1977; 60: 273–278
12 Auld PAM, Nelson NM, Cherry KB, Rudolph AJ, Smith LA. Measurement of thoracic gas volume in newborn infant. J Clin Invest 1963; 42: 476–483
13 Milner AD, Saunders RA, Hopkin IE. Is air-trapping important in the maintenance of the functional residual capacity in the hours after birth? Early Hum Dev 1978; 2: 97–105
14 Boon AW, Ward-McQuaid JMC, Milner AD, Hopkin IE. Thoracic gas volume, functional residual capacity and air-trapping in the first six hours of life: The effects of oxygen administration. Early Hum Dev 1981; 5: 157–161
15 Thibeault DW, Wong MM, Auld PAM. Thoracic gas volume changes in premature infants. Pediatrics 1967; Vol. No. 40: 403–409

16 Saunders RA, Milner AD, Hopkin IE. Longitudinal studies of infants with the Wilson-Mikity Syndrome: clinical, radiological and mechanical correlations. Biol Neonate 1978; 33: 90–99
17 Olinsky A, Bryan MH, Bryan AC. Influence of lung inflation on respiratory control in neonates. J Appl Physiol 1974; 36: 426–429
18 Boon AW, Milner AD, Hopkin IE. Physiological responses of the newborn infant to resuscitation. Arch Dis Child 1979; 54: 492–497
19 Greenough A, Morley LJ, Davis JA. Provoked augmented inspirations in ventilated premature babies. Early Hum Dev 1984; 9: 111–117
20 Greenough A, Morley LJ, Davis JA. Respiratory reflexes in ventilated premature babies. Early Hum Dev 1983; 8: 65–75
21 Greenough A, Morley LJ, Davis JA. Interaction of spontaneous aspiration with artificial ventilation. J Pediatr 1983; 103: 769–773
22 Greenough A, Wood S, Morley LJ, Davis JA. Pancuronium prevents pneumothoraces in ventilated premature babies who acutely expire against positive-pressure inflation. Lancet 1984; i: 1–3
23 Field D, Milner AD, Hopkin IE. High and conventional rates of positive-pressure ventilation. Arch Dis Child 1984; 59: 1151–1154
24 Greenough A, Morley CJ, Pool J. Fighting the ventilator—are fast rates an effective alternative to paralysis? Early Hum Dev 1986; 13: 189–194
25 Greenough A, Greenall F, Gamsu H. Synchronous respiration: Which ventilation rate is best? Acta Paediatr Scand 1987; 76: 713–718
26 Milner AD, Boon AW, Saunders RA, Hopkin IE. Upper airway obstruction and apnoea in preterm babies. Arch Dis Child 1980; 55: 22–25
27 Butcher-Puech MCE, Henderson-Smart DJ, Holley D, Lacey JL, Edwards DA. Relationship between apnoea duration and type and neurological status of preterm infants. Arch Dis Child 1985; 60: 953–958
28 Gerhardt T, Bancalari E. Apnoea of prematurity. 1. Lung function and regulation of breathing. Pediatrics 1984; 74: 58
29 Martin RJ, Carlo WA, Robertson SS. Biphonic response of respiratory frequency to hypercapnia in preterm infants. Pediatr Res 1985; 19: 791–796
30 Rigatto H, Harapesi Z, Leagy FN, et al. Ventilatory response to 100% and 15% O_2 during wakefulness and sleep in preterm infants. Early Hum Dev 1982; 7: 1–4
31 Henderson-Smart DJ, Pettigrew AG, Campbell DJ. Clinical apnoea and brain stem neural function in preterm babies. N Engl J Med 1983; 308: 353–357
32 Martin RJ, Miller MJ, Carlo WA. Pathogenesis of apnoea in preterm infants. J Pediatr 1986; 109: 733–741
33 Mathew OP, Roberts JL, Thach BT. Pharyngeal airway obstruction in preterm infants during mixed and obstructive apnoea. J Pediatr 1982; 100: 964–968
34 Knill R, Bryan AC. An intercostal-phrenic intubitory reflex in human newborn infants. J Appl Physiol 1976; 40: 352–356
35 Gerhardt T, Bancalari E. Apnoea of prematurity: II Respiratory reflexes. Pediatrics 1984; 74: 63–66
36 Milner AD, Saunders RA, Hopkin IE. Apnoea induced by airflow obstruction. Arch Dis Child 1977; 52: 379–382
37 Miller MJ, Carlo WA, Martin RJ. Continuous positive pressure selectively reduces obstructive apnoea in preterm infants. J Pediatr 1985; 106: 91–97

Surfactant therapy for very premature babies

C J Morley
Department of Paediatrics, University of Cambridge, Cambridge, UK

> Fifteen randomised trials of surfactant therapy for babies have been published. They have used six surfactant preparations. Some are from animal lungs or human amniotic fluid, some are synthetic. They have been given either at birth as a prophylaxis for neonatal respiratory distress syndrome or as rescue treatment for babies in respiratory failure. They have mainly used single doses varying from 25 mg to 200 mg. The outcome of these trials is varied but all surfactant preparations show beneficial effects and the only apparent side effect is an increase in the incidence of patent ductus arteriosus with some natural surfactants. The effects are too varied to show that one is better than another. However, the overall benefits in the first 24 hours are an improvement in oxygenation and a reduction in ventilatory pressure. The longer term effects are a reduction in pneumothoraces, periventricular haemorrhage, bronchopulmonary dysplasia and death.

The prospect of surfactant therapy for premature babies is now reaching an exciting stage. In the late 1950's it was shown that premature babies were deficient in pulmonary surfactant and that this was closely associated with respiratory distress syndrome (RDS) and hyaline membranes in the lungs of those babies who died.[1] In the following 20 years there was a surge of research into the biochemistry, physiology and biophysics of pulmonary surfactant with the ultimate goal of increasing our knowledge so that surfactant could be manipulated in the fetus and newborn premature baby to reduce the severity of the RDS and possibly prevent the disease. In the last 10 years this knowledge has been used to develop at least seven different preparations of surfactant for clinical trials to hopefully prevent premature babies developing severe RDS.

SURFACTANT PREPARATIONS FOR TREATING PREMATURE BABIES

The surfactant preparations can be divided into two main groups. Firstly, surfactants derived from natural sources such as animal lungs or human amniotic fluid and secondly artificial or synthetic surfactants.

Natural surfactants

Four natural surfactants have been made by different techniques.

1. *Surfactant TA*, developed in Japan, is made from homogenised cow lungs.[2-4] It is extracted with chloroform/methanol and ethyl acetate. To achieve optimum physical properties small amounts of dipalmitoylphosphatidylcholine (DPPC), palmitic acid and triglyceride are added. It contains 84% phospholipids and about 1% protein. Most of the protein is a 600 M_r (6 kDa) surfactant apoprotein. It is a freeze dried preparation and when used for endotracheal instillation 100–120 mg is sonicated for 5 minutes with 3–4 ml saline.

2. *Calf lung surfactant (CLSE)*[5-7] is made by washing surfactant out of the lungs of dead calves with physiological saline. This material is then extracted and purified by precipitation with acetone. The final material contains 90–97% phospholipid and 1% protein which is mainly low molecular weight apoprotein. It is sterilised by flash autoclave. Before use 90 mg are vortexed with 3 ml of physiological saline.

3. *Porcine surfactant (Curosurf)*[8,9] is harvested from minced pig lungs, extracted and purified by washing, chloroform-methanol extraction, liquid-gel chromatography and passed through a 0.2 µm filter. It consists of 99% polar lipids—mainly phospholipids and 1% hydrophobic proteins which have a molecular weight of less than 15 000 M_r (15 kDa). It is used as a suspension of 80 mg/ml at 200 mg/kg.

4. *Human amniotic fluid surfactant*[10,11] is produced by collecting clean amniotic fluid at elective caesarian sections for term deliveries. The surfactant is then extracted and purified by centrifugation and passage through a 20 µm filter. Approximately 3 deliveries are needed to produce one dose of surfactant. It is used as 60 mg suspended by vortexing with 3.5 ml of 0.6% saline.

Artificial surfactants

Three artifical surfactants have been used to treat babies.

1. In Belfast a surfactant was made from DPPC (1 g) and human high density lipoprotein (HDL) (4 ml) mixed in with 150 ml 0.9% sodium chloride, sterilised by irradiation and given as a 3–5 ml dose into the endotracheal tube at birth.[12]

2. An artificial surfactant (ALEC) has been made in Cambridge from two pure sterile phospholipids, DPPC and unsaturated phosphatidylglycerol (PG) in a ratio of 3:1.[13-19] It contains no protein. It has been used in trials both as a powder and as a suspension of 50 to 100 mg in 1 ml cold saline.

3. The third artifical surfactant (Exosurf)[20] has been made in California and consists of DPPC (13.5 mg/ml), tyloxapol (1.0 mg/ml) and hexadecanol 1.5 mg/ml). This is used in a dose of 7 ml/kg instilled into the endotracheal tube at birth.

INTERPRETATION OF CLINICAL TRIALS

There have been several preliminary studies of surfactant therapy which have not included a control group. This obviously makes accurate interpretation of the surfactant effect rather difficult. However, the major surfactants have now been tested by controlled studies. Only the results of these latter trials will be presented.

There are now 15 reports of controlled clinical trials with surfactant therapy in premature babies. They can be subdivided into 9 trials of surfactant treatment given to babies at birth called 'prophylactic treatment'[5-7,9,11,12,15-19] and 6 trials of surfactant given when the babies have obvious RDS requiring oxygen treatment and ventilation, called 'rescue treatment'.[9,10,19,21-23] The basic data about the gestational age of the babies, number of babies, surfactant used and entry criteria for the trials are shown in Table 1.

Comparison of the results from prophylactic trials where all babies at risk of developing RDS entered the trials with rescue trials where only babies with established RDS were randomised are not satisfactory. Comparisons even within prophylactic or rescue trial groups are also difficult because the entry criteria for each trial was different. For example, in the prophylactic trials some randomised all babies below 35 weeks gestation, others concentrated on a high risk group of babies from 25 to 29 weeks

Table 1 Basic data on the different trials

Prophylactic trials

Author	Surfactant	Dose	Volume	Placebo	Number	Gestation	Excluded	Intubated
Enhorning	CLSE	75–100 mg	3–4 ml	none	72	25–29	Acute Deliv.	All
Shapiro	CLSE	90 mg	3 ml	NaCl	32	25–29	Acute Deliv.	All
Kwong	CLSE	90 mg	3 ml	NaCl	27	24–28	Acute Deliv.	All
Merritt	Human	60 mg	3 ml	Air	60	24–29	L:S > 1.9	All
Halliday	DPPC/HDL	30 mg	5 ml	none	100	25–33	L:S > 1.9	All
Wilkinson	ALEC	25 mg	powder	none	24	<32	L:S > 1.7	All
Morley	ALEC	25 mg	powder	none	129	25–35	None	All
Morley	ALEC	50–100 mg	1 ml	NaCl	341	23–34	None	Some
Ten Centre	ALEC	100 mg	1 ml	NaCl	328	25–29	None	Some

Rescue trials

Author	Surfactant	Dose	Volume	Placebo	Numbers	Birthweight or gestation	Inclusion	Time
Hallman	Human	60 mg	3.0 ml	none	45	<1500	RDS > 60% O_2	<10 h
Wilkinson	ALEC	25 mg	powder	none	24	<31 week	RDS L:S <1.8	?
Gitlin	Surf TA	100 mg	3.3 ml	NaCl	41	1000–1500	RDS > 40% O_2	<8 h
Raju	Surf TA	100 mg	3.3 ml	NaCl	30	751–1750	RDS > 50% O_2	<6 h
McCord	Curosurf	200 mg	2.5 ml	none	29	700–2000	RDS > 60% O_2	1–15 h
Fujiwara	Surf TA	120 mg	4.0 ml	none	91	750–1749	RDS > 60% O_2	>6 h

ALEC = Artificial lung expanding compound
Surf TA = Surfactant TA
CLSE = Calf lung surfactant extract

gestation. In the rescue trials some only include babies with low L:S ratio and phosphatidylgylcerol assays others do not measure the lung maturity. Some of these trials enrolled babies who were very ill, that is ventilated and receiving more than 60% oxygen, and others only required the babies to be in more than 40% oxygen. Some trials entered all babies born in the hospital even if they were compromised by asphyxia, haemorrhage, infection or had very prolonged rupture of the membranes whereas others excluded such babies.

The dose of surfactant used in different trials has varied from 25 mg to 200 mg. Surfactants were used in varying physical states from pure phospholipid powder to lyophilized surfactant extract sonicated or suspended in volumes up to 8 ml of saline to form a milky fluid. Some trials have used no placebo for the controls, others have used air or equal volumes of saline. Most trials have tried to 'blind' the neonatal unit staff from whether the baby received surfactant or was a control. Although this keeps the staff guessing none of the trials can be assuredly blind. The number of doses has varied from one dose at birth up to four doses in the first 24 hours.

OUTCOMES OF THE TRIALS

When assessing the efficacy of surfactant different outcomes have been stressed by different trials. Some have emphasised an acute improvement in oxygenation while others have concentrated on a reduction in mortality, bronchopulmonary dysplasia (BPD) or periventricular haemorrhage (PVH). So far there are no published clinical trial data on the efficacy of Exosurf.

Despite early beliefs that all babies with RDS were surfactant deficient and therefore surfactant treatment would cure them, not all babies respond to treatment. Fujiwara has reported that in babies weighing < 1000 g when observing the effect of Surfactant TA on oxygenation; 64% had an immediate and sustained response, 20% relapsed and 16% had a poor or no response. He felt that the factors tending to lead to an unsatisfactory response were; PDA, cardiogenic shock or persistent fetal circulation. In retrospect it is not surprising that these very immature babies, who suffer from so many compounding diseases and complications should not always respond to surfactant therapy. Perhaps it is more surprising that so many do respond.

The major univariate outcome measures of the trials are shown below in the tables as 95% confidence intervals. This allows the difference between the treated and control babies to be seen with the variation in that difference due to the number of babies in the trial. Only the trials accurately reporting the data are included. Where possible most results are calculated for babies less than 30 weeks gestation.

Mortality

Mortality is a crude but important measure of surfactant treatment. Where possible the mortality has been calculated for babies under 30 weeks gestation and shown in Table 2. The overall trend is that surfactant treatment reduces mortality. No surfactant increased the mortality. In the rescue groups the confidence intervals are wide but Raju's trial of surfactant TA[23] and the trial of porcine surfactant[9] produced significant reductions in mortality. In the prophylactic group, there were significant reductions with Enhorning's calf surfactant,[5] human surfactant[11] and ALEC powder[15,16] and suspension.[17,18] It is not possible to compare the effects of different preparations. On average there was a 65% reduction in mortality. This might be spuriously high because some of the trials were stopped when a significant difference in mortality was noted. Even at a lesser effect surfactant therapy would be the single best therapy to improve neonatal mortality.

Periventricular haemorrhage

Table 3 shows the effect of different surfactant preparations on all grades of periventricular haemorrhage. Overall, surfactant treatment appears to reduce the incidence. The rescue trials with a significant effect are McCord's trial with porcine surfactant[9] and Fujiwara's with Surfactant TA.[23] However, there is a wide variation in effect of Surfactant TA with no effect in Gitlin's trial,[21] a possible but not significant effect in Raju's trial[22] and a significant reduction shown by Fujiwara.[23] This demonstrates the difficulties of small trials showing the true effect. In the prophylactic trials, significant reductions in PVH were shown by Halliday's artificial surfactant,[12] ALEC suspension in the Cambridge–Nottingham trial,[17] ALEC powder[15,16] and Enhorning's calf surfactant.[5] With wide confidence intervals and different trial designs it is difficult to say that one surfactant has a better effect than another.

Table 2 Effect on different surfactant trials on mortality

Author	Surfactant	Gestation or weight	Controls n	Surfactant n	95% CI for improvement in mortality per 100 babies	Refs
Prophylactic trials						
Enhorning*	CLSE	25–29	33	39	3 to 33	5
Kwong**	CLSE	24–28	13	14	−16 to 32	6
Morley**	ALEC dry	23–29	34	28	18 to 56	15, 16
Wilkinson*	ALEC dry	<32	12	12	−5 to 39	19
C-N Trial**	ALEC	25–29	67	69	1 to 31	17
Ten Centre*	ALEC	25–29	149	159	4 to 22	18
Halliday**	DPPC+HDL	27–29	14	16	−15 to 51	12
Merritt*	Human	24–29	29	31	14 to 58	11
Rescue trials						
Hallman**	Human	<1500	23	22	−12 to 36	10
Wilkinson*	ALEC	<32w	12	12	−30 to 30	19
Gitlin*	Surf TA	1000–1500	23	18	−18 to 32	21
Raju*	Surf TA	751–1750	13	17	3 to 69	22
McCord*	Curosurf	701–2000	15	14	−1 to 65	9
Fujiwara*	Surf TA	750–1750	41	50	−7 to 22	23

Data calculated where possible for babies less than 30 weeks gestation because deaths are rare in more mature babies
* = Neonatal Mortality
** = Overall Mortality
ALEC = Artificial lung expanding compound
CLSE = Calf lung surfactant extract
Surf TA = Surfactant TA

Table 3 Effect of different surfactant trials on the incidence of periventricular haemorrhage

Author	Surfactant	Gestation or weight	95% CI for improvement in PVH per 100 babies	Refs
Prophylactic trials				
Enhorning	CLSE	25–29	10 to 56	5
Kwong	CLSE	24–28	−36 to 36	6
Morley	ALEC dry	23–29	7 to 55	15, 16
Morley	ALEC	23–34	3 to 17	17
Ten Centre	ALEC	25–29	−1 to 17	18
Halliday	DPPC+HDL	27–33	2 to 22	12
Merritt	Human	24–29	−9 to 27	11
Rescue trials				
Hallman	Human	<1500	−9 to 49	10
Gitlin	Surf TA	1000–1500	−32 to 30	21
Raju	Surf TA	751–1750	−15 to 57	22
McCord	Curosurf	701–2000	28 to 88	9
Fujiwara	Surf TA	750–1749	1 to 35	23

ALEC = Artificial lung expanding compound
CLSE = Calf lung surfactant extract
Surf TA = Surfactant TA

Pneumothorax

Babies with the most severe RDS are at risk of developing a pneumothorax and have a poorer outcome. The effect of the different trials is shown in Table 4. As surfactant therapy lowers surface tension it was thought that it might lead to overdistension of the lungs and increase the incidence of pneumothoraces. Surprisingly therefore, the overall trend from the trials is for surfactant treatment to reduce the incidence of pneumothoraces. The chance of a deleterious effect with any surfactant is small. The rescue trials all produce a significant but varied reduction in pneumothoraces. In the prophylactic trials, the effect is to reduce the incidence of pneumothoraces but it is a smaller effect because the incidence of pneumothoraces tends to be lower. Halliday's trial showed an insignificant increase in pneumothoraces.[12] Human surfactant[11] and ALEC powder[15,16] were the only ones to produce a significant reduction.

Patent ductus arteriosus

In the first non-randomized trial of Fujiwara[2] patent ductus arteriosus (PDA) occurred in 9 out of 10 babies and it looked as

Table 4 Effect of different surfactant trials on the incidence of pneumothorax

Author	Surfactant	Gestation or weight	95% CI for improvement in pneumothorax per 100 babies	Refs
Prophylactic trials				
Enhorning	CLSE	25–29	−2 to 38	5
Kwong	CLSE	24–28	−28 to 46	6
Morley	ALEC dry	23–29	18 to 60	15, 16
Morley	ALEC	23–34	−6 to 10	17
Ten Centre	ALEC	25–29	−7 to 13	18
Halliday	DPPC+HDL	27–33	−23 to 7	12
Merritt	Human	24–29	0 to 36	11
Rescue trials				
Hallman	Human	<1500	4 to 46	10
Gitlin	Surf TA	1000–1500	15 to 65	21
Raju	Surf TA	751–1750	2 to 70	22
McCord	Curosurf	701–2000	29 to 89	9
Fujiwara	Surf TA	750–1749	21 to 55	23

ALEC = Artificial lung expanding compound
CLSE = Calf lung surfactant extract
Surf TA = Surfactant TA

Table 5 Effect of different surfactant trials on the incidence of patent ductus arteriosus

Author	Surfactant	Gestation or weight	95% CI for improvement in PDA per 100 babies	Refs
Prophylactic trials				
Enhorning	CLSE	25–29	−11 to 35	5
Kwong	CLSE	24–28	−54 to 18	6
Morley	ALEC dry	23–29	−33 to 11	15, 16
Morley	ALEC	23–34	−7 to 7	17
Ten Centre	ALEC	25–29	−12 to 8	18
Halliday	DPPC+HDL	27–33	−25 to 6	12
Merritt	Human	24–29	−9 to 27	11
Rescue trials				
Hallman	Human	<1500	−12 to 36	10
Gitlin	Surf TA	1000–1500	−26 to 36	21
Raju	Surf TA	751–1750	−80 to −16	22
McCord	Curosurf	701–2000	−53 to 19	9
Fujiwara	Surf TA	750–1749	−20 to −9	23

ALEC = Artificial lung expanding compound
CLSE = Calf lung surfactant extract
Surf TA = Surfactant TA

though this may be a major side effect of surfactant therapy. Animal experiments have also suggested that it might be a complication of surfactant therapy. Table 5 shows the incidence of PDA in both the prophylactic and rescue trials. Overall, it shows that surfactant therapy might increase the tendency to PDA. The trials which showed a significant increase in the incidence of PDA were Raju's[22] and Fujiwara's[23] trial of bovine Surfactant TA. No trial showed a significant reduction in PDA.

Time in oxygen

One of the difficulties with assessing the effect of surfactant therapy on time in oxygen or time receiving ventilation is that more surfactant treated babies survived and so there is not an even balance between the groups. With more survivors it is possible that the surfactant treatment could result in babies receiving respiratory support for a longer time. Not all the trials give the time babies received oxygen. Those that do show a very wide variation within each group. In the majority there was no difference.

Changes in oxygenation

The severity of RDS is reflected in the level of inspired oxygen required to maintain normal arterial oxygenation. Table 6 shows a comparison of the effect of different surfactant preparations on oxygenation over the first 3 days. This shows the percentage improvement in oxygenation caused by surfactant. If there was no improvement the value would be zero. The larger the percentage change the better the effect of surfactant. Although surfactant therapy improves oxygenation the effect is only demonstrable in most trials for the first 72 hours.

Table 6 Percentage difference in oxygenation between treated and controls in the first 3 days

Trial	1 hour	24 hours	48 hours	72 hours	Reference
		Prophylactic trials			
Enhorning	22%	31%	30%	20%	5
Kwong	14%	31%	26%	—	6
Merritt	27%	38%	35%	32%	11
Morley	11%	21%	19%	27%	17

Trial	Before	24 hours	48 hours	72 hours	Reference
		Rescue trials			
Hallman	0	45%	56%	29%	10
Gitlin	−21%	69%	71%	9%	21
Raju	11%	25%	44%	38%	22

In four of the prophylactic trials there is some beneficial effect within an hour of birth which increases at 24 hours and by 72 hours the effect is waning except for the artifical surfactant which is still improving.

In three rescue trials oxygenation is expressed as a percentage improvement in the arterial-alveolar oxygen concentration. All three trials show an acute improvement which also diminished by 72 hours. Note the different effect when the same surfactant is used in different trials.

Time receiving ventilation

Few of the trials show this result. Those that do show a modest improvement from surfactant treatment for the survivors.

Changes in airway pressure

Not all the trials show results of the airway pressure changes in ventilated babies after surfactant treatment. Those that do show a consistent improvement in the first three days. Taking account of the different babies in the trials there is little difference between the surfactants. The mean pressure difference over the controls is shown in Table 7.

Bronchopulmonary dysplasia

The incidence of BPD is not reported in all the trials. Table 8 shows that surfactant therapy significantly reduces the incidence

Table 7 Mean airway pressure difference (cm H_2O) between treated and controls in the first 3 days

Trial	1 hour	24 hours	48 hours	72 hours	Reference
		Prophylactic trials			
Merritt	−2.9	−2.0	−2.9	−2.9	11
Morley*	−3.5	−4.3	−4.2	−3.5	17

Trial	Before	24 hours	48 hours	72 hours	Reference
		Rescue trials			
Gitlin	0.5	−4.2	−2.6	−3.0	21
Hallman	0.2	−1.2	−1.0	−0.1	10
Raju	−1.0	−5.2	−3.4	−2.8	22
Fujiwara	−0.3	−4.0	−4.3	−2.9	23

*= change in mean peak inspiratory pressure

Table 8 Incidence of bronchopulmonary dysplasia in survivors

Study	SA Used	Infants No. SA	C	95% CI for improvement in BPD in survivors	Ref
Enhorning	CLSE	39	33	4 to 42	5
Kwong	CLSE	14	13	5 to 67	6
Merritt	Human	31	29	7 to 67	11
Morley	ALEC	55	43	0 to 30	17
Hallman	Human	22	23	2 to 60	10
Raju	Surf TA	17	13	−41 to 47	22
Gitlin	Surf TA	18	23	−18 to 46	21

SA = Surfactant
C = Controls   ALEC = Artificial lung expanding compound
CLSE = Calf lung surfactant extract
Surf TA = Surfactant TA

of BPD in the survivors in all the trials except those with Surfactant TA.[21,22]

Dose of surfactant

Although the doses of surfactant used in these trials vary (from 25 mg to 200 mg) they are all very much larger, by as much as 10 fold, than the amount needed to form a surfactant layer on the inside of completely surfactant deficient lungs. It is difficult to understand why such comparatively large doses should be required for therapy when surface balance studies of each surfactant suggest that much smaller doses of the surfactant would reach the surface rapidly, spread fast to completely cover the surface and be replenished quickly. It is possible that a large proportion of the exogenous surfactant is absorbed into the lungs and some is inhibited by exuded plasma proteins. The reason such a high dose of surfactant has been chosen is that experiments have shown this to give the best effect. Animal experiments suggested that about 50 mg/kg was the optimal dose. Secondly, as most trials were only using one dose they did not want to miss a therapeutic effect by giving too small a small dose. A recent Japanese trial (3) randomised babies weighing between 750 and 1750 g to a high dose 120 mg/kg and a low dose 60 mg/kg. Both treatments improved oxygenation and decreased ventilatory requirements with the best effect from the high dose. In the low dose infants the improvement in oxygenation was not sustained in a significant proportion. This suggested that for Surfactant TA the babies on the high dose had a better outcome. However, for other surfactants the appropriate dose of each surfactant is not known and is one of the many factors in surfactant therapy which needs to be elucidated.

Most trials have used only one dose and it is surprising that this has had an effect which can be measured in some babies for days. In animal experiments repeat doses have been used and not shown to be consistently effective although one study suggests that repeated small doses may benefit babies. It has been postulated that a major factor determining the loss of surfactant efficacy is the exudation of large amounts of serum proteins onto the airway surface. This inhibits surfactant function and may also diminish the effect of repeated doses. The place of repeated doses still needs to be clarified.

CONCLUSION

The overview of all the trials of surfactant therapy must be that it is beneficial to very premature babies less than 30 weeks gestation. The main benefits are an improvement in oxygenation and a reduction in ventilator pressures and a reduction in mortality, intraventricular haemorrhages and possibly some reduction in the incidence of BPD in the survivors. The only major side effect shown to date is in the rescue trials where there was an increase in PDA in babies treated with natural surfactant.

Prophylactic surfactant treatment has been shown to be beneficial and apparently harmless, even though some babies who would not develop RDS were treated. It would therefore seem appropriate in future to treat all babies at reasonable risk of developing RDS at birth. In practical terms this means all babies of less than about 30 weeks gestation because they have at least a 25% chance of requiring assisted ventilation. All premature babies who need intubating at birth for resuscitation should probably also be treated because asphyxia increases their risk of RDS. Rescue treatment can then be given to babies who subsequently develop serious RDS and require ventilation or who are transferred into neonatal intensive care units from other hospitals for ventilation.

One of the main concerns about using natural surfactant preparations in very premature babies is the foreign protein introduced into their lungs to which they may become sensitised. However, the evidence to date is that antibodies to this protein cannot be detected after the babies have been treated.

Even though there are still problems to be sorted out about dose regimes and techniques of delivery, it is to be hoped that surfactant will be available for treating babies in the very near future.

These trials have shown that although surfactant therapy reduces the severity of RDS and its complications, the majority of the babies still suffer from the disease. This may give us an indication about the underlying factors causing RDS. It strongly suggests that surfactant deficiency is not the only aetiological factor in this disease and we should now turn our attention to improving other compounding problems such as structural immaturity and protein leak onto the lung surface. There is some suggestion from preliminary animal experiments that TRH to the mother and surfactant to the baby may further improve lung function.[24]

One of the exciting areas of surfactant research at the moment is investigation of the role of surfactant associated apoproteins.[25-27] There seem to be at least three very low molecular weight hydrophobic proteins which appear to be associated with surfactant. Although at least one of them may be important for surfactant spreading their exact function is still to be elicited. It is possible that further generations of artificial surfactant may contain both synthesised apoproteins and phospholipids.

Although it has been suggested that artificial surfactant is not as effective as natural surfactant the clinical trials of artificial surfactant ALEC on the respiratory problems, complications and outcome of very premature babies have shown that babies under 30 weeks can be treated with this surfactant made from two phospholipids and it significantly reduces the incidence of complications and improves the babies' outcome. This artificial surfactant does not contain apoproteins and yet is still effective. This is important because experiments have suggested that only surfactants which contain apoproteins are likely to be effective.[27]

There is no evidence that any surfactant preparation has any major therapeutic advantage over any other because the trials are not easily comparable. In consequence the decision about which surfactant should be used will depend upon its possible side effects, its ease of preparation and delivery, its availability and its price. It may be that in future, clinical trials will be undertaken to compare two or three surfactant preparations. However, it will be extremely difficult to obtain answers with any degree of accuracy because several hundred very premature babies would be required confidently to show a difference, or lack of it, in any of the major outcomes like death, handicap, intraventricular haemorrhage, pneumothorax, BPD or time on ventilation.

REFERENCES

1 Avery ME, Mead J. Surface properties in relation to atelectasis and hyaline membrane disease. Am J Dis Child 1959; 97: 517–523
2 Fujiwara T, Chida S, Watabe Y, Maeta H, Morita T, Abe T. Artificial surfactant therapy in hyaline membrane disease. Lancet 1980; i: 55–59
3 Konishi M, Fujiwara T, Takeuki Y, et al. Surfactant replacement therapy in neonatal respiratory distress syndrome. Eur J Pediatr 1988; 144: 20–25
4 Tanaka Y, Takei T, Kanazawa Y, Seida K, Masuda K, Kiuchi A, Fujiwara T. Preparation of surfactant from minced bovine lung, chemical composition and surface tension properties. J Jap Med Soc Biol Interface 1982; 13: 27–34
5 Enhorning G, Shennan A, Possmayer F, Dunn M, Chen CP, Milligan J. Prevention of neonatal respiratory distress syndrome by tracheal instillation of surfactant. A randomized clinical trial. Pediatrics 1985; 76: 145–153
6 Kwong SM, Egan EA, Notter RH, Shapiro DL. Double-blind clinical trial of calf lung surfactant extract for the prevention of hyaline membrane disease in extremely premature infants. Pediatrics 1985; 76: 585–592
7 Shapiro DL, Notter RH, Morin FC, Deluga KS, Golub LM, Sinkin RA, Weiss KI, Cox C. Double blind, randomized trial of calf lung surfactant extract administered at birth to very premature infants for prevention of respiratory distress syndrome. Pediatrics 1985; 76: 593–599
8 Noack G, Berggren P, Curstedt T et al. Severe neonatal respiratory distress syndrome treated with isolated phospholipid fraction of natural surfactant. Acta Paediatr Scan 1987; 76: 687–705
9 McCord FB, Curstedt T, Halliday HL, et al. Surfactant treatment and the incidence of intraventricular haemorrhage in severe respiratory distress syndrome. Arch Dis Child 1988; 63: 10–16
10 Hallman M, Merritt TA, Jarvenpaa AL, Boynton B, Mannino F, Gluck L, Moore T, Edwards D. Exogenous human surfactant for treatment of severe respiratory distress syndrome: A randomized prospective clinical trial. J Pediatr 1985; 106: 963–969
11 Merritt TA, Hallman M, Bloom BT, Berry C, Benirschke K, Sahn D, Key T, Edwards D, Jarvenpaa AL, Pohjavuori M, Kankaanpaa K, Kunnas M, Paatero H, Rapola J, Jaaskelainen J. Prophylactic treatment of very premature infants with human surfactant. N Engl J Med 1986; 315: 785–790
12 Halliday HL, McClure G, Reid M, Lappin TRJ, Meban C, Thomas PS. Controlled trial of artificial surfactant to prevent respiratory distress syndrome. Lancet 1984; i: 476–478
13 Bangham AD, Morley CJ, Phillips MC. The physical properties of an effective lung surfactant. Biochim Biophys Acta 1979; 573: 552–556
14 Bangham AD, Miller NGA, Davies RJ, Greenough A, Morley CJ. Introductory remarks about Artificial Lung Expanding Compounds (ALEC). Colloid and Surfaces 1984; 10: 337–347
15 Morley CJ, Bangham AD, Miller N, Davis JA. Dry artificial surfactant and its effect on very premature babies. Lancet 1981; i: 64–68
16 Morley CJ. The Cambridge experience of artificial surfactant. In: Walters DV, Strang LB, Geubelle F, eds. Physiology of the fetal and neonatal lung. Lancaster: MTP Press, 1987: Ch. 18, pp. 255–272
17 Morley CJ, Greenough A, Miller N, et al. Randomized trial of artificial surfactant (ALEC) given at birth to babies from 23 to 24 weeks gestation. Early Hum Dev 1988; (in press)
18 Ten Centre Study Group. Ten centre trial of artificial surfactant (artificial lung expanding compound) in very premature babies. Br Med J 1987; 294: 991–996
19 Wilkinson A, Jenkins PA, Jeffrey JA. Two controlled trials of dry artificial surfactant: early effects and later outcome in babies with surfactant deficiency. Lancet 1985; ii: 287–291

20 Durand DJ, Clyman RI, Heymann MA, et al. Effects of a protein-free, synthetic surfactant on survival and pulmonary function in preterm lambs. J Pediatr 1985; 107: 775–780
21 Gitlin JD, Soll RF, Parad RB et al. Randomized controlled trial of exogenous surfactant for the treatment of hyaline membrane disease. Pediatrics 1987; 79: 31–37
22 Raju TNK, Vidyasagar D, Bhat R, et al. Double-blind controlled trial of single-dose treatment with bovine surfactant in severe hyaline membrane disease. Lancet 1987; i: 651–656
23 Fujiwara T, Konishi M, Ogawa Y, et al. Surfactant replacement for respiratory distress syndrome. A multicentre clinical trial. Jap J Pediatr 1987; 40: 549–568 (in Japanese)
24 Ikegami M, Jobe AH, Pettanzano A, Seidner SR, Berry DD, Ruffini L. Effects of maternal treatment with corticosteroids, T_3, TRH, and their combinations on lung function of ventilated preterm rabbits with and without surfactant treatments. Am Rev Respir Dis 1987; 136: 892–898
25 Takashihi, A, Fujiwara T. Proteolipid in bovine lung surfactant: its role in surfactant function. Biochem Biophys Res Commun 1986; 135: 527–532
26 Curstedt T, Jornvall H, Robertson B, Bergman T, Berggren P. Two hydrophobic low-molecular-mass protein fractions of pulmonary surfactant. Characterisation and biophysical activity. Eur J Biochem 1987; 168: 255–262
27 Suzuki Y, Curstedt T, Grossman G, et al. The role of low molecular weight (< 15 000 Daltons) apoproteins of pulmonary surfactant. Eur J Respir 1986; 69: 336–345

Development of renal function

Neena Modi
Department of Paediatrics and Neonatal Medicine, Royal Postgraduate Medical School, Hammersmith Hospital and Queen Charlotte's Hospital, London

> The improved survival of extremely immature infants, developments in ventilator techniques and advances in the understanding of neurological morbidity have brought neonatal medicine to the point where other organ systems are beginning to be studied in detail. Present knowledge of renal function in the extremely immature infant has mainly arisen from extrapolation from studies on immature animals and older human infants. There has been very little direct study of extremely immature infants in the first days of life and less of the human fetus *in utero*. This paper will attempt to review the information available relating to the development of renal function in the extremely immature infant. Although investigations on animal models will be touched on, it is intended to concentrate here on features relating directly to the human fetus and neonate.

ANATOMICAL DEVELOPMENT

The development of human renal function and the definitive kidney proceeds with the formation of the three excretory organs, the pronephros, mesonephros and metanephros. The pronephros has no excretory role, merely giving rise to the mesonephric duct; it arises at around the third week of gestation and involutes over the following fortnight. The functional significance of the mesonephric kidney varies greatly between different mammalian species. The mesonephros comprises primitive tubules and glomeruli and in the human fetus, degenerates by the twelfth week.[1] There is overlap between the development of the mesonephros and the metanephros, with the first definitive nephrons arising from the metanephros in the fifth week and becoming functional by eight weeks. Nephrons are formed in a centrifugal manner with the first in the innermost region of the cortex. At 22 weeks all nephrons are juxtamedullary.[2] By 35 weeks gestation each kidney contains the full complement of one million nephrons.[3] Birth does not accelerate nephrogenesis.[4]

The renal blood supply is established by the ninth week and arises from the aorta at the level T12–L2, a relationship that is constant between 24 and 44 weeks.[5] The morphological development of the kidney is accompanied by a changing distribution of intrarenal blood flow. In the immature puppy kidney, relative perfusion is highest in the juxtamedullary nephrons.[6] In the lamb, the intrauterine environment is also characterized by a relatively low renal blood flow and high renal vascular resistance.[7,8] The kidneys of fetal rhesus monkeys receive approximately 2.7% of the combined ventricular output.[9] Rudolf et al,[10] studying the circulation of the previable human fetus demonstrated a decrease in cardiac output to the kidneys, from a mean of 6% in fetuses of under 50 g to around 3% in fetuses of over 151 g.

Tubular function has begun by the ninth week and by the fourteenth week the loops of Henle are functioning. However, even at term there is still an anatomical underdevelopment of the proximal tubules.[11] The largest, most mature juxtamedullary glomeruli possess the longest proximal tubules. During postnatal life the tubules lengthen, increasing absorptive and secretory capacity.

Kidney length increases from a mean of 31 mm at 24 weeks gestation to 36 mm at 32 weeks and 41 mm at term[12] (Fig. 1).

Little is known of the development of fetal renal sympathetic innervation. Although studies of the fetal lamb suggest that sympathetic function is not established till late in gestation,[13] Zimmerman[14] describes innervation of the distal convoluted tubules in 13–16 week gestation human fetuses.

INTRAUTERINE RENAL FUNCTION

Though the placenta is the major regulatory organ of the fetus and intact renal function is not necessary for fetal development, fetal renal function may influence fetal outcome. The most obvious example is the effect of reduced urine production on amniotic fluid volume and resultant fetal malformation; it is also probable that derangements in fetal regulation of extracellular fluid volume are responsible for some instances of poly- and oligohydramnios.

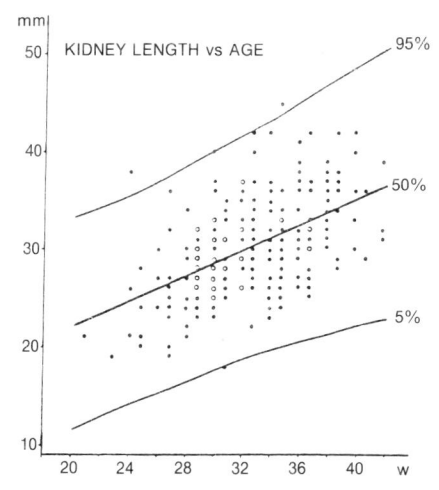

Fig. 1 Renal length v. gestational age: experimental values and polynomial regression, 5th and 95th percentiles (Reproduced from Radiology, with permission of the publishers.[12]).

Urine production

The human fetus begins urine production at around five weeks gestation. Kurjak et al,[15] using the method devised by Campbell et al,[16] observed an increase in urine production from about 2 ml h^{-1} (4.5 ml kg^{-1} h^{-1}) at 20 weeks gestation to about 12 ml h^{-1} (6 ml kg^{-1} h^{-1}) at 32 weeks and 26 ml h^{-1} at 39 weeks (8 ml kg^{-1} h^{-1}). Urine production then declines abruptly.[17] The factors regulating fetal urinary output in the human are poorly understood. The maternal administration of frusemide normally results in fetal diuresis. However, the stressed fetus of an abnormal pregnancy may show no response to maternal frusemide and is more likely to have a lower urine production rate[17] even when renal function is normal.[18] This may be due to the increased level of antidiuretic hormone shown to occur in the stressed human infant at birth[19] and in the fetal lamb subjected to hypovolaemic[20] or asphyxial[21] stress. Vasopressin is present in the human fetal pituitary by 11 weeks gestation.[22] There may be other hormonal influences on fetal urine production. Aldosterone affects electrolyte handling in the fetal lamb in a manner similar to the adult response.[23] However cortisol, while having little renal effect on the adult sheep kidney except at high levels, results in increased fetal urinary flow and the increased excretion of sodium, potassium and chloride.[24]

Between 34–40 weeks, the human fetus swallows between 200 and 600 ml of amniotic fluid daily.[25] However, there is no clear relationship between fetal urinary output, swallowing and amniotic fluid volume. Van Otterlo et al,[26] studying 67 normal pregnancies from 36–41 weeks gestation and 16 diabetic pregnancies between 28–40 weeks, found no relationship between the rate of fetal urine production and amniotic fluid volume. However, a low urine flow rate was found with oligohydramnios with growth retardation of the fetus. Similarly, congenital malformations that prevent the ingestion of anmiotic fluid are not invariably associated with polyhydramnios.[27] Wladimiroff and Campbell[17] found no correlation between fetal weight and voiding rate.

Though unnecessary for intact development, the fetal kidney does respond appropriately to regulate water and electrolyte imbalance. Maternal polyhydramnios and neonatal hyponatraemia have been described in association with prolonged maternal ingestion of chlorothiazide.[1] It is likely that the fetal kidney responded to salt depletion by increasing urine output in an attempt to correct the fetal sodium and water imbalance. In the chronically catheterized fetal sheep preparation, the maternal infusion of hypertonic saline has been shown to produce peaks in fetal vasopressin before and at peak fetal sodium concentration. This suggests that there was a rapid fetal to mother flow of water following maternal hypertonic saline administration and a combined volume-osmolar stimulus to the fetus.[28] A strong correlation has been shown between maternal plasma volume and amniotic fluid volume when fetal malformations and diabetic pregnancies are excluded. The same authors[29] also present evidence to suggest that fetal endocrine responses influence maternal plasma volume.

Tubular function

Gersh[30] has studied the morphological differentiation of the thick and thin limbs of the loops of Henle in several animal species and correlated this with evidence of tubular function. On the basis of morphological criteria thus determined, he concluded that function was possible in human loops of Henle in the metanephros at thirteen weeks.

Fetal urine is an ultrafiltrate of fetal serum and is hypotonic throughout gestation, made so by selective reabsorption of sodium and chloride. A concentration of sodium in fetal urine exceeding

100 mmol l^{-1} and osmolality exceeding 210 mosmol kg^{-1} has been shown to be predictive of impaired renal function and poor fetal outcome.[31] The healthy fetus is thus capable of considerable retention of sodium, an obvious corollary to the demands of growth. The fetus at term also excretes a large amount of sodium, approximately 8 mmol kg^{-1} d^{-1}—this is of course in the face of an *ad libitum* intake via the placenta and is more than twice the amount such an infant is likely to receive from breast milk. The fetus must therefore have the capacity to increase tubular reabsorption of sodium still further, a response that comes into play following birth and the removal of transplacental supplies.

The infant *in utero* is in a state of relative water diuresis, excreting around 20% of filtered water and forming urine with a low urea and creatinine urine to plasma ratio (approximately 5). There is virtually no phosphate or glucose in fetal urine, despite the fact that fetal serum has a higher concentration of inorganic phosphate than maternal serum[32] demonstrating that these two discrete transport mechanisms are functional in the fetal kidney.

Glomerular filtration

Glomerular filtration depends upon ultrafiltration pressure (the balance between hydrostatic pressure across the glomerular membrane and the osmotic pressure of non filtered colloids), renal plasma flow and the ultrafiltration coefficient (a function of total capillary surface area and permeability per unit area). The development of these factors during gestation has not been studied to any great extent in the human fetus.

A mean glomerular filtration rate (GFR) of 2.66 ml min^{-1} (SD ± 1.47) has been estimated in term infants *in utero* in the six hours prior to delivery[15] using ultrasound measurement of fetal urine production rate, cord blood creatinine and creatinine concentration in first voided urine. Other measurements of GFR have not been made in the human fetus *in utero* though attempts are being made to develop appropriate techniques.[33]

The results of animal studies cannot be extrapolated directly to the human fetus in view of variations in differentiation in relation to gestational age and the duration of intrauterine existence. An abrupt increase in GFR at the time of completion of nephrogenesis has been shown to occur in several mammalian species. The reasons for this are not known. Until this point, although there is a steady increase in absolute GFR, GFR factored by weight remains relatively stable.[34] In chronically catheterized fetal lambs GFR increases at the same rate as body weight.[34] In the dog nephrogenesis is not completed until three weeks after birth; in the human nephrogenesis is completed at 34 weeks gestation and GFR has also been shown to increase at this conceptional age.[35-37]

PERINATAL HOMEOSTASIS

The fetus *in utero* excretes a large volume of hypotonic urine of low sodium content. Following birth the infant enters a phase of relative oliguria. There is no evidence that GFR falls acutely in the first day following birth. GFR, when measured in the first day of life, correlates with gestational age when expressed in absolute terms (ml min^{-1}) but shows (if anything) a tendency to fall when expressed per kg of body weight (ml min^{-1} kg^{-1}).[38] This is similar to the pattern of development seen in the chronically catheterized sheep fetus,[34] but is in marked contrast to the postnatal change in GFR when a rise occurs which is disproportionately higher than the rise in body weight. The first urine formed postnatally is hypertonic to plasma with an increased concentration of urea, potassium and phosphate but not of sodium and chloride.[32] The change in urine volume thus appears to be brought about by a decrease in free water clearance. This may be mediated by the increased levels of arginine vasopressin (AVP) present in the neonate around delivery.[39]

The phase of relative oliguria is followed, after a variable period of hours to days, by a diuretic phase during which the extracellular space undergoes contraction. Sodium is the principal electrolyte of extracellular fluid and is of necessity lost during this contraction. In infants with respiratory disease the time of onset of diuresis is determined primarily by the onset of improvement in respiratory function. Though this association has been the subject of several investigations the underlying mechanisms have not been explained. Earlier suggestions that the diuresis represented an improvement in renal function consequent on improved oxygenation[40,41] were refuted when it was shown that the diuresis was not initiated subsequent to the improvement in respiratory function.[42-44] Certain authors[42-45] have concluded that the diuresis precedes the improvement in respiratory function. However, careful examination of their data reveals that they equally show that the **onset** of the diuretic phase in fact follows the **onset** of improvement in respiratory function and that continuing diuresis then accompanies continuing respiratory improvement.

The onset of diuresis appears to be the consequence of a change in renal sodium handling. In a study of 26 neonates of less than 34 weeks gestation with respiratory disease, a tendency to retain sodium changed to a tendency to excrete sodium at the point of improvement in respiratory function.[46] The change in sodium handling coincided with the onset of diuresis. Figure 2 shows the change in sodium handling with decreasing alveolar-arterial oxygen gradient in an individual infant. In other words until the point of improvement in respiratory function, the extremely preterm neonate continues to handle sodium as *in utero*, exhibiting a tendency to retention. The overall stimulus to retain sodium by the growing fetus and neonate is therefore temporarily overruled by a stimulus to excrete sodium.

These observations suggest that the trigger to diuresis and extracellular fluid volume contraction may be the release of a natriuretic agent brought about by a decrease in pulmonary vascular resistance and increased left atrial filling. The finding by Kojima et al.[47] that the level of atrial natriuretic peptide (ANP) rises during the diuretic phase of respiratory distress syndrome lends support to this hypothesis which is currently being investigated by the author. The clinical implications of these observations are that sodium supplements should not be provided to the sick preterm neonate until after the postnatal diuresis. The wide acceptance of recomendations that extremely immature infants require in excess of 3 mmol kg^{-1} d^{-1} [36,48] is probably responsible for inappropriately early supplementation leading to persistence of a relatively expanded extracellular space. An expanded extracellular fluid space acts as a stimulus for increased tubular excretion of sodium, as well as glucose and bicarbonate[49,50] and thus may be in part responsible for the pattern of abnormalities so often seen in sick low birth weight infants where hyponatraemia and the need for sodium supplementation occur in the face of clinical oedema and mild metabolic acidosis.

There are maternal influences on neonatal fluid and electrolyte balance: an expanded extracellular volume has been described in preterm neonates whose mothers had received intravenous fluids prior to delivery;[51] these infants, who were hyponatraemic, had an increased risk of developing pulmonary air leak, i.e. interstitial emphysema, pneumothorax, pneumomediastinum and pneumopericardium.[52]

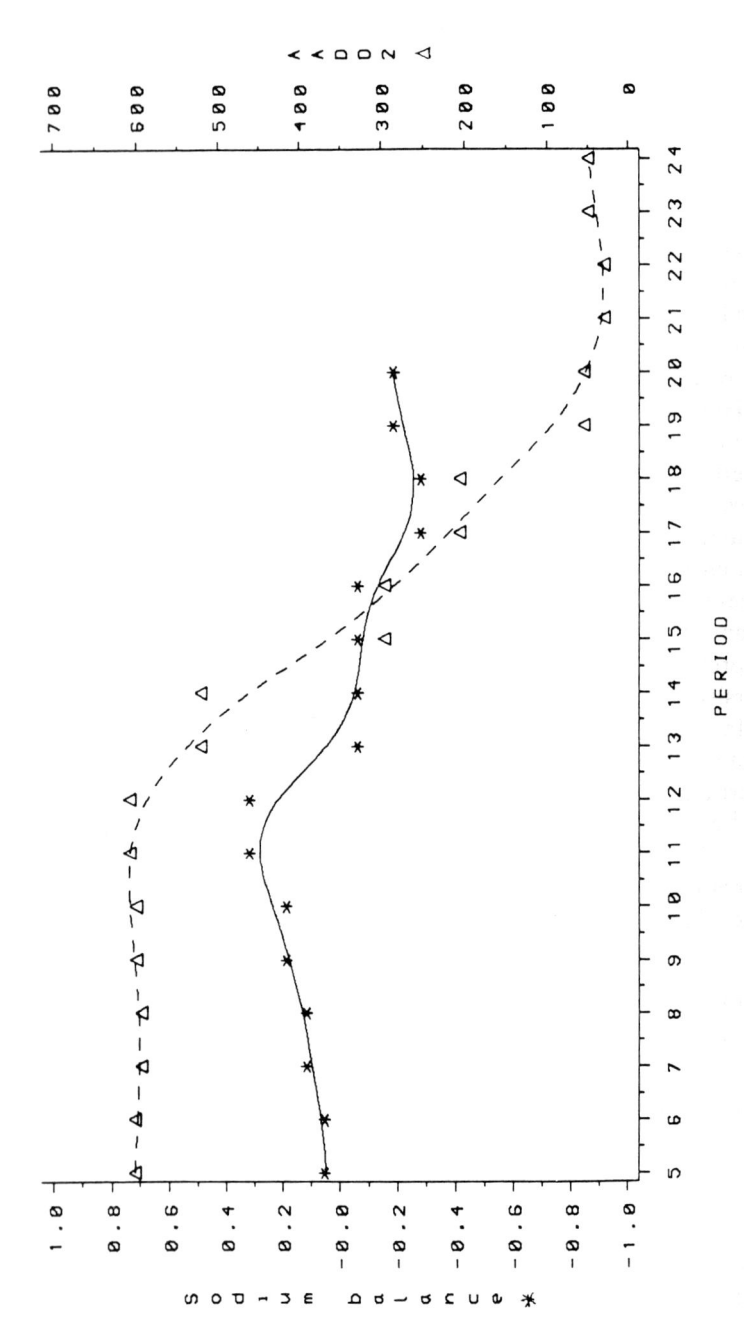

Fig. 2 Sodium balance (mmol kg^{-1}, d^{-1}) and AADO$_2$ (Torr) by time period (4 hourly blocks) in an individual infant[46].

NEONATAL RENAL FUNCTION

Urine flow rate

As discussed above, urine flow rate is low on the first day of life and rises subsequently. In the presence of a renal solute load of 15 mosmol kg^{-1} d^{-1} and an approximate maximum urinary concentration of 500–700 mosmol kg H$_2$O^{-1} solute retention might be expected to occur at a urine flow rate of less than 1 ml kg^{-1} d^{-1}.[53] Extremely immature infants have considerably smaller solute loads on the first day of life and in these infants a urine flow rate of less than 0.5 ml kg^{-1} h^{-1} on day one of life and 1 ml kg^{-1} h^{-1} thereafter should be regarded as abnormal.

High urine flow rates in the immediate newborn period are seen in infants with tubular damage, as a physiological response to fetal overhydration such as in maternal fluid overload and in the presence of polyhydramnios. The author has observed an infant who was noted to have a high intrauterine urinary flow rate and in whom polyhydramnios was present. This infant was born at 28 weeks gestation and developed moderately severe hyaline membrane disease; despite this she had a high urinary flow rate of approximately 7 ml kg^{-1} h^{-1} on the first day of life which persisted to five days.

In a study (Modi N, unpublished observations) of preterm infants of less than 1500 g birth weight, mean urine flow rate increased from 0.7 ml kg^{-1} h^{-1} on day one of life to 2.8 ml kg^{-1} h^{-1} on day four, 3 ml kg^{-1} h^{-1} on day six and then fell to 2.5 ml kg^{-1} h^{-1} on day seven. It has been estimated that the most immature preterm infants might achieve a maximum urine flow rate of around 7 ml kg^{-1} h^{-1}.[54]

Glomerular filtration rate

The pattern of development of GFR in the human infant born between 24 and 35 weeks gestation has been variably described. There is general agreement that GFR correlates with gestational and post conceptional age.[55] However, Fawer et al,[56] expressing their results per unit surface area, found GFR to increase rapidly up to the 35th week and then to level off to term. They explain this in terms of the development of new nephrons up to 35 weeks. Other workers describe a shallow gradient until 34 weeks gestation with GFR becoming abruptly steeper thereafter.[35,36] These authors expressed their results in absolute terms of ml min^{-1}. The author's own work, expressing GFR per kg body weight (Fig. 3), has shown only a small increase between 25 and 34 weeks. Leake and Trygstad,[38] studying infants on the first day of life, found GFR to (if anything) decrease slightly between 27 and 43 weeks when expressed per kg body weight. Examination of their data for absolute GFR reveals little change up to 34 weeks gestation and then a tendency to rising values.

The difficulties in interpreting measures of GFR in the neonate have, at least in part, been magnified by the inappropriate use of GFR 'corrected' for surface area. As long ago as 1952, McCance and Widdowson[57] questioned the use in paediatric practice of surface area to standardize GFR. It would be logical to relate GFR to the size of the fluid pool affected by the kidney. In the neonate all fluid compartments are changing fairly rapidly and correlate closely with body weight. Coulthard and Hey[58] have argued elegantly in favour of weight as the best standard for GFR. Surface area to weight ratio changes little in adulthood whereas it falls dramatically during the first weeks of life in keeping with the rapid weight gain of the infant. An adult with a GFR of 80 ml min^{-1} m$^{2-1}$ filters approximately 2 ml min^{-1} kg^{-1}. To achieve a GFR of 80 ml min^{-1} m$^{2-1}$ a 28 week gestation infant of surface area of 0.1 m^2 would need to filter 8 ml min^{-1} kg^{-1}. Such an infant actually filters around 0.5 ml min^{-1} kg^{-1} with a full term baby filtering up to 1.6 ml kg^{-1} min^{-1}. GFR is generally held to be extremely low in the very preterm infant. However, the magnitude of difference between the baby of 28 weeks gestation and the adult is thus closer to fourfold rather than sixteenfold.

The increase in GFR at the time of completion of nephrogenesis has been mentioned above. A second abrupt increase occurs after the first day of life. There is then a continuing rise over the first few postnatal weeks which is more gradual in the preterm infant.[59,60] There is evidence to suggest that this postnatal increase is a consequence of a decrease in renal vascular resistance and increased renal blood flow.[61] Renal blood flow is low and renal vascular resistance high during the last trimester of gestation in fetal lambs,[7,8] in comparison to values in the adult animal. In the immediate postnatal period renal blood flow in newborn lambs is similar to fetal values. Though renal blood flow does not therefore appear to change immediately following birth, there is subsequently a significant increase in keeping with the increase in GFR referred to above.

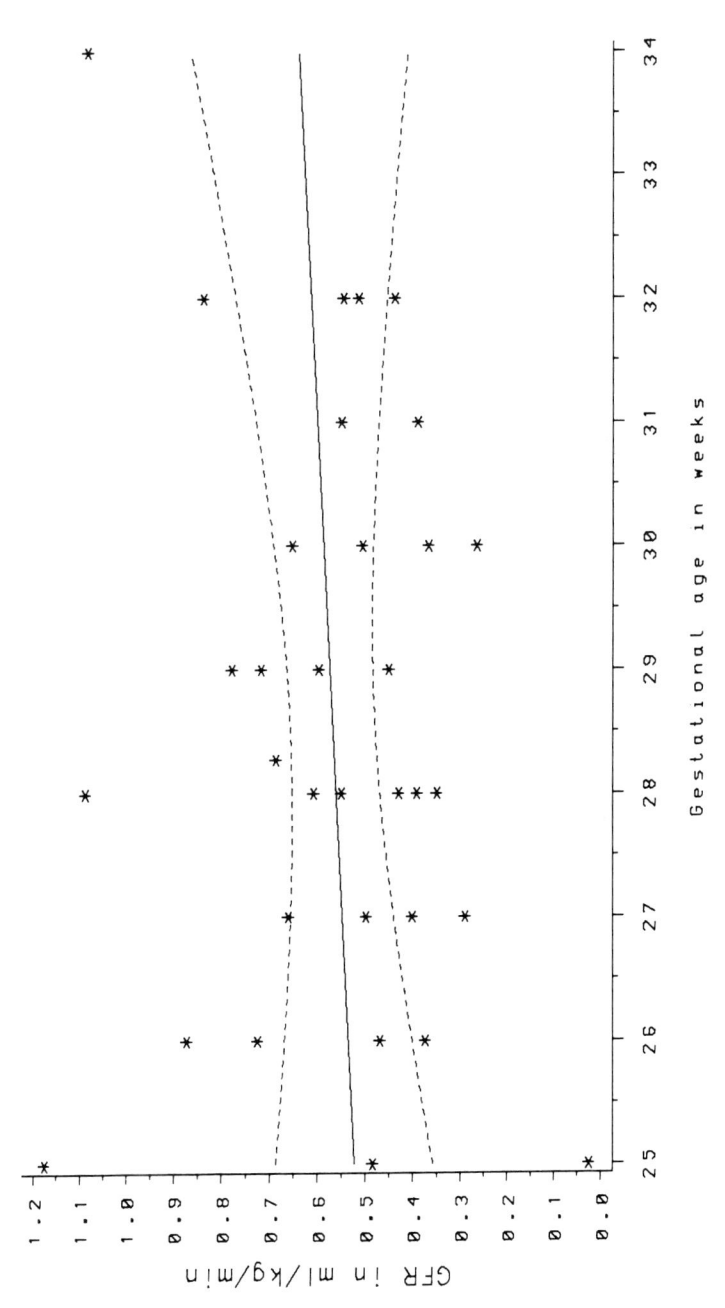

Fig. 3 Regression of glomerular filtration rate on gestational age, with 95% confidence limits for regression line (N. Modi, unpublished observations).

Very few measurements of GFR have been made in the less than 28 week gestation infant. In a study of very low birth weight babies in the first week of life, from 25–34 weeks gestation, receiving intensive care (Modi N, unpublished observations), GFR varied widely but clustered around 0.3–0.7 ml min^{-1} kg^{-1} (Fig. 3). These values are similar to those obtained by other workers studying well infants.[35,38,55,56,62]

A further problem in the definition of 'normal' values for GFR in the extremely immature infant lies in the wide variation in between baby values. This is hardly surprising given the physiological adaptations that are occurring and the numerous clinical influences on GFR. In infants with hyaline membrane disease, GFR has been variably reported as both decreasing and remaining unchanged.[42,45] Given current methods of management, this variation probably reflects the degree of hypoxaemia rather than the actual disease process. The author's data shows a tendency to falling GFR with increasing alveolar-arterial oxygen gradient but with wide variation in absolute values. Hypercapnia causes a decrease in renal blood flow and increase in renal vascular resistance in the fetal lamb.[63]

Sodium

Sodium handling in the immature infant is characterized by three features: urinary sodium losses are high, the natriuretic response to a salt load is blunted and there is a net stimulus to conserve sodium—a prerequisite for growth. The maturation of sodium handling is reflected in the ontogeny of the renin-angiotensin-aldosterone system (RAAS), the prostaglandins and possibly atrial natriuretic peptide.

The first step in the process of sodium reabsorption occurs in the proximal tubule. Here the reabsorption of sodium and water is isotonic and governed by both active and passive forces. Physical factors affecting peritubular capillary fluid resorption influence sodium transport at the proximal tubule.[64] These factors have not been studied in the human, preterm neonate. However, animal studies do not suggest that proximal tubular reabsorption is responsible for the sodium retention that characterizes the infant.[65] Coulthard and Hey[54] have estimated distal sodium delivery in babies under 34 weeks gestation to be between 17 and 20% of the glomerular filtrate, a similar value to that reported by Rodriguez-Soriano J et al.[66] Micropuncture studies of 'late proximal' tubules at various stages of maturation also suggest that the fraction of filtrate reabsorbed is no greater than in the adult nephron.[67] The sodium retention of infancy must therefore be presumed to be due to enhanced reabsorption at the distal tubule.

The renin-angiotensin-aldosterone system rather than physical forces appear to be significant with regard to sodium reabsorption at the distal tubule. Aldosterone secretion is relatively elevated in the newborn.[68,69] As the action of aldosterone results in sodium absorption and postassium excretion, the urine potassium to sodium ratio is used as an index of aldosterone dependent distal tubular activity. This ratio is postively correlated with conceptional age[36] but shows no relationship to aldosterone excretion rate in the most immature infants.[59] These observations are explained by postulating a limited responsiveness of the distal tubule to aldosterone in extremely immature infants which increases with maturation and which is accelerated by birth. The retention of sodium during growth and the blunted natriuretic response of the preterm neonate to a saline infusion is thus believed to be due to the high level of activity of the RAAS. Conversely the high renal sodium losses of the extremely immature infant appear to be due in part to the limited responsiveness of the distal tubule to aldosterone stimulation.[65] Sulyok et al.[70] have shown that though preterm infants, in response to negative sodium balance, are able to augment plasma renin activity to values above those found in full term infants, their adrenals fail to respond adequately.

In the fetus *in utero* a urinary sodium concentration in excess of 100 μmol l^{-1} is predictive of poor renal function,[31] yet postnatally such levels are often seen in the presence of ostensibly normal function. An increased GFR, such as occurs in the postnatal period, without a concomitant increase in tubular resorptive capacity would explain this observation and has been used as evidence of functional glomerulotubular imbalance.[71,72] A morphological imbalance exists in the preponderance of glomerular over tubular development.[11] The postnatal urine flow rate after the period of initial oliguria is however similar to the intrauterine flow rate despite the increase in GFR. Tubular resorptive capacity for water therefore appears to have matured *pari passu* with glomerular filtration suggesting an alternative explanation for the high urinary sodium losses.

The possible role of atrial natriuretic peptide in the regulation of sodium handling in the preterm infant has been discussed above, in relation to the acute changes occurring in the immediate neonatal period and the 'physiological' reduction in extracellular fluid volume with loss of sodium and water. Tulassey et al.[73] have examined ANP concentrations in two groups of preterm babies fed differing sodium intakes between 1 and 5 weeks of age. They noted a steady increase in ANP concentration in the group receiving the higher intake and suggest that the continuing positive sodium balance seen in these infants is evidence of a relatively reduced natriuretic effect of ANP in the developing kidney.

In the newborn rat kidney both the total reabsorptive capacity of the proximal tubule and the activity of Na/K ATPase, the enzyme determining active sodium transport, increase postnatally.[74] Fractional sodium excretion (percentage excretion of filtered sodium) decreases with increasing gestational age. In infants below 30 weeks gestation the fractional sodium excretion is over 5% in the first three days of life in comparison to a value of 0.2% in full-term neonates.[62] Al-Dahhan et al.[36] have also shown sodium excretion to decrease postnatally in human infants and suggest that this is related to the increased activity of the RAAS that has been shown to occur shortly following birth.[70] In infants of 30–32 weeks gestational age the urinary Na/K ratio decreases from around 6 in the first postnatal week to 1 between 5–6 weeks.[69] The higher urinary Na/K ratio is taken as evidence of the reduced responsiveness to aldosterone, a possible consequence of low Na/K ATPase activity. In summary the sodium losses that characterize the extremely immature infant are a function of both proximal and distal tubular immaturity;[75] the sodium retention of growth is the consequence of the high level of activity of the RAAS.

The concentration of sodium in 'spot' urine specimens is often used to monitor the requirement for sodium supplementation. This is inappropriate in the extremely immature infant in the first week of life in the absence of a consideration of sodium balance and respiratory status. The obligatory loss of sodium during the physiological contraction in extracellular fluid volume has been referred to above. The author has examined 590 urine specimens from 34 babies of gestational age 25–34 weeks (mean = median = 28) during the first week of life. These infants were all receiving intensive care and required varying degrees of respiratory support. Urinary sodium concentration ranged from 8–220 mmol l^{-1} (mean = 85, median = 81).

Potassium

Potassium excretion in very low birth weight infants is generally between 1–2 mmol kg^{-1} d^{-1} [76,77] and the provision of 2 mmol kg^{-1} d^{-1} is considered appropriate maintenance. However stressed preterm neonates tend to develop negative potassium balance. Contributory factors may be increased prostaglandin synthesis and the frequent use of diuretics. Engle and Arant[77] describe a cumulative negative potassium balance by day 4 of life, of approximately 10% of total body potassium in nine preterm babies requiring ventilatory support. In this study the urinary excretion of potassium was significantly correlated with the urinary excretion of prostaglandin E$_2$.

Calcium and phosphate

Little is known of renal calcium and phosphate handling in the extremely immature infant. As mentioned above, phosphate is not present in fetal urine suggesting early maturation of tubular resorption. However during the first week of life the fractional excretion of phosphate is higher in preterm than in fullterm infants.[35] The relative expansion of the extracellular space has been cited as contributory but does not explain the apparent change in phosphate handling with the onset of postnatal existence. After the first week of life fractional phosphate excretion is low in both preterm and fullterm infants[78] and may be regarded as an appropriate response to growth. Parathormone has not been implicated in the phosphate retention of infancy; rather, it appears to be a consequence of the low GFR.[78]

Glucose

Renal glucosuria is common in immature infants in that glucosuria may be present despite increasing glucose reabsorption with filtered glucose load (N Modi, unpublished observations). This splay in the glucose titration curve may reflect differences in postnatal age and extracellular volume in addition to nephron heterogeneity in individual infants. In a study of glucose handling in 16 infants of less than 34 weeks gestation (mean = median = 28) who developed hyperglycaemia (blood glucose exceeding 10 mmol l^{-1}) during the course of routine clinical care, the mean glucose infusion rate was 8.9 mg kg^{-1} min^{-1}. The fraction of filtered glucose reabsorbed was 88.9%. Urine flow rate, fractional urine flow and ratio of urine output to fluid intake were statistically unchanged during increasing glucosuria (N Modi, unpublished observations). Similarly creatinine clearance was unchanged, confirming the observations of Stonestreet et al.[79] Unlike the situation in older infants, the immature kidney thus appears unable to hyperfiltrate in the presence of hyperglycaemia. The danger of hyperglycaemia to the extremely immature infant must lie in the associated hyperosmolality and not with the development of an osmotic diuresis.

Water

Water balance is maintained by altering urine volume and concentration. The ascending limb of the loop of Henle and the distal tubule function as the 'diluting' segments where reabsorption of solute takes place without water. The ability to form a concentrated urine is dependent on the hypertonic medullary interstitium established by the loop of Henle countercurrent system. The permeability to water of the distal tubule and collecting duct is controlled by the action of antidiuretic hormone.

It has been shown that the peak urine flow of mature infants given a water load is the same as that of adults when expressed per unit body water.[80] Coulthard and Hey[54] have also recently challenged the widely held view that newborns have a reduced capacity for water excretion. They demonstrated that healthy preterm (29 to 34 weeks) babies were able to cope with water intakes ranging from 96–200 ml kg^{-1} d^{-1} from the third day of life, sodium intake remaining constant. Other studies of the effect of varying fluid loads in tiny babies have failed to maintain a constant sodium intake. It is likely that the morbidity associated with increased fluid intakes is in fact attributable to the increased sodium load, mediated by failure to achieve a contraction in extracellular fluid volume.[81] Water and sodium should be prescribed independently and in particular, the use of 'fixed formula' parenteral solutions is ill advised.

Coulthard and Hey[54] describe a minimum osmolality of 45 mosmol kg^{-1} in a group of healthy infants, of less than 34 weeks gestation, receiving a liberal fluid intake. They estimate that the smallest babies are likely to have an upper limit of urine flow of around 7 ml kg^{-1} h^{-1}, with larger babies achieving double this rate. In contrast, the author, studying a group of babies of similar gestational and postnatal age who required ventilatory support, noted a minimum urine osmolality of 90 mosmol kg^{-1}.

Urine osmolality is known to increase and free water clearance to decrease in hypoxic fetal lambs.[82] However, the renal response to hypoxia appears to be gestation dependent. In lamb fetuses near term, hypoxia has been shown to result in a decreased renal blood flow, concomitant rise in plasma renin activity, increased AVP secretion, decreased heart rate and rise in mean arterial pressure. During the reactive hyperaemia seen following hypoxia urinary prostaglandin E and F_{2a} rose. In contrast, lamb fetuses of greater immaturity showed none of these responses other than a rise in AVP in only half the animals studied.[82]

Arginine vasopressin is present in the posterior pituitary of the eleven week old human fetus;[22] concentrations increase up to 28 weeks gestation with relatively little increase thereafter.[83] Nephron sensitivity to vasopressin increases with maturity.[84] High renal prostaglandin E production in the newborn may interfere with cyclic AMP production and so diminish the cellular action of vasopressin.[85] The immature medulla is characterized by a limited osmotic gradient, a consequence of short loops of Henle, low urea production and high blood flow through the vasa recta. There is evidence to suggest that the renal solute gradient is the most important factor limiting the renal response to vasopressin in that maximum urine osmolality achieved is higher during hypernatraemic dehydration.[84] Rees et al. have shown that osmotic and volume stimuli are able to stimulate the secretion of vasopressin in preterm infants from 26 to 35 weeks gestation. The maximum urine osmolality achieved was 550 mosmol kg^{-1}. In addition peaks of vasopressin secretion occurred in response to non-osmotic stimuli, resulting in inappropriately concentrated urine. Despite the immature response to AVP the preterm neonate is at frequent risk of developing the syndrome of inappropriate AVP secretion during, for example, deteriorating respiratory function, the development of pneumothoraces and large periventricular haemorrhage.[86]

Practical considerations

Early hyponatraemia is more likely to be the consequence of fluid overload, either maternal, iatrogenic and neonatal, or precipitated by inappropriate ADH secretion. Late hyponatraemia, in a well infant, is more likely to be due to sodium depletion. Consideration of the infant's weight, in addition to serum sodium concentration, will elucidate the problem.

Creatinine

The neonate's plasma creatinine concentration is elevated at birth. Though the level reflects the maternal concentration, it is also influenced by gestational age, with higher levels in preterm infants. Levels fall exponentially to plateau at around 37 weeks post conceptional age[87] The author has studied creatinine excretion in 31 babies during the first week of life (gestational age range 25–34, mean = median = 28); the mean creatinine coefficient was 71.2 µmol kg^{-1} d^{-1} (median = 71.4, range 18–184). The creatinine coefficient (creatinine excretion per unit body weight) is a reflection of the relative amount of muscle in the body.[88] In this group of preterm neonates creatinine coefficient was shown to have a stronger correlation with gestational age than with birth weight. This suggests that birth weight is a poor reflection of relative muscle mass and is in keeping with the parallel observation that body water content is both variable and strongly correlated with birth weight.

SUMMARY

The extremely immature infant is generally credited with extremely immature renal function. This belief notwithstanding, it is also true that renal function in the tiniest babies is sophisticated enough to meet homeostatic needs. Many problems hitherto attributed to 'immaturity' appear to be the consequences of extreme stresses, frequently iatrogenic.

REFERENCES

1 McCrory WW. Developmental Nephrology. Cambridge: Harvard University Press, 1972
2 Potter EL. Development of the human glomerulus. Arch Pathol 1965; 80: 241–255
3 McDonald MS, Emery JL. The later intrauterine and postnatal development of human glomeruli. J Anat 1959; 93: 331–341
4 Potter EL, Thierstein ST. Glomerular development in the kidney as an index of fetal maturity. J Pediatr 1943; 22: 695–706
5 Phelps DL, Lachman RS, Leake RD, Oh W. The radiologic localization of the major aortic tributaries in the newborn infant. J Pediatr 1972; 81: 336–339
6 Olbing H, Blaufox MD, Aschinberg LC et al. Postnatal changes in renal glomerular blood flow distribution in puppies. J Clin Invest 1973; 52: 2885–2895
7 Aperia A, Broberger O, Herin P, Joelsson I. Renal haemodynamics in the perinatal period. Acta Physiol Scand 1977; 99: 261–269
8 Robillard JE, Weismann DN, Herin P. Ontogeny of single glomerular perfusion rate in fetal and newborn lambs. Pediatr Res 1981; 15: 1248–1255

9 Behrman RE, Lees MH, Petersen EN et al. Distribution of the circulation in the normal and asphyxiated primate. Am J Obstet Gynaecol 1970; 108: 956–969
10 Rudolf AM, Heymann MA, Teramo K et al. Studies on the circulation of the previable fetus. Pediatr Res 1971; 5: 452–465
11 Fetterman GH, Shuplock NA, Philipp FJ, Gregg HS. The growth and maturation of human glomeruli and proximal convolutions from term to adulthood. Pediatrics 1965; 35: 601–619
12 Jeanty P, Dramaix-Wilmet M, Elkhazem N et al. Measurement of fetal kidney growth on ultrasound. Radiology 1982; 144: 159–162
13 Assali NS, Holm NW, Sehgal N. Regional blood flow and vascular resistance of the fetus in utero. Am J Obstet Gynaecol 1962; 83: 809
14 Zimmerman HD. Elektonenmikroskopische befunde sur innervation des nephron nach untersuchungen an der fetalen nachniere des menschen. Z Zellforsch 1972; 129: 65
15 Kurjak A, Krikinen P, Latin V, Ivankovic D. Ultrasonic assessment of fetal kidney function in normal and complicated pregnancies. Am J Obstet Gynaecol 1981; 141: 266–270
16 Campbell S, Wladimiroff JW, Dewhurst CJ. The antenatal measurement of fetal urine production. J Obstet Gynaecol Br Common 1973; 80: 680–686
17 Wladimiroff JW, Campbell S. Fetal urine production rates in normal and complicated pregnancy. Lancet 1974; i: 151–154
18 Harman CR. Maternal furosemide may not provoke urine production in the compromised fetus. Am J Obstet Gynaecol 1984; 150: 322–323
19 De Vane GW, Porter JC. An apparent stress induced release of AVP by human neonates. J Clin Endocrinl Metab 1980; 51: 1412–1416
20 Kelly RT, Rose JC, Meis PJ et al. Vasopressin is important for restoring cardiovascular homeostasis in fetal lambs. Am J Obstet Gynaecol 1983; 146: 807–812
21 De Vane GW, Naden RP, Porter JC, Rosenfeld CR. Mechanism of AVP release in the sheep fetus. Pediatr Res 1982; 16: 504–507
22 Levina SE. Endocrine features in development of human hypothalamus, hypophysis and placenta. Gen Comp Endocrinol 1968; 11: 151
23 Siegel SR, Oakes GK, Palmer S. Transplacental transfer of aldosterone and its effects on renal function in the fetal lamb. Pediatr Res 1981; 15: 163–165
24 Wintour EM, Coghlan JP, Towstowless M. Cortisol is natriuretic in the immature ovine fetus. J Endocrinol 1985; 106: R13–R15
25 Gitlin D, Kumate J, Morales C et al. The turnover of amniotic fluid in the human conceptus. Am J Obstet Gynaecol 1972; 113: 632–645
26 Van Otterlo LL, Wladimiroff JW, Wallenburg HCS. Relationship between fetal urine production and amniotic fluid volume in normal pregnancies and pregnancies complicated by diabetes. Am J Obstet Gynaecol 1977; 84: 205–229
27 Abramovitch DR, Garden A, Jandial L et al. Fetal swallowing and voiding in relation to hydramnios. Obstet Gynaecol 1979; 54: 15–29
28 Leake RD, Weitzman RE, Fisher DA. Maternal fetal osmolar homeostasis: fetal posterior pituitary autonomy. Pediatr Res 1977; 11: 408
29 Goodlin RC, Anderson JC, Gallagher TF. Relationship between amniotic fluid volume and maternal plasma volume expansion. Am J Obstet Gynaecol 1983; 146: 505–511
30 Gersh I. The correlation of structure and function in the developing mesonephros and metanephros. Contrib Embryol 1937; 26: 35
31 Golbus MS, Filly RA, Callen PW et al. Fetal urinary tract obstruction: management and selection for treatment. Sem Perinatol 1985; 9: 91–97
32 McCance RA, Widdowson EM. Renal functions before birth. Proc R Soc Lond [Biol] 1953; 141: 488–497
33 Glick PL, Harrison MR, Golbus MS et al. Management of the fetus with

congenital hydronephrosis. II. Prognostic criteria and selection for treatment. J Pediatr Surg 1985; 20: 376–387
34 Robillard JE, Kulvinskas C, Sessions C et al. Maturational changes in the fetal glomerular filtration rate. Am J Obstet Gynaecol 1975; 122: 601–606
35 Arant B. Developmental patterns of renal functional maturation compared in the human neonate. J Pediatr 1978; 92: 705–712
36 Al-Dahhan J, Haycock GB et al. Sodium homeostasis in term and preterm neonates. 1. Renal aspects. Arch Dis Child 1983; 58: 335–342
37 Engle WD, Arant BS. Renal handling of beta2microglobulin in the human neonate. Kidney Int 1983; 24: 358–363
38 Leake RD, Trygstad CW. Glomerular filtration rate during the period of adaptation to extrauterine life. Pediatr Res 1977; 11: 959–962
39 Alexander K, Leung C, McArthur RG et al. Circulating antidiuretic hormone during labour and in the newborn. Acta Paediatr Scand 1980; 69: 505–510
40 Cort RL. Renal function in the respiratory distress syndrome. Acta Paediatr 1962; 51: 313–323
41 Guignard JP, Torrado A, Mazouni SM, Gautier E. Renal function in respiratory distress syndrome. J Pediatr 1976; 88: 845–850
42 Engle WD, Arant BS et al. Diuresis and respiratory distress syndrome: physiologic mechanisms and therapeutic implications. J Pediatr 1983; 102: 912–917
43 Heaf DP, Belik J, Spitzer AR et al. Changes in pulmonary function during the diuretic phase of respiratory distress syndrome. J Pediatr 1982; 101: 103–107
44 Langman CB, Engle WD, Baumgart S et al. The diuretic phase of respiratory distress syndrome and its relationship to oxygenation. J Pediatr 1981; 98: 462–466
45 Costarino AT, Baumgart S, Norman ME, Polin RA. Renal adaptation to extrauterine life in patients with respiratory distress syndrome. Am J Dis Child 1985; 139: 1060–1063
46 Modi N, Hutton JL. Does respiratory function influence sodium handling in preterm, very low birth weight neonates? (Submitted for publication)
47 Kojima T, Hirata Y, Fukuda Y et al. Plasma atrial natriuretic peptide and spontaneous diuresis in sick neonates. Arch Dis Child 1987; 62: 667–670
48 Engelke SC, Shah BL, Vasan U, Raye JR. Sodium balance in very low birth weight infants. J Pediatr 1978; 93: 837–841
49 Arant BS. Non renal factors influencing renal function during the perinatal period. Clin Perinatol 1981; 8: 225–240
50 Robillard JE, Sessions C, Burmeister L et al. Influence of fetal extracellular volume contraction on renal absorption of bicarbonate in fetal lambs. Pediatr Res 1977; 11: 649–655
51 Rojas J, Mohan P, Davidson KK. Increased extracellular water volume associated with hyponatraemia at birth in premature infants. J Pediatr 1984; 105: 158–161
52 Mohan P, Rojas J, Davidson KK. Pulmonary air leak associated with neonatal hyponatraemia in premature infants. J Pediatr 1984; 105: 153–157
53 Ziegler EE, Fomon SJ. Fluid intake, renal solute load and water balance in infancy. J Pediatr 1971; 78: 561–568
54 Coulthard M, Hey EN. Effect of varying water intake on renal function in healthy preterm babies. Arch Dis Child 1985; 60: 614–620
55 Leake RD, Trygstad CW, Oh W. Inulin clearance in the newborn infant: relationship to gestational and postnatal age. Pediatr Res 1976; 10: 759–762
56 Fawer CL, Torrado A, Guignard JP. Maturation of renal function in fullterm and preterm neonates. Helv Paediatr Acta 1979; 34: 11–21
57 McCance RA, Widdowson EM. The correct physiological basis on which to compare infant and adult renal function. Lancet 1952; ii: 860–862

58 Coulthard MG, Hey EN. Weight as the best standard for glomerular filtration in the newborn. Arch Dis Child 1984; 59: 373–375
59 Aperia A, Broberger O, Herin P, Zetterstrom R. Sodium excretion in relation to sodium intake and aldosterone excretion in newborn preterm and fullterm infants. Acta Paediatr Scand 1979; 68: 813–817
60 Sevastik M, Herin P, Aperia A, Zetterstrom R. Postnatal development of renal function in very low birth weight infants (Abstr) Early Hum Dev 1986; 14: 135–136
61 Gruskin AB, Edelmann CM. Maturational changes in renal blood flow in piglets. Pediatr Res 1970; 4: 7–13
62 Siegel SR, Oh W. Renal function as a marker of human fetal maturation. Acta Paediatr Scand 1976; 65: 481–485
63 Beguin F, Dunihoo DR, Quilligan EJ. Effect of CO_2 elevation on renal blood flow in the fetal lamb in utero. Am J Obstet Gynaecol 1974; 119: 630–637
64 Giebisch G. Functional organisation of proximal and distal tubular electrolyte transport. Nephron 1969; 6: 260
65 Spitzer A. The role of the kidney in sodium homeostasis during maturation. Kidney Int 1982; 21: 539–545
66 Rodriguez-Soriano J et al. Renal handling of sodium in preterm and fullterm neonates: a study using clearance methods during water diuresis. Pediatr Res 1983; 17: 1013–1016
67 Spitzer A, Brandis M. Functional and morphologic maturation of superficial nephrons: relationship to total kidney function. J Clin Invest 1974; 53: 279
68 Dillon MJ, Gillin MEA, Ryness JM, De Swiet M. Plasma renin activity and aldosterone concentration in the human newborn. Arch Dis Child 1976; 51: 537–540
69 Sulyok E, Nemeth M, Tenyi I et al. Postnatal development of the renin-angiotensin-aldeosterone system in relation to electrolyte balance in premature infants. Pediatr Res 1979; 13: 817–820
70 Sulyok E, Nemeth M, Tenyi I et al. Relationship between maturity, electrolyte balance and the function of the renin-angiotensin-aldosterone system in newborn infants. Biol Neonate 1979; 35: 60–65
71 Aperia A, Broberger O, Elinder G et al. Postnatal development of renal function in preterm and fullterm infants. Acta Paediatr Scand 1981; 70: 183–187
72 Aperia A, Broberger O, Broberger U et al. Glomerular tubular balance in preterm and fullterm infants. Acta Paediatr Scand 1983; Suppl 305: 70–76
73 Tulassay T, Rascher W, Seyberth HW et al. Role of atrial natriuretic peptide in sodium homeostasis in premature infants. J Pediatr 1986; 109: 1023–1027
74 Larsson L, Aperia A, Elinder G. Structural and functional development of the nephron. Acta Paediatr Scand 1983 (Suppl) 305: 56–60
75 Sulyok E, Varga E, Gyory K et al. On the mechanisms of renal sodium handling in newborn infants. Biol Neonate 1980; 37: 75–79
76 Guignard JP, John EG. Renal function in the tiny premature infant. Clin Perinatol 1986; 13: 377–401
77 Engle WD, Arant BS. Urinary potassium excretion in the critically ill neonate. Pediatrics 1984; 74: 259–264
78 Brodehl J, Gellisen K, Weber HP. Postnatal development of tubular phosphate reabsorption. Clin Nephrol 1982; 17: 163–171
79 Stonestreet BS, Rubin L, Pollak A et al. Renal functions of low birth weight infants with hyperglycaemia and glucosuria produced by glucose infusions. Pediatrics 1980; 66: 561–567
80 McCance RA, Naylor MJB, Widdowson EM. The response of infants to a large dose of water. Arch Dis Child 1954; 29: 104–109
81 Stonestreet BS, Bell EF, Warburton D, Oh W. Renal response in low birth

weight neonates: results of prolonged intake of two different amounts of fluid and sodium. Am J Dis Child 1983; 137: 215–219
82 Robillard JE, Weitzman RE et al. Developmental aspects of the renal response to hypoxaemia in the lamb fetus. Circ Res 1981; 48: 128–138
83 Schubert F, George JM, Rao MB. Vasopressin and oxytocin content of human fetal brain at different stages of gestation. Brain Res 1981; 213: 111–117
84 Svenningsen DW, Aronson AS. Postnatal development of renal concentration capacity as estimated by DDAVP test in normal asphyxiated neonates. Biol Neonate 1974; 25: 230–241
85 Joppich R, Scherer B, Weber PC. Renal prostaglandins: relationship to the development of blood pressure and concentrating capacity in preterm and fullterm healthy infants. Eur J Pediatr 1979; 132: 253–259
86 Rees L, Brook CGD, Shaw J, Forsling M. Hyponatraemia in the first week of life in preterm infants. I. Arginine vasopressin secretion. Arch Dis Child 1984; 59: 414–422
87 Trompeter RS, Al-Dahhan J, Haycock GB et al. Normal values for plasma creatinine concentration related to maturity in normal term and preterm infants. Int J Pediatr Nephrol 1983; 4: 145–148
88 Novak LP. Age and sex differences in body density and creatinine excretion of high school children. Ann NY Acad Sci 1963; 110: 545

The immature skin

N Rutter
Department of Child Health, University of Nottingham, Nottingham UK

The infant below 28 weeks gestation is born with an immature skin with a poorly formed epidermal barrier, although rapid postnatal maturation occurs over the first two weeks of life. This leads to a high transepidermal water loss with consequent difficulties in fluid balance and temperature control, accidental poisioning from percutaneous absorption of chemicals, and superficial damage from use of adhesives in neonatal care. Percutaneous respiration occurs more readily than at term and may be of benefit. Immaturity of the dermis and the associated skin appendages is not of major clincial significance.

The skin of an infant below 28 weeks gestation is substantially different from the skin of a more mature infant, structurally and functionally. The consequences of these differences are mainly hazardous and need to be recognised by those who manage such infants. The skin consists of three layers, each with a different function: epidermis, dermis and subcutaneous layer. Most attention will be paid to the epidermis since it is the least developed with the most serious consequences.

STRUCTURE

Epidermis

From 18 weeks gestation the fetal periderm starts to regress and is shed into the amniotic fluid as the underlying epidermis develops a stratified horny layer.[1,2] By 26 weeks the periderm has disappeared and the stratum corneum covers the whole skin surface but the third trimester is required for its maturation. Before 28 weeks the epidermis is thin and has only two or three cell layers[3]—the poorly developed stratum corneum shows little keratinization (Fig. 1). By 32 weeks epidermal development is largely complete

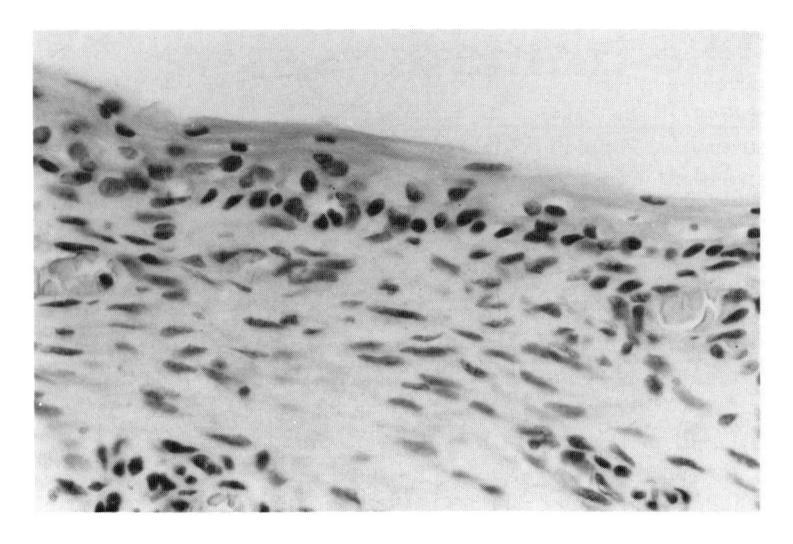

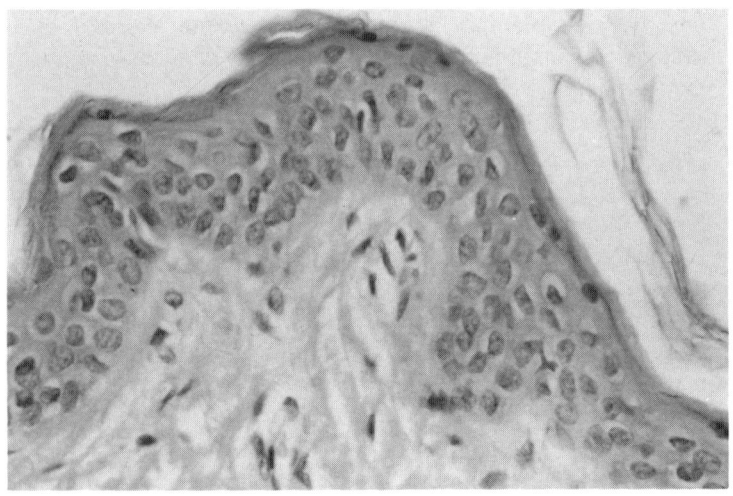

Fig. 1 Effect of maturity on development of the epidermis. Both photomicrographs are from abdominal skin at autopsy, magnification × 100. The upper is from an infant of 26 weeks gestation, one day old, with a thin epidermis and little development of kerantinized stratum corneum. The lower is from an infant of 40 weeks gestation who died during labour. (Reproduced from *Clinics in Perinatology* with permission).[4]

and the epidermis of a term infant is virtually indistinguishable from that of an adult.[3]

The effect of birth on the immature epidermis is remarkable. There is an enormous acceleration of maturation so that by two weeks of age even the most immature infant has the epidermal development of a term infant (Fig. 2). This hastened maturation resembles the epidermal healing which occurs in the adult after superficial burns or stripping of the stratum corneum with adhesive tape, and is presumably stimulated by the change from a fluid

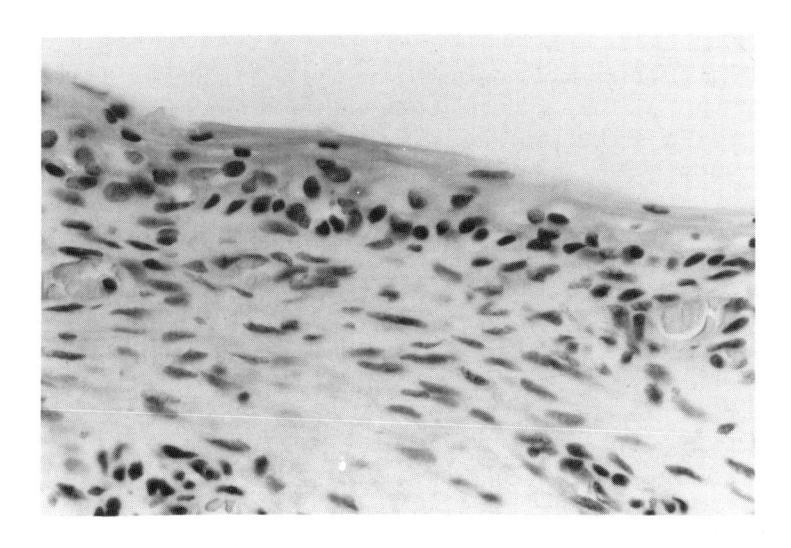

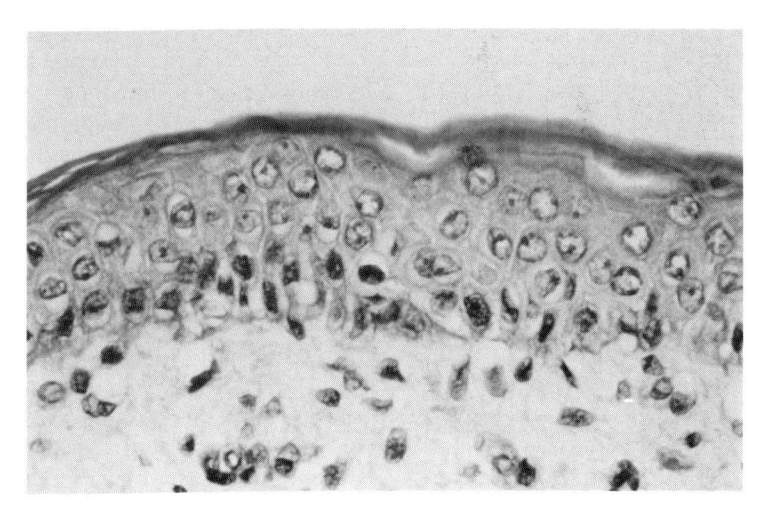

Fig. 2 Effect of postnatal age on development of the epidermis. The upper is the same as shown in Figure 1, from an infant of 26 weeks gestation, one day old. The lower is from an infant of 26 weeks gestation, 16 days old, showing a mature epidermis. (Reproduced from *Clinics in Perinatology* with permission).[4]

to a gaseous environment. It is not known how it is mediated. Epidermal growth factor can produce epidermal maturation when given in pharmacological doses to animals,[5,6] but appears not to be important in the human newborn.[7]

Dermis and subcutaneous layer

Sweat glands, sebaceous glands, hair follicles, capillaries and nerve endings are fully formed by the end of the second trimester. Scanning electron microscopy shows differences in the arrangement of collagen and elastic fibres of the preterm dermis compared with the mature dermis.[2] The subcutaneous layer is barely present before 28 weeks gestation and only develops as an adipose organ in the third trimester.

FUNCTION

Epidermis

The stratum corneum with its overlapping plates of dead cells filled with the fibrous protein keratin gives skin its barrier properties. The body's contents are preserved and protected from an adverse physical and chemical environment. Body water is conserved and potentially harmful chemicals and bacteria are kept out. The epidermal barrier of an infant below 28 weeks gestation is functionally immature but from 32 weeks onwards it functions in a similar way to that of an adult. The following aspects of epidermal barrier function will be considered: the conservation of water, the percutaneous absorption of chemicals, gas exchange across the skin and damage to the barrier layer resulting from practices in neonatal management.

Conservation of body water

Body water diffuses through the epidermis along a water vapour pressure gradient and is lost to the atmosphere. This transepidermal water loss (TEWL) is not under physiological control but is determined by the effectiveness of the epidermis as a barrier to water diffusion and the environmental conditions of temperature, relative humidity and air speed. Together with respiratory water loss TEWL makes up insensible weight loss.

TEWL is low from 32 weeks gestation to term (approximately

8 g m^{-2} h^{-1}), even lower per unit area of skin than in the adult. Before 32 weeks it rises exponentially and is particularly high before 28 weeks gestation (Fig. 3).[8,9,11] At 24 weeks, values can be 10 times greater per unit area than at term. The rapid structural

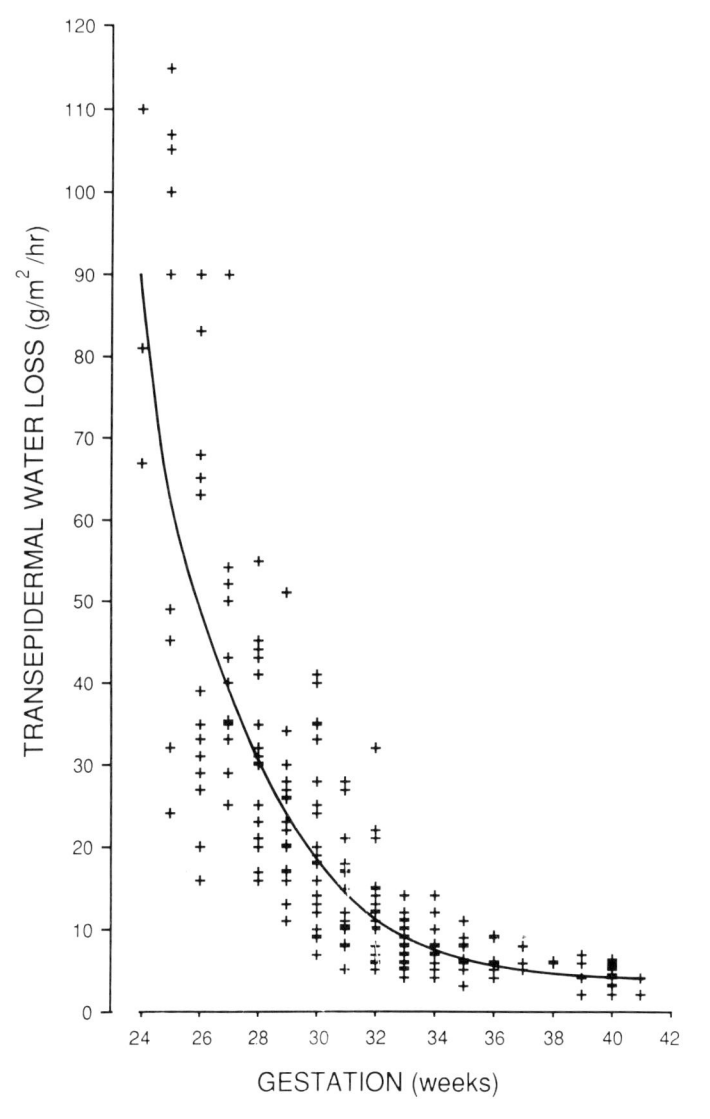

Fig. 3 The effects of gestation on transepidermal water loss. Measurements were made from abdominal skin and carried out in the first few days of life.

maturation of the immature epidermis after birth is mirrored by rapid functional maturation. By about two weeks of age the very immature infant has rates of TEWL which are similar to those found in a term infant.[8,10,11] Thus the clinical problems which result from a high TEWL are largely confined to infants born before 28 weeks gestation during the first two weeks of life.

TEWL is also influenced by environmental factors, ambient humidity being the most important. There is a linear inverse relationship between TEWL and relative humidity. TEWL is high under the usual low humidity conditions found in a neonatal unit (30 to 40% relative humidity) but falls to zero as the relative humidity approaches 100%.[9] TEWL increases as skin and environmental temperature increase although the effect is not great over the range of temperatures a preterm infant encounters. It increases with forced convection when an increase in airspeed disrupts the boundary layer of still air next to the skin,[12,13] as occurs when infants are nursed naked in incubators or under radiant warmers. It also increases with exposure of the skin to radiant energy, as occurs under phototherapy or a radiant warmer,[14] an effect which is independent of temperature, airspeed or humidity.

The consequences of a high TEWL are difficulties in fluid balance and temperature control.

Fluid balance

Infants below 28 weeks gestation have a proportionally higher body water content than term infants (86% compared with 75% at term and 58% in the adult), a result of a higher extracellular fluid volume. A high insensible weight loss is a consequence of a high TEWL but because of the complexity of factors which influence TEWL, it cannot be accurately predicted in an immature infant. Very few investigators have examined insensible weight loss in infants born before 28 weeks gestation—results are largely reported by birth weight and range from 40 to 150 ml/kg/24 hours in infants weighing below 1.25 kg to 10 to 15 ml/kg/24 hours at term.[15-18] Because of difficulty in predicting fluid needs the immature infant is easily depleted or overloaded with water. Too little fluid results in high weight loss, clinical dehydration, oliguria, hypernatraemia and impaired excretion of drugs. Too much fluid results in weight gain (or absence of the usual weight loss), exacerbation of oedema, worsening of respiratory distress, delayed closure of the ductus arteriosus and hyponatraemia.

Temperature control

Six hundred calories of heat are lost with every ml of water which evaporates from the skin. The infant below 28 weeks gestation is already vulnerable to cold stress because of a low heat producing mass, a relatively large surface area and lack of subcutaneous tissue insulation. A high TEWL makes hypothermia inevitable unless there is a powerful supplementary heat source or steps are taken to reduce evaporative losses.

Management of the infant below 28 weeks gestation is greatly simplified if steps are taken to reduce TEWL towards levels found in the term infant. This is achieved by adding humidity to the air surrounding the infant, either by humidification of the incubator[19] or by use of a waterproof covering which produces a humid microclimate next to the skin.[20-22] The infant can be draped with a thin polyethylene sheet or nursed in a small polyethylene tent, methods which are both suitable for use under a radiant warmer. Normothermia is thereby maintained and extremes of fluid balance are avoided. Monitoring of fluid balance is particularly important in the infant below 28 weeks gestation and is mandatory if nursed under a radiant warmer. Accurate daily or more frequent weighing, measurement of plasma sodium and osmolality, and measurement of urine concentration by osmolality or specific gravity are all guides to the fluid requirements of an immature infant.

Percutaneous absorption

The epidermis provides an effective barrier against harmful agents unless it is damaged or diseased. Minute amounts of topically applied drugs are absorbed through the intact skin of a child or adult but if the skin is extensively burned or the epidermis is affected by widespread disease, systemic absorption of topical agents occurs and may be of clinical significance. The newborn infant from 32 weeks gestation has an epidermis which similarly resists percutaneous absorption but topically applied agents may still have a systemic effect since the agent may be applied to a much higher proportion of the total body surface than in a child or adult but the volume of distribution of the drug will be low. If there is skin damage or disease, the risk of accidental toxicity is much greater.

The infant below 28 weeks gestation has a poor barrier to

percutaneous absorption.[23] In vivo and in vitro studies have shown that the rate of absorption of topically applied agents may be several orders of magnitude higher than rates found in mature infants.[4] Drug absorption correlates well with epidermal structural maturation and with measured TEWL, so that by two weeks of age the rate of absorption of topical agents per unit area of skin is similar to term levels.[23] However, the high surface area to body mass ratio in these tiny infants means that toxicity can occur even though percutaneous absorption is slight.

Hazards

Methaemoglobinaemia from percutaneous absorption of aniline dye used to mark nappies was described over 100 years ago.[24] In current practice it is toxicity from percutaneous absorption of topical antiseptics which is particularly worrying in the very immature infant. Hexachlorophene was routinely used for bathing newborn infants to prevent staphylococcal infection but it took several years for toxicity to be recognised.[25-27] It is readily absorbed through the immature skin and leads to a vacuolar myelinopathy with neurological illness and sometimes death. Iodine is readily absorbed and can lead to goitre and hypothyroidism.[28] Alcohol (methyl, ethyl or isopropyl) evaporates quickly before much absorption can take place, but if evaporation is prevented by occlusion, absorption can cause haemorrhagic necrosis of the dermis and systemic toxicity.[29,30] Chlorhexidine is the most commonly used antiseptic in the newborn—although it is undoubtedly absorbed it is not known to have any adverse effects. It should be used very sparingly and in aqueous rather than alcoholic solution. Topical antibiotic sprays must be avoided in the immature newborn because they contain the ototoxic aminoglycoside neomycin.

The extremely immature infant is commonly ill in the immediate newborn period with multiple organ system failure. It is therefore easy to ascribe illness and death to immaturity without considering the possibility of accidental poisoning from percutaneous absorption of topical agents. This can be reduced if staff on neonatal units periodically review all the various agents which they apply to a preterm infant's skin, asking themselves whether the agents could be absorbed or whether their use is really necessary. Any low molecular weight chemical which is soluble in water or lipid will be readily absorbed through the immature skin—topical application is equivalent to oral or intravenous administration.

Percutaneous gas exchange

Although the mature epidermis is relatively impermeable to gases, small amounts of oxygen are absorbed and carbon dioxide excreted via the skin. This gas exchange has been widely studied in adults and accounts for about 1% of total respiration. From 32 weeks gestation to term the epidermis is no more permeable to gases than in the adult and percutaneous respiration is similarly unimportant. Before 32 weeks and especially before 28 weeks gestation the epidermis is about six times more permeable to oxygen and carbon dioxide (Fig. 4), but gas exchange correlates well with TEWL and structural maturation of the epidermis—gas exchange therefore falls with postnatal age and reaches term values by three weeks.[31] Oxygen absorption is greatly enhanced by increasing the ambient oxygen concentration and it has been estimated that if an immature infant is surrounded by oxygen at 95% concentration (but still continues to breath air), up to 20% of the resting oxygen requirements and a similar proportion of carbon dioxide excretion can be met percutaneously.[32] Percu-

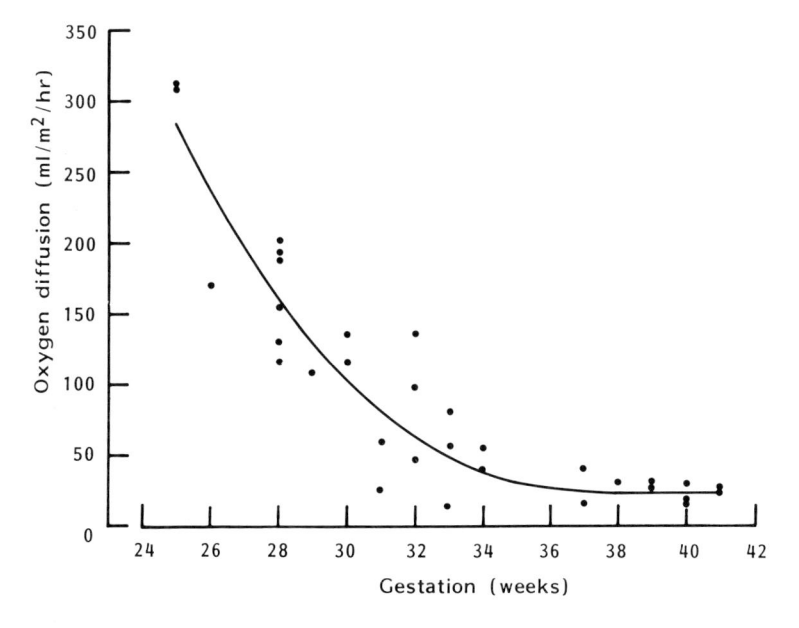

Fig. 4 The effect of gestation on diffusion of oxygen through the skin—similar changes are seen with carbon dioxide excretion. Measurements were made from abdominal skin and carried out in the first few days of life.

taneous oxygen delivery before 28 weeks gestation results in a clinically significant increase in arterial oxygen tension of 5 to 15 mmHg (Fig. 5).[33]

Clinical significance

Immaturity of the lungs leads to inadequate pulmonary gas exchange in infants below 28 weeks gestation. Poor oxygenation is usually the greatest clinical problem—carbon dioxide excretion is easier to achieve, perhaps because the percutaneous route is playing a significant role. Percutaneous oxygen delivery is well worth trying if there is persistent pulmonary hypertension and an infant remains hypoxaemic in spite of ventilation with pure oxygen. It may allow the inspired oxygen concentration and ventilation pressures to be reduced with a consequent lessening of iatrogenic lung damage. If percutaneous oxygen is given it is important to monitor arterial Po_2 carefully—an infant might appear to be pink because of well saturated cutaneous blood yet be centrally hypoxaemic.

Epidermal damage

When adhesive tape is removed from the skin, it strips off the most superficial layer of the stratum corneum. If the epidermis is mature and the stratum corneum has several cell layers, a single stripping has a negligible effect on epidermal barrier function. Repeated stripping is necessary to produce a significant increase in TEWL. A single stripping however has a marked effect on the barrier properties of the immature epidermis with only two or three cell layers.[23] There is a large increase in TEWL and percutaneous drug absorption through the damaged area and a strong theoretical possibility of bacterial penetration leading to systemic sepsis. The more immature the infant, the greater is the likelihood of illness and the more monitoring is required. ECG electrodes, transcutaneous gas probes and the fixing of indwelling venous and arterial lines all involve the use of adhesives—in an infant below 28 weeks gestation, up to 15% of the total surface area can be traumatized by stripping each day.

Steps need to be taken to reduce epidermal damage in these delicate infants. The minimum amount of skin should be involved and probes should be chosen with an adhesive which causes the least damage. Karaya gum ECG electrodes for example do not

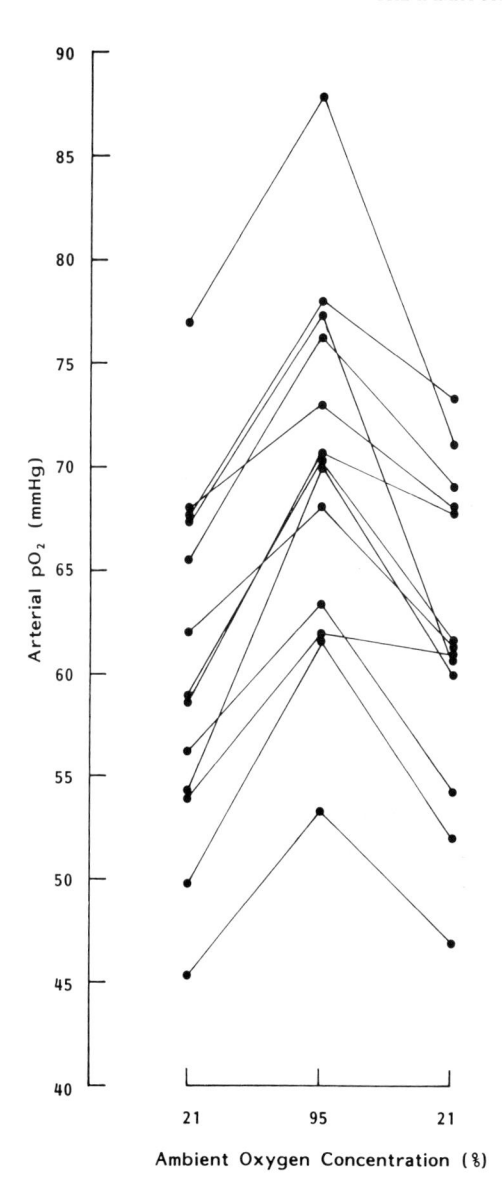

Fig. 5 The effect on arterial oxygen tension of surrounding intubated, ventilated infants with 95% oxygen (each infant is at first in air, then surrounded by 95% oxygen, then in air again). Six of the thirteen infants were below 28 weeks gestation and they tended to show the greatest increase in arterial oxygen tension. (Reproduced from Lancet with permission)[33]

strip the epidermis on removal.[34] A spray-on copolymer dressing can be used under transcutaneous gas electrodes to reduce the damage caused by heating the skin and by adhesive stripping—care has to be taken though to ensure that it does not interfere with normal function of the electrode.[35] Strongly adhesive tape of the type used in adults is very damaging to the immature skin and should be avoided—occasionally it can cause damage down to the basal layer of the epidermis with consequent permanent scarring. There is a need for the development of monitoring techniques which do not involve sticking probes to the skin of immature infants.

Dermis

Although the sweat glands are fully formed by 25 weeks gestation and are present in much greater density than in a child or adult, they do not function in the early newborn period. Thermal sweating occurs from birth after 36 weeks gestation but takes up to two weeks or more to appear in the preterm infant.[36,37] When sweating first appears in the preterm infant it occurs at fewer sites, with less intensity and in response to a greater heat stress than in a mature infant. The impaired sweat response is presumably due to neurological immaturity. Clinically it is of little importance since cold stress is a far more common threat to the infant below 28 weeks gestation. The ability to regulate skin blood flow is impaired in very immature infants. Cutaneous blood vessels react to topically applied vasoconstrictors[23] but less well to changes in core or ambient temperature. This together with the lack of subcutaneous insulation makes the infant below 28 weeks gestation in effect poikolothermic—core temperature and surface temperature are similar and drift up and down according to the ambient temperature.

Finally, although there are microscopic differences in the collagen and elastin fibres of the dermis of an infant below 28 weeks gestation compared with a term infant, this does not seem to be associated with clinical problems. The skin appears to stretch and recoil without difficulty. Furthermore, healing of wounds is usually rapid and effective. Infants below 28 weeks gestation who survive to childhood have varying numbers of scars resulting from venepuncture, extravasation of intravenous fluids, chest drains and heel pricks but these reflect the enormous number of invasive procedures the infants are subjected to. Thoracotomy and laparotomy scars heal readily and are cosmetically no different to the scars produced by surgery in older infants and children.

REFERENCES

1 Holbrook KA. Human epidermal embryogenesis. Int J Dermatol 1979; 18: 329–356
2 Holbrook KA. A histological comparison of infant and adult skin. In: Maibach HI; ed. Neonatal skin. New York: Marcel Dekker, 1982: pp. 3–31
3 Evans NJ, Rutter N. Development of the epidermis in the newborn. Biol Neonate 1986; 49: 74–80
4 Rutter N. Percutaneous drug absorption. Clinics in Perinatology 1987; 14: 911–930
5 Cohen S, Elliot GA. The stimulation of epidermal keratinisation by a protein isolated from the submaxillary gland of the mouse. J Invest Dermatol 1963; 40: 1–5
6 Thorburn GD, Waters MJ, Young IR, Dolling M, Buntinc D, Hopkins PS. Epidermal Growth Factor: a critical factor in fetal maturation? In: 'The Fetus and Independent Life'. Ciba Found Symp 1981; 86: 172–198
7 Evans NJ, Rutter N, Gregory H. Urinary excretion of epidermal growth factor in the newborn. Early Hum Dev 1986; 14: 277–282
8 Rutter N, Hull D. Water loss from the skin of term and preterm babies. Arch Dis Child 1979; 54: 858–868
9 Hammarlund K, Sedin G. Transepidermal water loss in newborn infants III Relation to gestational age. Acta Paediatr Scand 1979; 68: 795–801
10 Hammarlund K. Sedin G, Stromberg B. Transepidermal water loss in newborn infants VII Relation to postnatal age in very preterm and full term appropriate for gestational age infants. Acta Paediatr Scand 1982; 71: 360–374
11 Hammarlund K, Sedin G, Stromberg B. Transepidermal water loss in the newborn. VIII. Relation to gestational age and postnatal age in appropriate and small for gestational age infants. Acta Paediatr Scand 1983; 72: 721–728
12 Clark RP, Cross KW, Goff MR, Mullen BJ, Stothers JK, Warner RM. Neonatal natural and forced convection. J Physiol 1978; 284: 22–23
13 Thompson MH, Stothers JK, McLellan NJ. Weight and water loss in the neonate in natural and forced convection. Arch Dis Child 1984; 59: 951–956
14 Wheldon AC, Rutter N. The heat balance of small babies nursed in incubators and under radiant warmers. Early Human Dev 1982; 6: 131–143
15 Fanaroff AA, Wald M, Gruber HS, Klaus MH. Insensible water loss in low birth weight infants. Pediatrics 1972; 50: 236–245
16 Wu PYK, Hodgman JE. Insensible water loss in preterm infants: changes with postnatal development and non-ionizing radiar.t energy. Pediatrics 1974; 54: 704–712
17 Bell EF, Weinstein MR, Oh W. Heat balance in premature infants: comparative effects of convectively heated incubator and radiant warmer with and without plastic heat shield. J Pediatr 1980; 96: 460–465
18 Baumgart S, Engle WD, Fox WW, Polin RA. Radiant warmer power and body size as determinants of insensible water loss in the critically ill neonate. Pediatr Res 1981; 15: 1495–1499
19 Harpin VA, Rutter N. Humidification of incubators. Arch Dis Child 1985; 60: 219–224
20 Baumgart S, Engle WD, Fox WW, Polin RA. Effect of heat shielding on convection and evaporation and radiant heat transfer in premature infants. J Pediatr 1981; 99: 948–956
21 Baumgart S, Fox WW, Polin RA. Physiologic implications of two different heat shields for infants under radiant warmers. J Pediatr 1982; 100: 787–790

22 Baumgart S. Reduction of oxygen consumption, insensible water loss, and radiant heat demand with use of a plastic blanket for low birthweight infants under radiant warmers. Pediatrics 1984; 75: 89–99
23 Harpin VA, Rutter N. Barrier properties of the newborn infant's skin. J Pediatr 1983; 102: 419–425
24 Rayner W. Cyanosis in newly born children caused by aniline marking ink. Br Med J 1886; 1: 294–295
25 Kopelman AE. Cutaneous absorption of hexachlorophene in low birthweight infants. J Pediatr 1973; 82: 972–975
26 Powell H, Swarner O, Gluck L, Lampert P. Hexachlorophene myelinopathy in premature infants. J Pediatr 1973; 82: 976–981
27 Shuman RM, Leech RW, Alvord ED. Neurotoxicity of hexachlorophene in the human. Pediatrics 1974; 54: 689–695
28 Chabrolle JP, Rossier A. Goitre and hypothyroidism in the newborn after cutaneous absorption of iodine. Arch Dis Child 1978; 53: 495–498
29 Schick JB, Milstein JM. Burn hazard of isopropyl alcohol in the neonate. Pediatrics 1981; 68: 587–588
30 Harpin VA, Rutter N. Percutaneous alcohol absorption and skin necrosis in a preterm infant. Arch Dis Child 1982; 57: 477–479
31 Evans NJ, Rutter N. Percutaneous respiration in the newborn infant. J Pediatr 1986; 108: 282–286
32 Cartlidge PHT, Rutter N. Percutaneous respiration in the newborn infant. Biol Neonate 1987; 52: 301–306
33 Cartlidge PHT, Rutter N. Percutaneous oxygen delivery to the preterm infant. Lancet 1988; i: 315–317
34 Cartlidge PHT, Rutter N. Karaya gum ECG electrodes for preterm infants. Arch Dis Child 1987; 62: 1281–1282
35 Evans NJ, Rutter N. Reduction of skin damage from transcutaneous oxygen electrodes using a spray-on dressing. Arch Dis Child 1986; 61: 881–884
36 Harpin VA, Rutter N. Sweating in preterm babies. J Pediatr 1982; 100: 614–619
37 Hey EN, Katz G. Evaporative water loss in the newborn baby. J Physiol 1969; 200: 605–619

Thermal control in very immature infants

David Hull
Department of Child Health, Queen's Medical Centre, Nottingham, UK

> Infants born at term have a full range of thermoregulatory responses and if provided with appropriate thermal insulation (swaddled) can maintain thermal stability over the environmental temperature range within the home. By contrast infants born before 28 weeks gestation not only lose heat rapidly because of very high rates of transepidermal water loss, they also have little or no thermoregulatory control. If they are to survive and flourish, they must initially be incubated like an egg and then the environment must be adjusted as they mature. It is an exacting task which is central to modern intensive neonatal care.

The progress of our understanding of the thermoregulatory control in the newborn has been signposted by a series of reviews in the British Medical Bulletin.[1-6] The full term human infant has a full complement of thermoregulatory responses, albeit ill-tested and of relatively limited capacity. Thus they make vasomotor and posturial changes to fluctuations in environmental temperature which influence the rates of heat loss.[7] On exposure to hot environments most newborn infants begin to sweat, most evidently on the forehead and thus to some extent increase heat loss.[8] Whereas on cold exposure the term infant can increase metabolic rate and thus heat production. Given average values, and assuming that the events sweating, postural adjustment, vasoconstriction and thermoregulatory thermogenesis occur in sequence and do not overlap, Wheldon[9] calculated that the average term infant weighing 3.5 kg, naked in an incubator would gain thermal control over the ambient temperature range 26°C to 36°C, and that the infant would feel comfortable, that is, within the thermoneutral range, between 32.5–34°C.

Similar studies as those used to produce the above calculations have been made by many investigations on infants born before 36 weeks gestation. The usual gestation band studied is 32–36 weeks in the first days of life, and 28–36 weeks in those infants thriving between 2–3 weeks of life. There is very little data on infants born under 28 weeks gestation in the first 2 weeks of life.

THE EFFECTS OF SIZE ALONE

The resting metabolic rate of the immature infant is similar to that of the term infant when expressed per kg body weight, and it rises more slowly after birth. It follows that the rate of heat production per unit surface area will be less. Similarly the tissue resistance of an immature infant with its thin skin and little subcutaneous fat will also be less, thus, even if a 1 kg 28 week gestation infant had thermoregulatory responses of the same order as those of the term infant, the range of thermal control would be much reduced (31–36°C) and the range of comfortable temperature higher and narrower (35.0–35.5°C) (Fig. 1).

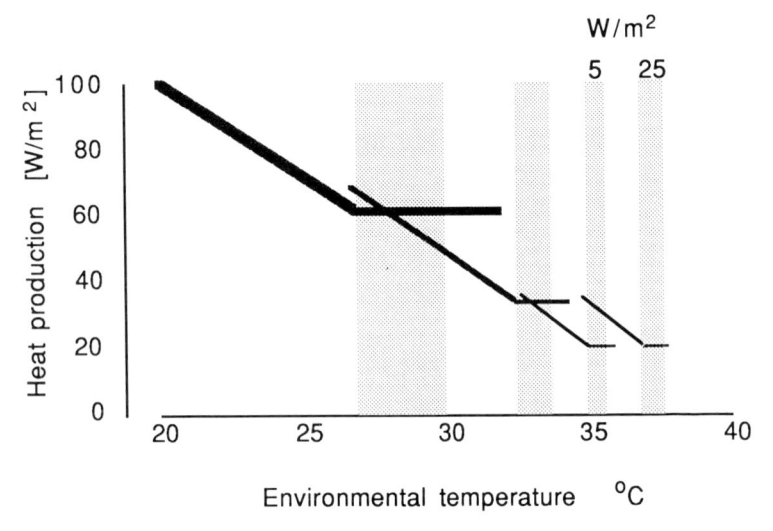

Fig. 1 This diagram illustrates the relationship between the environmental temperature and the metabolic rate of a seated adult [■■■], a healthy naked term infant who has the capacity to double the metabolic rate on cold exposure [━━], and an infant weighing 1 kg assuming that the capacity for thermogenesis on cold exposure is the same as the term infant [———]. Two plots are shown, one for an immature infant with a water-tight skin, and one with a moderate rate of transepidermal water loss (Wheldon 1982).

TRANSEPIDERMAL WATER LOSS

There is, however, another factor which has a major effect on thermoregulation in infants under 28 weeks gestation. At this gestation the skin is only 2 to 3 cells thick and contains little keratin so that it leaks.[10-13] This has many consequences (see Rutter, this issue), one is the leaking water evaporates from the skin causing the heat transfer by evaporative water loss. Under usual nursery conditions this exceeds the infant's total rate of heat production. This has the consequence of making the environmental temperature ranges at which the infant might be able to achieve thermal comfort and stability even higher (Fig. 1).

THERMOREGULATORY RESPONSES

The calculated curves in Figure 1 assume that the infant makes some thermoregulatory responses. Clearly for the very immature infant postural adjustments and vasomotor changes, even at an optimistic interpretation are not going to have much impact if the infant is to be isolated and nursed with little or no clothing. So, the thermoneutral range will be very narrow.

Thermoregulatory thermogenesis

In human newborn infants as in many mammals shivering does not appear to occur on cold exposure and it is probable that most of the extra heat produced on cold exposure occurs in brown adipose tissue. It has been known since the turn of the century that multilocular fat appears before unilocular fat and that such tissue is present in infants born on the edge of viability (24–27 weeks). Figures 2a, b show electronmicrographs of an adipocyte from an infant born at 22 weeks gestation. The cell is multilocular and the cytoplasm contains mitochondria of moderate size and complexity, both features consistent with it being a precursor of a brown adipocyte. So, it is possible that the end organ of thermoregulatory thermogenesis is present in an infant of 24–28 weeks gestation.

Putting the infants to the test is more difficult. In a very limited study[14] it was found that infants of this gestation in the first week of life did not have higher metabolic rates when their body temperatures fell below 36.5°C than those who were above it. There was no evidence of increase in heat production when the infants were cool. It seems unlikely that they attempt it, though it

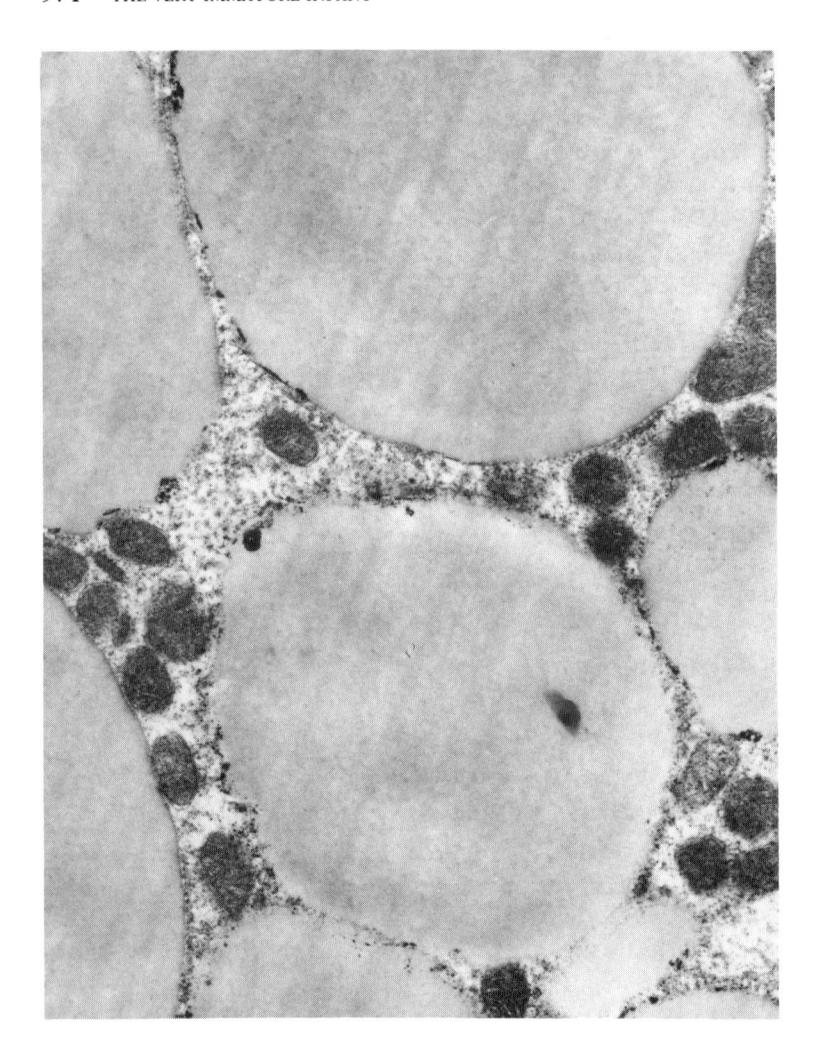

Fig. 2a Electron micrograph of brown adipose tissue from a 22 week fetus. **b** At low power the many fat vacuoles can be seen with numerous mitochondria lying in the cytoplasm. (× 15,000.)

is possible that they were unable to sustain it or alternatively they did not have the respiratory reserve to achieve it. Thus on current knowledge it must be assumed for practical purposes that the under 28 week infant makes no attempt to maintain thermal stability by thermogenesis.

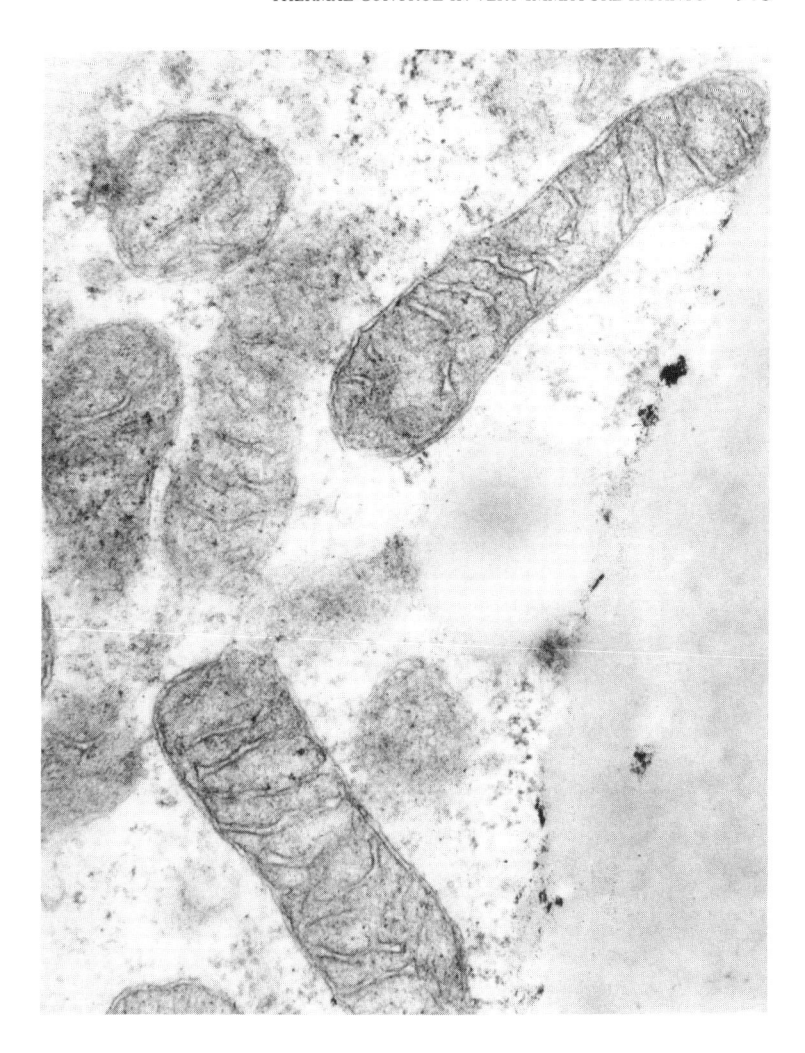

Fig. 2b At higher power the mitochondria can be seen to be moderately complex in structure. (× 50,000.)

Sweating

Likewise infants under 28 weeks do have sweat glands. Given the high transepidermal water loss, it would be difficult to establish that they did not work in hot environments, however there is other evidence to suggest that it is unlikely that they do so.

Term babies sweat, at least most of them do, in environmental conditions which push their deep body temperature above 38.0°C.[18] At earlier and earlier gestation Harper & Rutter[15] found that fewer infants began to sweat and at fewer sites and that no babies in the first 7 days of life born under 32 weeks gestation could be shown to sweat. Thus it seems most unlikely that infants under 28 weeks gestation would do so.

CHANGES AFTER BIRTH

Birth itself induces some very interesting changes. From the limited data available it would seem that the resting metabolic rate of infants under 28 weeks gestation increases only slowly after birth. The measures were made on the healthy infants who required no respiratory support, so presumably they are the fittest. By comparison with other animals it is those that are the most lively after birth (e.g., sheep) that have a rapid increase in resting metabolic rate and those that are least active (e.g., rabbit) that do not. The preterm infant is less 'active' than a term infant so its slow rise in metabolic rate is not unexpected. Dysmature infants have a much sharper rise in resting rate expressed per kg than infants of similar weight but earlier gestation.[3]

On the other hand the skin matures in advance of what it would do *in utero*, keratin is produced so that it quickly becomes watertight, this will reduce evaporative heat loss and increase at least to some extent, thermal insulation. It also appears to accelerate sweat gland activity so that the capacity to sweat develops at an earlier post conceptual age than it would have done otherwise.[15] Whether there is accelerated development in brown adipose tissue and the capacity for non-shivering thermogenesis is not known. Nor it is known whether thermogenesis develops to the extent that it is seen in term infants, whether there is a shift in the timing from non-shivering to shivering thermogenesis. Studies on prematurely delivered lambs would suggest that birth induces a premature peaking of the contribution of brown adipose tissue.[16]

In practical terms these changes can be monitored by recording the incubator air temperature required to maintain the infant's rectal temperature at 37.0°C (Fig. 3).[17]

INCUBATION AND POIKILOTHERMY

The easiest way to maintain thermal stability in infants under 28 weeks gestation under 7 days of age is to incubate them like an

Air and body temperatures of immature infants [Chellappah 1980]

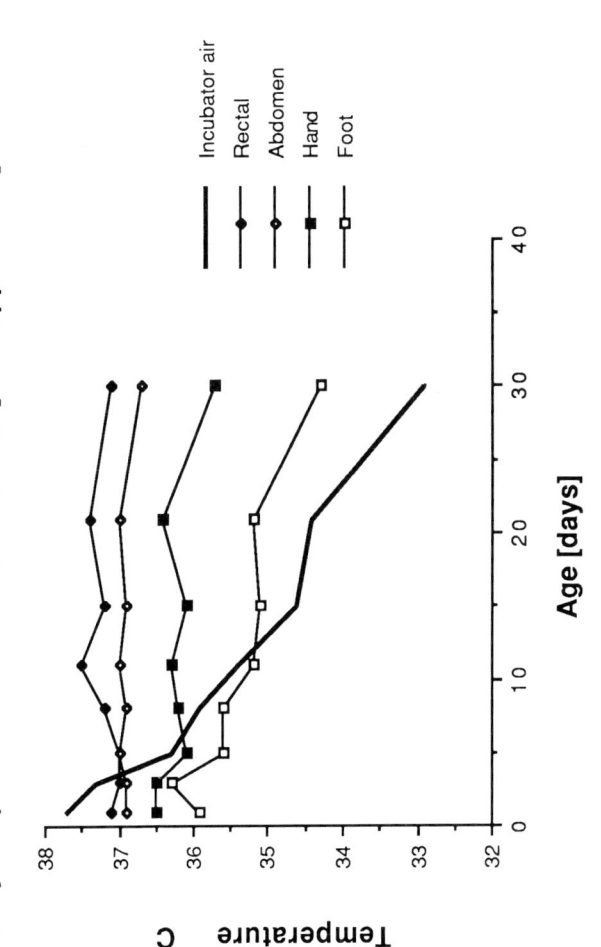

Fig. 3 Changes with post-natal age of the incubator air temperature and the rectal and surface temperatures of very immature infants. The figures are the average taken from ten infants. Over the same period the rate of transepidermal water loss fell on average from 22 to 8 g water m^{-2}h^{-1} (Chellappah 1980).

egg.[18] If an air environment is used, then the air temperature and surrounding surface temperatures would have to be at or a little above the desired temperature for the infant, and the air would have to be close to 100% saturation. That seems to be an unreasonable and very testing requirement, but in effect many newborn mammals are nursed in such conditions. It is also tempting to conclude that the infant under 28 weeks gestation is poikilothermic, implying that it tolerates its body temperature moving up and down with ambient conditions. There is no justification for reaching that conclusion either. Again there are newborn mammals for whom their size and thermal insulation is such that in isolation, any thermoregulatory responses would severely compromise survival. For example, mice develop thermoregulatory thermogenesis in the first 3 days of life, in hamsters it occurs in the second week (Fig. 4).[19,20] But, both show behavioural thermoregulation and under natural conditions seek ambient conditions which maintain their deep body temperatures around 38°C.

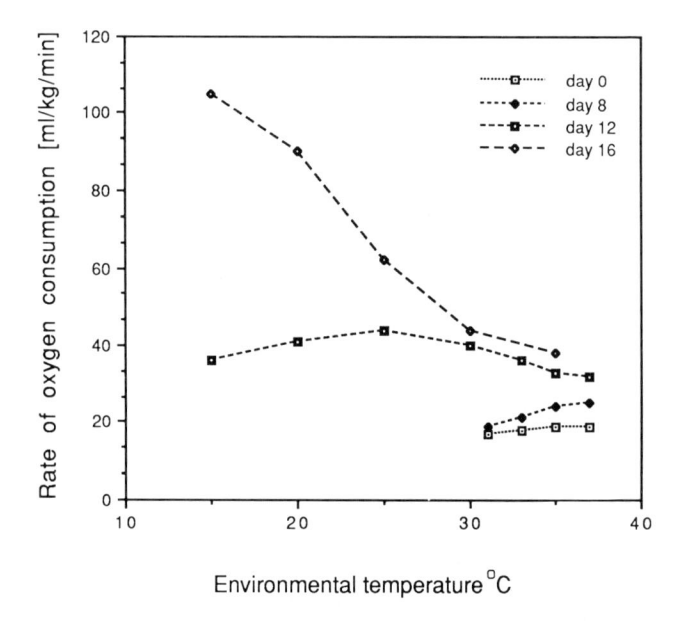

Fig. 4 The rate of oxygen consumption of hamsters on the day of birth (day 0) and 8, 12 and 16 days later. Note not only the development of cold induced thermogenesis but also the rise in the resting metabolic rate.[20]

There is evidence in the rabbit that the environmental conditions that they experience in the first days of life, do, for a short period 2–4 days determine what they perceive as a 'comfortable' temperature. Whether this phenomenon operates in man is not known.[21] The possibility that we might 'condition' very immature infants by the environments in which we elect to nurse them must not be forgotten.

HEAT EXCHANGES

The physical channels of heat transfer to and from a body in a given environment are radiation, convection, conduction and evaporation. In a living, breathing being, evaporative heat exchanges are divided into a fairly fixed loss from the respiratory tract and a variably and to some extent controllable evaporation from insensible water loss and sweating, from the skin surfaces. If all the body temperatures remain constant then the net rate of heat loss equals the rate of heat production. The relative contribution of the various modes of heat transfer will depend on the environment as well as the infant. Thus in a term infant on the second day of life when the skin has dried out, naked but for a nappy and lying in an incubator, in essence a plastic box with warm air circulating through it, and at a resting metabolic rate, the three principal modes of heat loss are radiation, convection and evaporation in that order, with little contribution from conduction (Fig. 5). For immature infants ranging from 28–35 weeks gestation at 3–13 days of life, the distribution is similar, but for an infant of 28 weeks weighing 1.08 kg age 3 days the position was very different (Fig. 5).[22] This was to be expected given the known high transepidermal water losses. In all three examples the infants were nursed at incubator settings that maintained their temperatures constant at about 37.0°C. This illustrates the considerable advantages of nursing very immature infants in environments which achieve high humidities immediate around the infant.[23] Attempts to reduce water loss by applying water resistant creams to the skin, whilst they achieve their primary objective make the infants more difficult to handle and probably more subject to skin infections and reactions. It is easier to cover the infants with sheets to create a micro-environment of 100% humidity, or alternatively to humidify the whole of the incubator space.[24]

The partition of heat transfer under radiant warmers is very

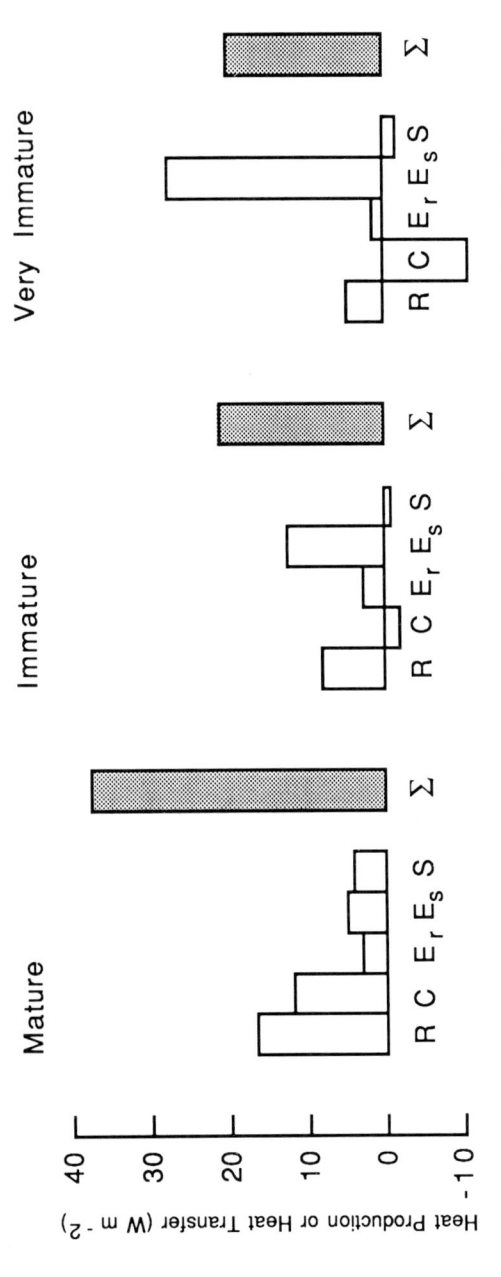

Fig. 5 The heat exchanges in full term, 32 week and under 28 week prematurely born infants nursed in an incubator. The infants were nursed so that their rectal temperatures were around 37°C. The very immature infant gained heat by convection and the surrounding air was warmer than the infants surface temperature. (R = Radiation, C = Convection, E = Evaporation divided into that from the respiration tract[r] and that from the skin surface[s], and S = Heat storage and the shaded column on the right gives the net sum of the heat exchanges). Data from Wheldon and Rutter 1982.

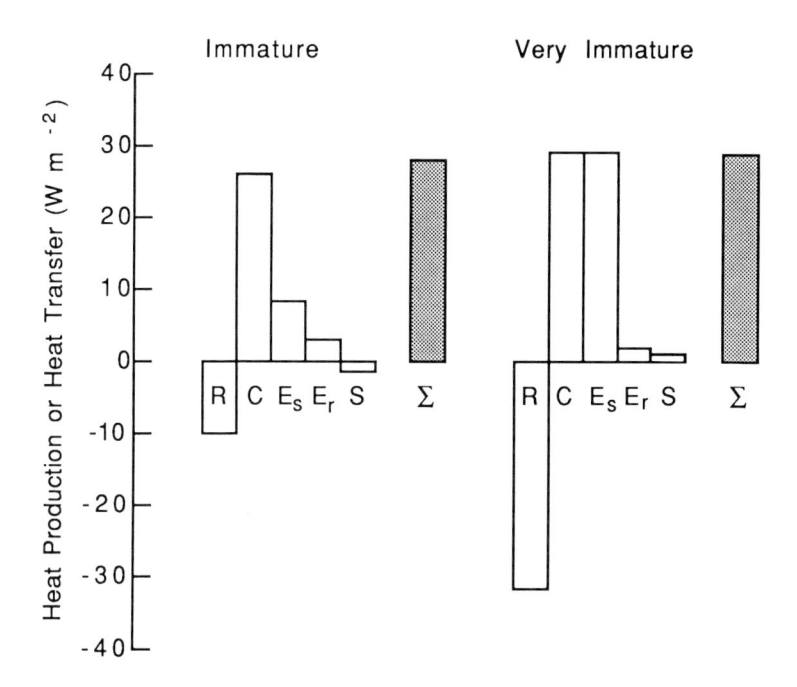

Fig. 6 The heat exchanges of a 32 week and an under 28 week infant nursed under a radiant warmer. Large radiant heat gain is required by the very immature infant to maintain body temperature. (The symbols are the same as those for Fig. 5). Data from Wheldon and Rutter 1982.

different (Fig. 6). In infants between 28–35 weeks gestation at 3–13 days there is a small net radiant heat gain to counterbalance the high convective heat losses. For the very immature infant there has to be a high net radiant heat gain to counteract the high evaporative as well as convective heat losses. This must be an unpleasant experience, it seems always to be associated with increased water loss and a higher resting metabolic rate; the precise mechanism of this reaction is uncertain.[25]

CONCLUSION

Keeping immature newborn sick infants comfortable is essential for their well-being and survival. One example of the many potential problems is illustrated by the serial body and incubator air temperature recordings of an infant of 25 weeks gestation who was placed immediately on arrival into an incubator set at 38°C in air mode. The rectal temperature at 20 minutes of age was 35°C

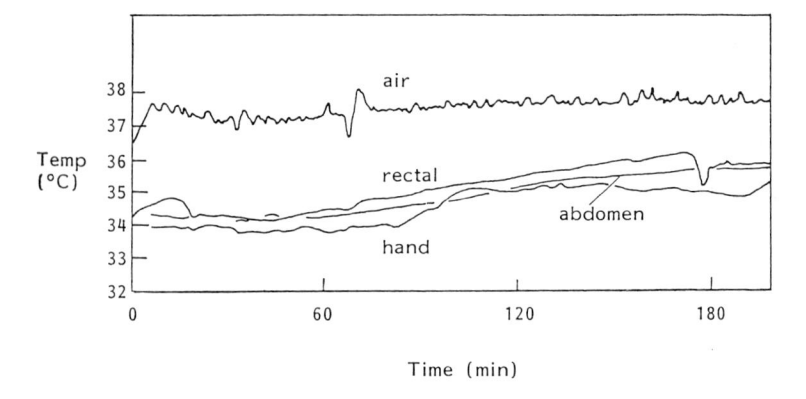

```
           38 ─                  air
                 ╱╲╱╲╱╲╱─╲╱╲─╱╲╱╲─╱─────╱╲─╱╲╱╲╱╲╱╲─╱╲╱╲╱╲╱
           37 ─
Temp       36 ─                  rectal
(°C)       35 ─
           34 ─                                    abdomen
                                  hand
           33 ─
           32 ─────┴──────────────┴──────────────┴──────────────┴
                  0              60             120            180

                                 Time (min)
```

Fig. 7 Incubator air temperature and rectal and surface temperatures of an infant of 25 weeks gestation on the first day of life after lung ventilation had commenced and an umbilical arterial line inserted. The infant had been covered by a plastic bubble blanket after the procedures but remained cold. The blanket was removed 5 minutes before the recording shown. Only after removal of the blanket did the infants temperature begin to rise, the blanket was acting to keep the infant cool (from Chellappah 1980).

indicating that even after taking this precaution the infant had cooled rapidly. By one hour artificial ventilation was required, at three hours an umbilical catheter had been inserted and an x-ray taken. At 4 hours of age his abdominal skin temperature was only 34.5°C, he was covered by a plastic bubble blanket, the incubator air temperature was still set at 38°C. Only when the plastic blanket was *removed* did he gain warmth from environment (Fig. 7). However, sufficient is now known about the thermoregulating responses and physical characteristics over the critical early weeks of life, and modern incubators have the capacity, that situations rarely arise where thermal comfort cannot be achieved.

REFERENCES

1 Hill JR. The newborn animal and environmental temperature. Br Med Bull 1961; 17: 164–167
2 Mount LE. Basis of heat regulation in homeotherms. Br Med Bull 1966; 22: 84–87
3 Scopes JW. Metabolic rate and temperature control in the human baby. Br Med Bull 1966; 22: 88–91
4 Hull D. The structure and function of brown adipose tissue. Br Med Bull 1966; 22: 92–96
5 Alexander G. Body temperature control in mammalian young. Br Med Bull 1975; 31: 62–68
6 Hey E. Thermal neutrality. Br Med Bull 1975; 31: 69–74

7 Harpin VA, Chellappah G, Rutter N. Responses of the newborn infant to overheating. Biol Neonate 1983; 44: 65–76
8 Rutter N, Hull D. Response of term babies to a warm environment. Arch Dis Child 1979; 54: 178–183
9 Wheldon AE. Heat exchange between the newborn baby and the environment. Ph D Thesis 1982; University of Nottingham
10 Fanaroff AA, Wald M, Gruber HS, Klaus MH. Insensible water loss in low birthweight infants. Pediatrics 1972; 50: 236–245
11 Rutter N, Hull D. Water loss from the skin of term and preterm babies. Arch Dis Child 1979; 54: 858–868
12 Hammarlund K, Sedin G. Transepidermal water loss in newborn infants III: Relation to gestational age. Acta Paediatr Scand 1979; 68: 795–801
13 Okken A, Jonxis JHP, Rispens P, Zijlstra WG. Insensible water loss and metabolic rate in low birthweight infants. Paediatr Res 1979; 1072–1075
14 Wheldon AE, Hull D. Incubation of very immature infants. Arch Dis Child 1983; 58: 504–508
15 Harper VA, Rutter N. Sweating in preterm babies. J Paediatr 1982; 100: 614–618
16 Alexander. Premature lambs
17 Chellappah G. Aspects of thermoregulation in term and preterm newborn babies. Ph D Thesis 1980; University of Nottingham
18 Hull D, Wheldon AE. Incubation of very immature infants. Arch Dis Child 1983; 58: 504–508
19 Vinter J, Hull D, Elphick MC. Onset of thermogenesis in response to cold in newborn mice. Biol Neonate 1982; 42: 145–151
20 Edson JL, Hull D, Elphick MC. The development of cold-induced thermogenesis in hamsters. J Dev Physiol 1981; 3: 387–396
21 Hull J, Hull D, Vinter J. The preferred environmental temperature of newborn rabbits. Biol Neonate 1986; 50: 323–330
22 Wheldon AE, Rutter N. The heat balance of small babies nursed in incubators and under radiant warmers. Early Hum Dev 1982; 6: 131–143
23 Harpin VA, Rutter N. Humidification of incubators. Arch Dis Child 1985; 60: 219–224
24 Brice JEH, Rutter N, Hull D. Reduction of skin water loss in the newborn II: Clinical trial of two methods in very low birthweight babies. Arch Dis Child 1981; 56: 673–675
25 Oritz A, Knudson RP, Alden ER, Toews WH. Oxygen consumption of infants under infrared radiant energy warmers. Paediatr Res 1977; 11: 539 (Abs. 1004)
26 Marks KH, Gunther RC, Rossi JA, Maisels MJ. Oxygen consumption and insensible water loss in premature infants under radiant heaters. Pediatrics 1980; 66: 228–232
27 Bell EF, Weinstein MR, Oh W. Heat balance in premature infants: comparative effects of convectively heated incubator and radiant warmer, with and without plastic heat shield. J Paediatr 1980; 96: 460–465
28 Williams PR, Oh W. Effects of radiant warmer on insensible water loss in newborn infants. Am J Dis Child 1974; 128: 511–514

Growth and nutrition of the very preterm infant

Jonathan C L Shaw
Department of Paediatrics, University College London, The Rayne Institute, London

> The poor energy reserves of the very preterm infant results in a survival time in starvation of less than 5 days. Total parenteral nutrition may therefore be life saving. The *in utero* growth of the fetus has become by default the reference standard for the growth of the preterm infant. Requirements of nutrients, however, are determined not only by growth rate but also by the maturity of the infant. Thus water requirements depend on rate of insensible water loss, GFR, renal solute load and arginine vasopressin secretion. Protein requirements **are** determined mainly by the high growth rate, and possibly in part by immaturity of biosynthetic pathways, whereas sodium requirements are determined mainly by the immaturity of the renal tubules. The rate of mineralisation of the skeleton may yet prove to be limited by the intestinal absorption of calcium. Since growth involves a positive non metabolisable base (NB) balance, and the renal control of the plasma concentration of NB is immature, attention must be paid to the NB concentration of the diet.

The Committee on Nutrition of the European Society of Paediatric Gastroenterology and Nutrition (ESPGAN) has recently published it's recommendations for the nutritional requirements of preterm infants.[1] It and other publications dealing with the same subject should be consulted as a source of references.[2-5] The ESPGAN Committee was aware of the difficulties of making a single set of requirements that met the needs of all low birthweight infants from 500 to 2500 g birthweight, and it made no recommendations as to the nutritional management of preterm infants before the establishment of full oral feeding. Nutrition of the very low birthweight infant however must begin with the provision of nutrients, rather than the introduction of a complete diet, and should therefore be deemed to begin from the time of birth. Since there is little published data dealing specifically with infants of less than 28 weeks gestation the particular nutritional predicament of these infants has to be inferred from the results of studies consisting predominantly of infants of more than 28 weeks gestation.

REFERENCE STANDARDS FOR GROWTH AND NUTRITION

Growth of the fetus *in utero*

In order to evaluate both the growth and the nutritional requirements of preterm infants the growth of the fetus *in utero* has, by default, become the ultimate reference standard. From data on the composition of the human fetus[6,7] *in utero* accumulation rates of different nutrients have been calculated.[8,9] These estimates lack precision but they help to identify substances such as calcium and phosphorus or iron, that may be provided in the diet in amounts very different from the intrauterine accumulation rate, and they enable differences between *in utero*, and postnatal weight gain and chemical growth, to be identified and evaluated, though not all such differences are necessarily harmful to health.

Weight gain *in utero*

Though the weight gain of the fetus *in utero* can be described by logistic equations based on models of inhibited growth,[10] the weight gain from 24 and to at least 35 weeks gestation is adequately described by a single exponential equation (Fig. 1),[11,12] from which can be calculated the specific growth rate. Table 1 shows a comparison of specific growth rates derived from different data. Those of Lubchenko et al (1963)[13] were from infants delivered in Denver, Colorado at an altitude of 1800 m, whereas in the others the infants were born at or near sea level. The specific growth rates and the final birth weights were lowest in the Denver study. Different socioeconomic class, and the exclusion of fetuses thought to be abnormally large may have contributed but the main factor was probably the higher altitude.[14]

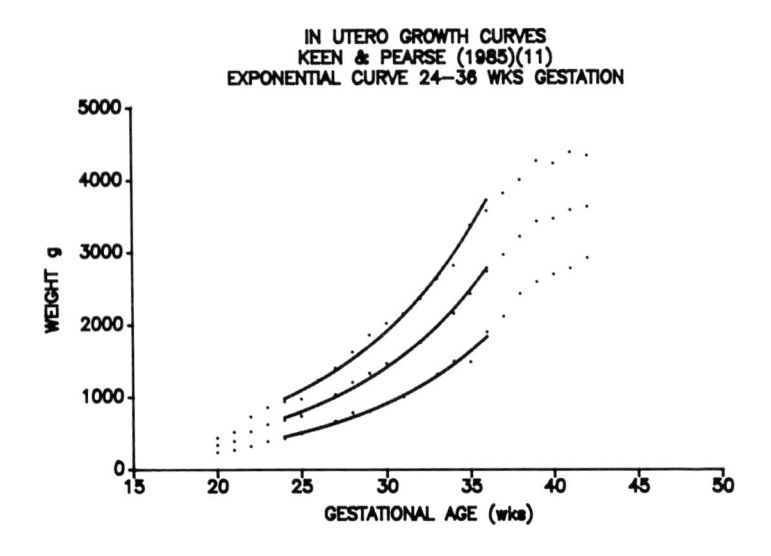

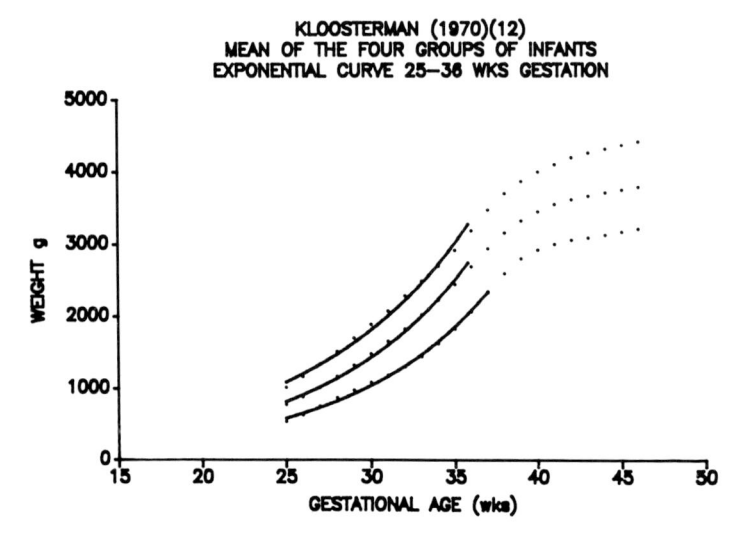

Fig. 1 Intrauterine growth data[11,12] to which has been fitted single exponential curves using least squares linear regression analysis

There is no significant difference between the specific growth rates before and after 28 weeks gestation, so these data probably represent the best estimate at present available for the specific growth rate of the fetus *in utero*. Since the growth rate of the full

Table 1 Comparison of specific growth rates for fetuses growing along different percentiles. The specific growth rates were calculated from the parameters of a simple exponential regression line ($\ln Y = \ln Y_0 \cdot e^{kt}$) fitted to the published data between 24 and 36 weeks gestation

Author	10% g kg^{-1} d^{-1}	50% g kg^{-1} d^{-1}	90% g kg^{-1} d^{-1}
Lubchenko et al (1963)[13]	15.6	14.4	12.8
Kloosterman (1970)[12]			
♀ Infants of primiparae	16.4	16.1	13.9
♀ Infants of multiparae	17.8	16.3	15.0
♂ Infants of primiparae	15.7	15.8	14.5
♂ Infants of multiparae	16.4	16.2	15.2
Kloosterman, average	16.6	16.1	14.6
	−2SD	MEAN	+2SD
Keen & Pearse (1985)[11]	16.6	16.2	15.9

term infant is 6.0 g kg^{-1} d^{-1} over the first month the nutritional requirements of the fetus will be greater. When comparing *in utero* and postnatal growth rates one must remember that because of the irreversible loss of sodium and water following birth (*vide infra*) the denominator of the specific growth rate is no longer the same, which makes interpretation of such comparisons rather uncertain.

Survival time in starvation

Table 2 gives the energy reserves as fat and the estimated survival time in starvation for infants of different birth weights.[15] No great precision is claimed for these estimates but they show that if a very immature infant is not to die of starvation, adequate nutrition must be started as soon after birth as possible—a 10% glucose infusion on its own is not sufficient.

ENERGY

The energy requirements of preterm infants on full oral feeding are stated to be 543 (range 460–690) kJ kg^{-1} d^{-1} (130 (range 110–165) kcal kg^{-1} day^{-1}).[1] It is difficult, however, even for the most robust infant, to establish full oral feeding in under a week or ten days so the short survival time in starvation even on a 10% glucose infusion constitutes the principal argument for introducing intravenous feeding (*vide infra*) as soon after birth as possible in infants under 1000 g birthweight.

Table 2 Energy reserves and survival time in starvation and semi starvation of infants of different birthweight[15]

Birth Weight	Fat g kg^{-1}	Fat kJ kg^{-1}	Estimated survival time days Water only	10% glucose
3.5 kg	150	5643	33	80
2.0 kg	60	2257	12	30
1.0 kg	23	865	4	11
0.5 kg	12	451	2	5

WATER

Water requirement is not determined so much by rate of growth but by the, renal solute load, renal concentrating ability, and above all in the infant of less than 28 weeks gestation in the first days of life by the glomerular filtration rate (GFR) and insensible water loss.

Water for growth

If the growth of the fetus is taken to be about 16 g kg^{-1} d^{-1} (Table 1), and about 70% of this is water, then the water needed for growth is about 11 ml kg^{-1} d^{-1}. Water of oxidation of infant feeds is said to be about 11.5 ml 418 kJ^{-1} (100 kcal^{-1}),[1] or 13.5 ml kg^{-1} d^{-1} at 502 kJ (120 kcal) kg^{-1} d^{-1}. The water of oxidation should therefore be sufficient to supply the requirements for growth.

Insensible water loss

The characteristics of the fetal epidermis and its permeability to water have been dealt with elsewhere in this issue (see Chapter by N Rutter). It is impracticable regularly to measure the evaporative water losses at the bedside and as a result disorders of water balance are common in the very low birthweight infant. The evaporation of water also interfers seriously with the thermoregulation of the infant. The very low birthweight infant consists of more than 80% water[6] (specific heat 4.18 J g^{-1} °C^{-1}). Therefore the loss of 4.18 kJ kg^{-1} (1.0 kcal kg^{-1}) from the body would reduce the body temperature by approximately 1.0°C. The heat of vaporisation of water at 37°C is 2.41 kJ g^{-1} so the evaporation of 2 g kg^{-1} of water could cause a drop of body temperature of 1.0°C.

Rates of evaporate water loss vary from 2–6 ml kg^{-1} h^{-1} equivalent to a heat loss of 116–347 kJ kg^{-1} d^{-1}. Whether this heat comes from the body or the environment is immaterial, the result is an unmeasurable consumption of heat at the surface of the infant which makes thermoregulation difficult, the energy consumption of the infant uncertain, and the accurate regulation of water intake almost impossible. It is essential therefore to humidify the environment—using either a perspex body box or polyethylene sheet. If a paper hygrometer kept permanently next to the baby records a relative humidity of over 80%, evaporative water losses should not be excessive. After about 48–72 hours of age the evaporative water losses decline, and the control of humidity can be gradually relaxed.

Water requirements

An intake of water of 65–100 ml kg^{-1} d^{-1} on day one, depending on the control of evaporative water losses, is usually recommended rising by steps to an intake of 180 ml kg^{-1} d^{-1} (range 150–200 ml kg^{-1} d^{-1}) on day 7.[1]

Because the GFR is low following birth (see N Modi, this issue) the minimum water intake in the first few days of life is determined by the evaporative water loss, and only later on by the renal solute load. Once full feeding has been established, provided the renal solute load is in the region of 13 mosmol kg^{-1} d^{-1} the urine osmolality will be in the range of the infant's ability to concentrate and dilute his urine (i.e. 60–500 mosmol per kg H$_2$O).[1] However events shown to cause inappropriate release of arginine vasopressin—such as birth asphyxia, periventricular haemorrhage or pneumothorax[16]—may cause a reduction in urine volume necessitating a reduction of water intake until there is an adequate urine output with a satisfactory osmolality.

'Fluids' are often restricted in infants with patent ductus arteriosus (PDA) or in those thought to be in heart failure. It is however important to consider what is being restricted and why. Volume restriction reduces not only the intake of water but also of energy, sodium and other nutrients. If there is water overload due to failure of osmoregulation (e.g. due to inappropriate release of arginine vasopressin) then water should be restricted independently of other nutrients. If on the other hand the problem is one of volume regulation then it may be more appropriate to restrict sodium intake. The nutritional consequences of 'restricting fluid' are often ignored to the detriment of the infant's nutrition. The evidence that water overload causes PDA is unconvincing[17] nor is it clear that 'fluid restriction' is always a good treatment. When there is left to right shunt through the ductus, secondary changes in atrial volume are thought to cause the raised levels of atrial natriuretic peptide that have been reported,[18] and might also cause inhibition of the release of AVP.[16] In such circumstances the restriction of salt and water may not prove to be the best treatment. However, the changes in total body water and total body sodium have not been properly investigated.

Recommendations for water intake in the first week of life are only a guide. Regular accurate measurements of body weight and of plasma sodium are essential for the fine tuning of the sodium and water intake. As a general rule the occurrence of hyponatraemia during the first four days of life in a very low birth weight infant is likely to be due to retention of water in excess of sodium, often due to inappropriate release of arginine vasopressin, and should be treated with water restriction. Only after that time does sodium depletion become a more important cause of hyponatraemia[19] and should be treated with sodium supplementation (*vide infra*).

PROTEIN

Table 3 gives estimates of the rate of nitrogen and protein accumulation by the human fetus *in utero*.[20] The concentration of nitrogen rises from 14.6 kg^{-1} at 24 weeks gestation to 18.6 g kg^{-1} at 36 weeks gestation.[6,7] These data suggest that the immature fetus does not have a higher protein requirement than more mature fetuses.

The protein content of human breast milk and infant formulae

Breast milk

Recent analyses have shown that the protein concentration of mature human breast milk is 8.9 g l^{-1} [1.37 g 418 kJ^{-1} (100 kcal^{-1})]. Of this about 10% is secretory IgA, which is resistant to low pH and the action of proteolytic enzymes and is poorly absorbed. Since lacto ferrin and lysozyme are also poorly absorbed the available protein content of breast milk may be nearer 7.0 g l^{-1}.[21]

Table 3 Nitrogen accumulation by the fetus *in utero* growing along different percentiles.[20] The figures in brackets are estimates of protein accumulation in g kg^{-1} d^{-1}, calculated as nitrogen × 6.25

Gestation weeks	10th% Nitrogen mg kg^{-1} d^{-1}	50th% Nitrogen mg kg^{-1} d^{-1}	90th% Nitrogen mg kg^{-1} d^{-1}
24	267(1.67)	252(1.58)	226(1.41)
26	279	261	236
28	293	274	247
30	304(1.9)	284(1.78)	256(1.6)
32	315	294	265
34	325	305	274
36	342(2.14)	320(2.0)	289(1.81)

At 200 ml kg^{-1} d^{-1} mature breast milk would provide at most 1.8 g kg^{-1} d^{-1} [1.4 g 418 kJ^{-1} (100 kcal^{-1})]. Rönholm et al. (1986)[22] have recently shown that preterm infants increase in weight and length faster if fed mature human breast milk supplemented with human milk protein (protein intake 3.2 g kg^{-1} d^{-1}) than if fed breast milk alone (protein intake 1.8 g kg^{-1} d^{-1}). This tends to confirm that pooled mature breast milk contains insufficient protein for the optimal growth of preterm infants. Table 4 compares the composition of milk of mothers delivering preterm and fullterm infants.[23] In both the protein concentration is higher at birth and declines over the first 28 days, though the protein energy ratio of the early milk may not be optimal. The differences between preterm and fullterm milk have not been confirmed by every one.[1] Britton (1986)[24] for example showed no difference in the total protein of preterm and fullterm breast milk, but in preterm milk immunoglobulins comprised a higher proportion of the protein. He also found that the β-casein declined faster

Table 4 Comparison of the composition of fullterm and preterm milk[23]

Lactation Days	Energy kJ l^{-1}		Protein* g l^{-1}		Protein: Energy$^+$ g 418 kJ^{-1}		Sodium mmol l^{-1}		Chloride mmol l^{-1}	
	FT	PT	FT	PT	FT	PT	FT	PT	FT	PT
3	2010	2130	23	32	4.7	6.3	22	27	27	32
7	2550	2800	19	24	2.8	3.6	17	22	21	25
14	2680	3010	16	22	2.4	3.0	11	23	15	16
21	2880	2760	15	18	2.2	2.8	11	13	15	17
28	2930	2930	14	18	2.0	2.5	8	13	13	17

*The protein is calculated as nitrogen × 6.25 and is probably an overestimate
+ Protein energy has been expressed per 418 kJ because in most other texts it is expressed per 100 kcals and 1 kcal = 4.18 kJ

in preterm milk than in full term milk. The nutritional advantages of the protein in preterm milk as opposed to fullterm milk therefore seems still to be in question. However, an infant's own mother's milk, if produced in sufficient volume, is better than pooled mature donor breast milk.

Formulae

The protein content of fullterm formulae is usually between 15–20 g l^{-1} [2.2–2.8 g 418 kJ^{-1} (100 kcal^{-1})], and of preterm formulae 14–24 g l^{-1} [1.9–3.0 g 418 kJ^{-1} (100 kcal^{-1})].[1] The ESPGAN committee[1] recommended that formulae for preterm infants should contain 2.25–3.0 g protein 418 kJ^{-1} (100 kcal^{-1}). At 543 kJ kg^{-1} d^{-1} (130 kcal kg^{-1} d^{-1}) this would provide 2.9–4.0 g kg^{-1} d^{-1}. It is therefore apparent that both fullterm and preterm infant formulae would provide the estimated requirements if fed at an appropriate volume (i.e. up to 200 ml kg^{-1} d^{-1}).

Protein turnover measurements and protein requirements

Jackson et al. (1981)[20] studied infants of 31–33 weeks gestation fed pooled donor breast milk, using metabolic balance techniques and ^{15}N glycine to estimate nitrogen turnover. They found a mean protein retention of 1.6 g kg^{-1} d^{-1} and a mean protein turnover (synthesis + excretion) of 12.1 g kg^{-1} d^{-1}. They showed that the obligatory nitrogen losses were 67 mg N$_2$ kg^{-1} d^{-1} and that zero balance would have been likely on a protein intake of 0.6 g kg^{-1} d^{-1}. The net protein utilisation was 70%. Table 5 gives estimates of protein requirements utilising the accumulation rates in Table 3 and the coefficient of absorption and net protein utilisation given above. These estimates of optimal protein intake are higher than that provided by pooled donor breast milk, but correspond quite closely to the recommendations of ESPGAN[1] for formula fed preterm infants and to the amounts that would be provided by an infant's own mother if the milk were fed at 180–200 ml kg^{-1} d^{-1}.

Protein quality

It is possible that net protein utilisation might be increased and the total protein requirements reduced if the aminoacid composition of the protein was improved. Widdowson et al. (1979)[25] showed that the rate at which the human fetus lays down glycine falls from

Table 5 Estimated protein requirements and protein energy ratios of preterm infants at different gestations

Gest weeks	Percentile 10th% g kg^{-1} d^{-1}	50th% g kg^{-1} d^{-1}	90th% g kg^{-1} d^{-1}
24	3.0	2.9	2.6
30	3.3	3.1	2.9
36	3.7	3.5	3.2
	g 418 kJ^{-1}*	g 418 kJ^{-1}*	g 418 kJ^{-1}*
24	2.3	2.2	2.0
30	2.5	2.4	2.2
36	2.8	2.7	2.5

*at an intake of 543 kJ (130 kcal) kg^{-1} d^{-1}

about 288 mg kg^{-1} d^{-1} at 24 weeks gestation to about 152 mg kg^{-1} d^{-1} at 36 weeks gestation. Breast milk provides only 65 mg kg^{-1} d^{-1}. The very immature infant must therefore synthesise most of his glycine requirements from percursors such as serine. Protein turnover studies using ^{15}N glycine[20,26] have shown that when preterm infants are fed less than 500 mg N$_2$ kg^{-1} d^{-1} (approximately 3.1 g protein kg^{-1} d^{-1}) the urine ammonia, but not the urea was labelled by the ^{15}N glycine. This suggested that the requirements of protein synthesis within the liver used all the available glycine and led to the proposal that glycine might be growth limiting in those infants.[20] This could be due to immaturity of the enzymes of the glycine cleavage system or to a deficiency of the precursor such as serine. The excretion of 5-oxoproline in the urine may prove a useful measure of glycine sufficiency in preterm infants[27] and enable this problem to be further investigated.

SODIUM

Sodium in the fetal body

The concentration of sodium in the fetal body falls from about 94 mmol kg^{-1} at 25 weeks gestation (500 g body weight) to about 74 mmol kg^{-1} at term (3.5 kg body weight).[6,7] The daily rate of accumulation between 24 and 36 weeks gestation has been estimated at between 0.85–1.1 mmol kg^{-1} d^{-1}.[8,9]

Changes in body composition in the first week of life

Preterm infants weighing about 1000 g lose on average 12% of body weight in the first four days of life and about 13 mmol Na$^+$

kg^{-1}, so about 75% of the weight loss can be accounted for by isotonic loss of ECF.[28] Thus if there is no inappropriate water retention due to inappropriate secretion of arginine vasopressin[19] or water loss due to uncontrolled transepidermal evaporation, the plasma sodium should remain constant during the first four days of life. As far as it is possible to tell from the available data, the loss of ECF is irreversible and is not restored when growth is resumed.[29] Furthermore there is no relationship between the sodium intake in the first four days of life and the amount of sodium lost[28] indicating that the negative sodium balance and weight loss of the first four days cannot be prevented by the administration of sodium. From about the fourth day onwards the negative sodium balance declines and provided the sodium intake is maintained at about 6–7 mmol kg^{-1} d^{-1} sodium balance is restored at the end of the first week of life in most infants.

Sodium balance and late hyponatraemia

When growth is resumed sodium balance becomes positive and amounts of sodium close to the intrauterine accumulation rate are retained.[30] Nevertheless there is a high incidence of hyponatraemia[31] and the plasma sodium concentration has been shown to depend on the sodium intake.[31,32] The cause of the late hyponatraemia is therefore a failure of the renal and possibly endocrine control of the composition and volume of the ECF (see N Modi, this issue). Though the data of Sulyok et al.[33] suggests that renal tubular sodium reabsorption is under maximum stimulation following birth, the evidence indicates that the renal tubular sodium absorption rises more slowly after birth than the GFR, and the consequent high fractional sodium excretion results initially in a negative sodium balance, a contraction of the extracellular fluid volume and protective release of antidiuretic hormone.[34] If the sodium intake is insufficient, the plasma sodium concentration declines until the filtered sodium is equal to the renal tubular sodium reabsorption when a new steady state is reached. The role of artrial natriuretic peptide in these changes is still uncertain.[35]

With maturation of renal function (see Modi elsewhere in this issue) the incidence of hyponatraemia declines after about 32 weeks gestation and the sodium requirements fall. Thus French et al. (1982)[36] showed that infants of 34 weeks gestation could maintain a normal plasma sodium whether they were fed a full term formula providing 1.2 mmol kg^{-1} d^{-1} of sodium or a preterm formula providing 3.9 mmol kg^{-1} d^{-1}.

Sodium requirements of very low birthweight infants

During the first 24 hours of life there is no obligatory sodium requirement. The GFR is low, urine volume small (about 30 ml kg^{-1}), and intakes of 2.0 mmol Na^+ kg^{-1} d^{-1} result in positive balance. Nor is sodium really an obligatory nutrient during the next three days while there is isotonic loss of sodium and water, however, sodium is generally given in a 10% glucose and 0.18% saline from the second day. This may serve to prevent extreme changes in plasma sodium concentration due to changes in water balance, and provides a sufficient sodium intake of 4.5–6.0 mmol kg^{-1} d^{-1} for many infants during the second half of the first week of life. In the absence of disorders of water balance (due to uncontrolled evaporative water loss or inappropriate release of arginine vasopressin) the sodium intake should be adjusted to maintain the desired plasma sodium concentration (e.g. 130–135 mmol l^{-1}). Some infants with very immature renal tubular sodium conservation may require 8–12 mmol kg^{-1} d^{-1}. As they mature the sodium intake can be gradually reduced.

Dietary sources of sodium

The sodium concentration of pooled human breast milk is only 7 mmol l^{-1} and provides insufficient sodium for preterm infants. The milk provided by the infant's own mother contains a higher concentration of sodium during the first four weeks of lactation (see Table 4) and if used will diminish the frequency and severity of hyponatraemia.[32] The sodium concentration of fullterm formulae ranges from 7–13 mmol l^{-1}, and of preterm formulae from 14–26 mmol l^{-1}.[1] None of these milks contain enough sodium for all preterm infants and sodium supplements will be required for many of the smallest infants. Because sodium requirements decline with postnatal age, and some infants may require a restricted sodium intake because of heart failure, it is not recommended that the sodium content of formulae designed for preterm infants should contain more sodium than those designed for fullterm infants.[1]

CALCIUM AND PHOSPHORUS

Calcium and phosphorus in the fetus[6,7]

The amount of calcium in the fetus rises from 2.4 g (60 mmol) in a fetus weighing 500 g to 30.4 g (760 mmol) in a fetus weighing 3.5 kg. The rate of accumulation of calcium is in the region of 3.0–3.25 mmol kg^{-1} d^{-1}.[8,9] The amount of phosphorus rises from 1.5 g (48 mmol) in a fetus of 500 g to 16.7 g (539 mmol) in fetus of 3.5 kg. The rate of accumulation of phosphorus is about 2.1–2.4 mmol kg^{-1} d^{-1}.[8,9] Approximately 0.6 mmol kg^{-1} d^{-1} of phosphorus is required for soft tissue growth and the remainder is deposited in bone. This rapid deposition of bone mineral results in bones at term that are very dense and compact. Following birth as the bone grows there is extensive remodelling of bone with a reduction in the density of bone mineral referred to as the 'physiological osteoporosis of the suckling'.[37]

Breast milk and most formulae provide less calcium and phosphorus than the intrauterine accumulation rate. This matters very little for preterm infants of 34 weeks gestation or more because they have accumulated at least 500 mmol (20 g) of calcium in their skeleton[6] and their calcium and phosphate requirements will shortly decline. Infants of less than 28 weeks gestation however have only 125–150 mmol (5–6 g) of calcium in their bodies at birth so the cumulative deficit becomes considerable if the diet is deficient in calcium and phosphorus or the calcium and phosphorus cannot be absorbed.

Breast milk

Figure 2 shows a summary of calcium retention as a function of calcium intake in infants fed different milks.[5,38,39] Infants fed breast milk receive only about 1.5 mmol kg^{-1} d^{-1} of calcium and 1.0 mmol kg^{-1} d^{-1} of phosphorus. Of this about 50% of the calcium and about 90% of the phosphorus is absorbed. Infants fed breast milk cannot therefore mineralise their skeletons at an intrauterine rate. A recent study of fortification of preterm milk with protein and calcium and phosphorus revealed no increase in bone mineral concentration using photon absorptiometry.[40] However, sedimentation of the insoluble calcium salts cannot be ruled out (see below), and careful balance studies of fortified breast milk are required.

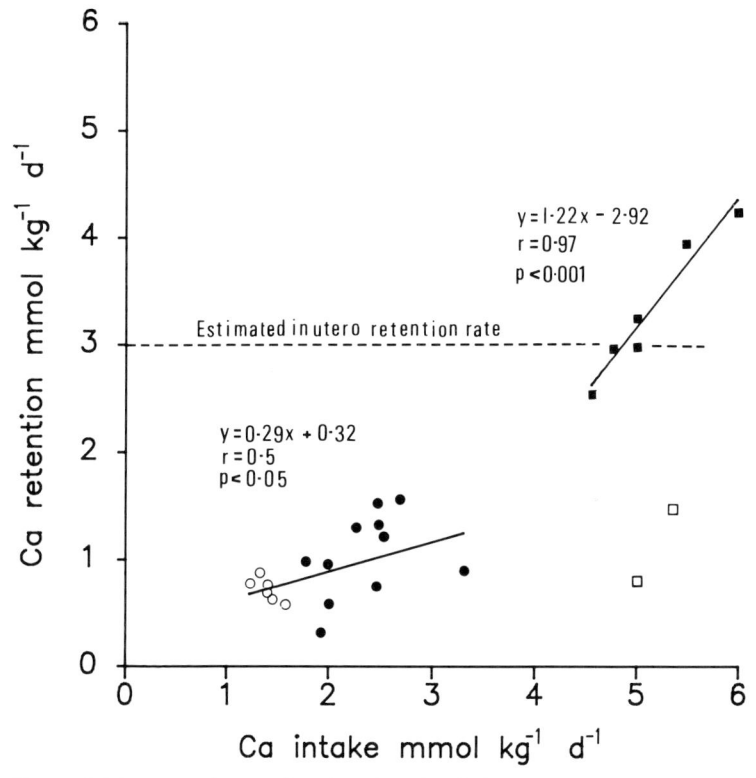

Fig. 2 Calcium retention as a function of calcium intake from published metabolic balance data[5,38,39] Breast milk ○ Cow milk □ Fullterm and preterm formulae ● High calcium USA preterm formulae ■

Formulae

Both full term formulae and those adapted for preterm infants (but without the large additions of calcium and phosphate discussed below) contain more calcium and phosphorus than breast milk and the results of balance studies in Figure 2 show that the mean calcium retention is increased but not above about 1.5 mmol kg^{-1} d^{-1} even in those infants fed cow milk with calcium intakes of over 5.0 mmol kg^{-1} d^{-1}. These milks therefore produce a valuable augmentation of calcium retention, and have been shown to reduce the incidence and severity of bone disease.[32]

BONE DISEASE OF PREMATURITY

As the baby grows the deficiency of calcium and phosphorous results in two related changes.

Osteopenia

There is a decline in the concentration of bone mineral causing radiolucent bones on X-ray.[41] This has been called the osteopenia of prematurity and the severity varies with the calcium and phosphorus content of the diet. Since a reduction of bone density follows normal full term birth it is not the presence of osteopenia but its magnitude that is important. In breast fed very immature infants the under mineralisation can be so severe that growth is impaired, the bones fracture and the ribs may become so flexible that they cannot function properly. It is less severe in infants fed formulae with a higher calcium and phosphorus content.

Phosphate depletion syndrome

This occurs particularly in infants fed breast milk.[42] It is precipitated when the demands of soft tissue growth for phosphorus (≈ 0.6 mmol kg^{-1} d^{-1}) leave insufficient to maintain the plasma phosphate concentration and thus ensure the full utilisation of the absorbed calcium. There is a low plasma phosphorus (<1.5 mmol l^{-1}), a high alkaline phosphatase, absent or low concentration of phosphorus (<0.1 mmol kg^{-1} d^{-1}) and a high concentration of calcium (e.g. 0.4 mmol kg^{-1} d^{-1}) in the urine, together with the changes of rickets in the growing ends of the long bones. Phosphate supplements of 0.3 mmol kg^{-1} d^{-1} given to infants fed breast milk have been shown to improve calcium retention, to eliminate the hypercalcuria,[43] and possibly to result in the healing of growing ends of the long bones. Phosphate supplements cannot however prevent the osteopenia. Higher intakes of phosphorus without additional calcium have been shown to result in the clearance of the superfluous phosphorus in the urine.[44] Phosphate depletion is rare in infants fed formula milks because of the higher phosphate content.

Vitamin D deficiency

If the infants are vitamin D deficient then the bone disease will be compounded by the changes of vitamin D deficiency rickets. Because of poor endowment at birth, malabsorption, rapid rate of growth, and possible immaturity of the biosynthetic pathways the vitamin D requirements of preterm infants are thought to be higher than those of full term infants. The ESPGAN committee recommended an intake in the range 800–1600 IU per day.[1] However many nurseries still give only 400 IU per day.[38,39]

High calcium and phosphorus formulae for preterm infants

The problem of osteopenia has led to attempts to mimic *in utero* accumulation rates by adding very large amounts of mineral to milks. Day et al. (1975)[45] supplemented SMA®–S26 with calcium lactate to provide calcium intakes in the region of 5.0 mmol kg^{-1} d^{-1}. They reported a rise in calcium absorption from 30% to 67% and retentions in the region of 3.0 mmol kg^{-1} d^{-1}. They did not however give additional phosphate and the phosphate retention was not correspondingly increased, so the new bone would have had the curious molar Ca:P ratio of about 5. The explanation was that the calcium lactate, being insoluble, had sedimented before it was given to the baby so that intake was overestimated. More recently some preterm formulae have been supplemented with large amounts of calcium and phosphate. In all these milks there is tendency for the extra mineral to sediment as it is insoluble[46] though the rate of sedimentation is said to have been reduced.[39] The results of balances using such milks are given in Figure 2. Though they show retentions comparable to the *in utero* accumulation rate the data are nevertheless very mystifying. They are quite different from all other data in ways that seem to show that the sedimentation problem may not have been overcome. First there is very little variation between different studies suggesting that something unusually reproducible is occurring. Secondly, the intercept on the x axis of 2.4 mmol kg^{-1} d^{-1} is consistent either with a considerable 'intake' before any calcium is absorbed or a massive endogenous loss of calcium, −2.92 mmol kg^{-1} d^{-1}. Thirdly the slope of the regression line is 1.2 which indicates the surprising fact that for a 1.0 mmol increment in dietary calcium 1.2 mmol are retained. Indeed if one subtracts the slope of the other regression line (0.29) one is left with a residual slope of 0.93—quite close to 1—which is what would be expected if the difference was due to sedimentation. The possibility that these results contain a major artefactual component due to sedimentation has not been convincingly ruled out, and so for the present they must be considered of uncertain significance.

Photon absorptiometry of bone has been used to determine whether the dietary calcium is being laid down in bone at intrauterine rates. Photon absorptiometry however, though a valuable tool, only measures an analogue of concentration and does not determine the size of the skeleton. It cannot therefore be used to learn how much calcium has been retained only whether bone mineral concentration has increased.

It seems to me to be unwise to feed such milks to very low birth weight infants at the present time. If the results are false then there is very little purpose and the effects of actually administering such large amounts of insoluble mineral unknown. If they are true then they seem to indicate a complete breakdown in the control of calcium absorption, and under such circumstances there must be some anxiety about where the calcium is being laid down.

The only way to be sure that the calcium and phosphorus intake is accurately known is to take samples for analysis from the milk that is actually to be used for the balance while it is being stirred to ensure homogeneity. Then all the unused milk, the milk residues and any in the delivery apparatus must be recovered at the end of every balance so that all unused milk can be pooled and analysed. It is then possible to discover by difference exactly how much calcium has gone into the infant. Errors in metabolic balances do not cancel themselves out but are additive and tend to overestimate retention and the higher the intake the greater the error. For example if milk is spilt and intake is overestimated by 10 ml, calcium retention in a breast fed infant will be overestimated by 0.08 mmol, but in an infant fed a high calcium milk the error will be 0.5 mmol. These errors are additional to any due to sedimentation.

NON METABOLISABLE BASE (NET BASE, NB)

For a more detailed discussion of the interaction of diet and acid base chemistry the interested reader should consult the following references.[1,47,48] Acids and bases are present in the body and in the diet in three forms carbonic acid, metabolisable acid and non metabolisable base (acid). The carbonic acid concentration of the diet is trivial and can be ignored. The metabolisable acids of the diet consist of titratable metabolisable acidic and basic groups on proteins and other lower molecular weight metabolisable organic compounds (e.g. lactic acid). Metabolisable acids confer on milks their acidity, they are readily disposed of by intermediary metabolism to carbon dioxide and water so they usually make a negligible contribution to acid base disturbances. Non metabolisable base (NB) on the other hand consists predominantly of inorganic acids and bases that cannot be disposed of by intermediary metabolism or pulmonary ventilation. They must be excreted in the urine and their concentration in the plasma is under specific renal control. They are absorbed from the diet, or formed within the body as end products of metabolism the most important of which is sulphuric acid produced from the oxidation of sulphur containing amino acids. The following general equation defines the concentration of NB in milk, plasma or indeed any biological medium (e.g. urine faeces or body tissue). The symbol c stands for concentration, and the symbol t for total amount.

$$cNB = (cNa^+ + cK^+ + 2cCa^{2+} + 2cMg^{2+})$$
$$- (cCl^- + 2ctSO_4^{2-} + 1.8ctP) \qquad [1]$$

(Note that 1.8 is the average negative charge per mole of phosphate at pH 7.4)

During growth the fetus, infant and child are all in positive balance for NB. The concentration of NB in the fetus rises from 140 mmol kg^{-1} at 23 weeks gestation to about 238 mmol kg^{-1} at 35 weeks gestation. This positive NB balance arises mainly from the incorporation of base into the hydroxyapatite mineral of bone.

$$10Ca^{2+} + 4.8HOP_4^{2-} + 1.2H_2PO_4^- + 2H_2O =$$
$$[Ca_3(PO_4)_2]_3 \cdot Ca(OH)_2 + 9.2H^+ \qquad [2]$$

Thus for each mmol of calcium laid down in the hydroxyapatite of bone 0.92 mmol of base is bound and 0.92 mmol H$^+$ are released into the ECF. From calculations of the rate of accumulation of calcium by the human fetus *in utero* it can be calculated that the fetal skeleton binds between 2.4–3.1 mmol NB kg^{-1} d^{-1}. *In utero* this is provided by the placenta but in the preterm infant it is provided by the diet. The NB retained can be determined after analysis of diet, urine and stool using equation [1] above as the difference between the NB absorbed and the NB in the urine.

Acid base disturbances of preterm infants

Preterm infants particularly the most immature are notably vulnerable to acid base disturbances of dietary origin. These occur because the renal mechanisms for reabsorbing NB (excreting non metabolisable acid) which control the concentration of NB in the plasma are immature and cannot adapt to extreme changes in the

NB in the diet. Thus Kildeberg[49] showed that preterm infants fed cow's milk developed a late metabolic acidosis. This was mainly due to the low NB intake due to the formation of sulphuric acid from oxidation of organic sulphur in sulphur containing amino acids. However the excretion of metabolisable acids in the urine may have interfered with renal NB reabsorption. Metabolic acidosis has been described in infants fed an earlier formulation of Nutramigen® in which the NB concentration was probably inadequate, though this was never established. Metabolic alkalosis has been described in infants fed chloride deficient formulae and breast milk. In these cases the alkalosis resulted from the high NB concentration of the milk, and the excessive renal NB regeneration stimulated by the demands of volume regulation in the absence of sufficient chloride.

There have been virtually no systematic studies of acid base balance in preterm infants using recently developed concepts.[46,47] So, though acid base disturbances are still common in the very low birthweight infant it is only possible to make general comments on the desirable acid base properties of the diet.

Milks should have a positive concentration of NB sufficient to provide for the observed rate of skeletal mineralisation and some to neutralise the sulphuric acid produced from the oxidation of sulphur containing amino acids. The concentration of sulphur containing amino acids should be sufficient for growth but not so high that the production of sulphuric acid is excessive. There should be sufficient phosphate in the diet to provide sufficient for skeletal growth, soft tissue growth, and some to give the urine an adequate buffer value. There must be sufficient chloride to satisfy the demands of volume regulation, otherwise there will be extra demand for renal NB regeneration and alkalosis.

TRACE METALS

Zinc

Zinc is an essential component of more than seventy metalloenzymes and many of which play a central role in the replication, transcription and repair of DNA during growth. Between 24 and 36 weeks gestation zinc accumulates in the fetus at a rate of about 3.8 $\mu mol\ kg^{-1}\ d^{-1}$, and the term infant contains about 1.01 mmol zinc.[50]

Zinc in milk

The concentration of zinc in breast milk falls from about 126 µmol l^{-1} in colostrum to 32 µmol^{-1} 2 months and to 12 µmol l^{-1} at 4–7 months of lactation. There are no differences between the zinc concentration of preterm and full term milk.[1] In the United Kingdom full term formulae contain from 32–70 µmol l^{-1} and preterm formulae contain between 96–113 µmol l^{-1}. In the USA some preterm formulae contain as much as 206 µmol l^{-1}.

Zinc absorption

Full term breast fed infants aged 5–8 days are in negative zinc balance, and preterm infants fed pooled pasteurised human donor breast milk (51 µmol Zn l^{-1}) were in negative balance for at least 40 days after birth.[51] When such infants pass term they will have less zinc in their bodies than a term infant. If they are then breast fed at a stage in lactation when the zinc concentration has declined to a low level they may develope zinc deficiency. Preterm infants fed formulae with a zinc concentration of 191 µmol l^{-1} are reported to be in positive balance.[52]

Zinc deficiency

Zinc deficiency is characterised by growth arrest, irritability, anorexia, alopecia, perioral and perineal dermatitis, vesicupustular lesions of the hands and feet, oesophagitis, diarrhoea, thymic atrophy and defects in cell mediated immunity.[50] Zinc deficiency has been reported as a late sequel to preterm birth. The infants were between 27–32 weeks gestation, the onset of symptoms occurred between 2–4.5 months of age, and most of them were breast fed.[1] In some the mother's milk had a very low zinc concentration 4–8.5 µmol l^{-1}. Symptoms disappeared within a few days on treatment with 15–61 µmol Zn kg^{-1} d^{-1}. The conditions causing zinc deficiency, namely low body stores at birth, rapid rate of growth, a negative balance after birth, and a declining concentration in breast milk make it important to be on the lookout for zinc deficiency in the very immature breast fed infant. Nevertheless proven zinc deficiency is very rare, particularly in formula fed infants receiving more that 11 µmol kg^{-1} d^{-1}.

Copper

Copper accumulates in the fetal body at a rate of about 0.8 μmol kg^{-1} d^{-1} and at term the fetus contains about 228 μmol of copper of which about half is present in the liver where it forms a reserve. Copper is a component of several enzymes such as tyrosine oxidase, lysyl oxidase and the cytosol superoxide dismutase.[53]

Copper in milk

The mean concentration of copper in breast milk is about 7.9 μmol l^{-1} and it declines little if at all during lactation. There are no significant differences between the copper concentration of preterm and full term milk. The copper concentration in infant formulae rarely exceeds that of breast milk and some have very low levels. At the present time most infant formulae available in the UK contain a minimum of 6.3 μmol l^{-1}, but Milumil® contains 4.1 μmol l^{-1} and Preaptamil® a formula designed for preterm infants contains curiously only 1.6 μmol l^{-1}.[54]

Copper absorption

Seven of ten full term infants fed breast milk were in negative balance for copper aged 5–8 days. Preterm infants fed pooled pasteurised donor breast milk are also in negative balance following birth but the majority are in positive balance by the 40th day of life.[51] Infants fed formulae with a higher copper content do not always achieve a positive copper balance.[52]

Copper deficiency[54]

The full syndrome of copper deficiency includes psychomotor retardation, hypopigmentation, sideroblastic anaemia and neutropenia ($<1.0 \times 10^9$ l^{-1}), bone disease with changes in the growing bone ends, and fractures. The plasma copper is usually less than 6.3 μmol l^{-1} and the caeruloplasmin is less than 0.13 g l^{-1}. The median age at diagnosis was 3.0 months and no case has been reported in a preterm infant less than 2.2 months. Response to treatment was prompt with doses of copper between 9–12.6 μmol kg^{-1} d^{-1}. Copper deficiency has never been described in any infant fed exclusively on breast milk. It has mainly been described in infants fed copper deficient TPN, and low copper formulae.

Table 6 Composition of total parenteral solution and daily intake of different substances. Maximum rate of administration 150–180 ml kg^{-1} d^{-1}

		Composition Litre^{-1}	Daily intake kg^{-1} d^{-1} at: 150 ml kg^{-1} d^{-1}	180 ml kg^{-1} d^{-1}
Glucose	g	100.00	15.00	18.00
Amino acids	g	16.60	2.50	3.00
Sodium	mmol	27.00	4.00	5.00
Potassium	mmol	19.00	2.90	3.40
Calcium	mmol (mg)	5.90(236)	0.89(35)	1.06(42)
Phosphorus	mmol (mg)	6.50(202)	0.98(30)	1.17(36)
Ca:P	mmol (mg)	0.91(1.17)		
Magnesium	mmol	1.10	0.16	0.19
Chloride	mmol	31.00	4.60	5.50
Zinc	μmol	15.40	2.31	2.77
Copper	μmol	4.70	0.70	0.85
Net Base	mmol	17.3	2.60	3.10
Energy	kJ	1845.00	277.00	333.00
Intralipid 20%* (15 ml kg^{-1} d^{-1})	kJ	8400.00	126.00	126.00
Total energy	kJ kg^{-1} d^{-1}		403.00	459.00
	kcal kg^{-1} d^{-1}		96.00	110.00
Water soluble vitamins				
Solivito	1.0 ml kg^{-1} d^{-1}			
Fat soluble vitamins				
Vitlipid infant 1.0 ml kg^{-1} d^{-1} to a maximum of 4.0 ml d^{-1}				

*Note that Intralipid 20%, will supply an additional 0.23 mmol (7.0 mg) kg^{-1} d^{-1} of phosphorus

There is therefore no case for supplementing breast milk with copper, and formulae for preterm infants should provide about 1.9 µmol Cu kg^{-1} d^{-1}. Though copper deficiency is rare subclinical deficiency may pass unrecognised because of difficulties in diagnosis.

TOTAL PARENTERAL NUTRITION

Total parenteral nutrition plays a very important part in the management of many infant's of less than 28 weeks gestation. For the infant of very low birth weight the technique of percutaneous insertion of a fine silicone rubber catheter into the right atrium of the heart has proved very successful.[8] It enables nutrition to start as soon after birth as possible, and saves the baby from the trauma of repeated peripheral infusions. It seems particularly useful when weaning the very immature infant from the ventilator. It avoids the need for nasogastric or orogastric tubes which may obstruct a valuable amount of the infants' airway, at a time when the baby is on the brink of respiratory failure. Though the technique of catheter insertion and incidence of complications has not changed in our department since it was first described, the composition of the TPN solution has changed a little. The current composition is given in Table 6. The aim was not precisely to mimic intrauterine accumulation rates but to provide nutrients in sufficient quantity to foster growth without risking metabolic overload. In particular the concentration of calcium and phosphorus because of their insolubility cannot be much further increased,[55] so the bones cannot mineralise at an intrauterine rate.

REFERENCES

1 Committee on the Nutrition of the Preterm Infant. European Society of Paediatric Gastroenterology and Nutrition. Nutrition and Feeding of Preterm Infants. Oxford: Blackwell Scientific Publications, 1987
2 American Academy of Pediatrics: Committee on Nutrition. Nutritional Needs of Low Birth Weight Infants. Pediatrics 1977; 60: 519–530
3 Canadian Paediatric Society: Committee on Nutrition. Feeding the Low Birth Weight Infant. Can Med Assoc J 1981; 124: 1301–1311
4 American Academy of Pediatrics: Committee on Nutrition. Nutritional Needs of Low Birthweight Infants. Pediatrics 1985; 75: 976–986
5 Tsang RC, ed. Vitamin and Mineral Requirements in Preterm Infants. New York: Marcel Decker, 1985
6 Widdowson EM, Dickerson JWT. Chemical composition of the body. In: Comar CL, Bronner F, eds. Mineral Metabolism. New York: Academic Press, 1961; Vol 2: Ch 17

7 Kelly HG, Sloan RE, Hoffman W, Saunders C. Accumulation of nitrogen and six minerals in the human fetus during gestation. Hum Biol 1951; 23: 61–74
8 Shaw JCL. Parenteral nutrition in the management of sick low birth weight infants. Pediatr Clin North Am 1973; 20: 333–358
9 Ziegler EE, O'Donnell AM, Nelson SE, Fomon SJ. Body composition of the reference fetus. Growth 1976; 40: 329–341
10 Bonds DR, Mwape B, Kumar S, Gabbe SG. Human fetal weight and placental weight growth curves: A mathematical analysis from a population at sea level. Biol Neonat 1984; 45: 261–274
11 Keen DV, Pearse RG. Birth weight between 14 and 42 weeks gestation. Arch Dis Child 1985; 60: 440–446
12 Kloosterman GJ. On intrauterine growth. Int J Gynaecol Obstet 1970; 8: 895–912
13 Lubchenko LO, Hansman C, Dressler M, Boyd E. Intrauterine growth as estimated from live born birth-weight data at 24 to 42 weeks of gestation. Pediatrics 1963; 32: 793–800
14 Yip R. Altitude and birthweight. J Pediatr 1987; 111: 869–876
15 Heird WC, Driscoll JM, Schullinger JN, Grebin B, Winters RW. Intravenous alimentation in pediatric patients. J Pediatr 1972; 80: 351–372
16 Rees L, Brook CGD, Shaw JCL, Forsling ML. Hyponatraemia in the first week of life in preterm infants. Part I. Arginine vasopressin secretion. Arch Dis Child 1984; 59: 414–422
17 Lorenz JM, Kleinman LI, Kotagal U, Reller MD. Water balance in very low birthweight infants: relationship to water and sodium intake and effect on outcome. J Pediatr 1982; 101: 423–432
18 Andersson S, Tikkanen I, Pesonen E, Meretoja O, Hynynen M, Fyhrquist F. Atrial natriuretic peptide in patent ductus arteriosus. Pediatr Res 1987; 21: 396–398
19 Rees L, Shaw JCL, Brook CGD, Forsling ML. Hyponatraemia in the first week of life in preterm infants. Part II Sodium and water balance. Arch Dis Child 1984; 59: 423–429
20 Jackson AA, Shaw JCL, Barber A, Golden MHN. Nitrogen metabolism in preterm infants fed human donor breast milk: the possible essentiality of glycine. Pediatr Res 1981; 15: 1454–1461
21 Räihä NCR. Nutritional proteins in milk and the protein requirement of normal infants. Pediatrics 1985; 75: 136–142
22 Rönholm KA, Perheentupa J, Siimes MA. Supplementation with human milk protein improves growth of small premature infants fed human milk. Pediatrics 1986; 77: 649–653
23 Gross SJ, David RJ, Bauman L, Tomarelli RM. Nutritional composition of milk produced by mothers delivering preterm. J Pediatr 1980; 96: 641–644
24 Britton JR. Milk protein quality in mothers delivering prematurely: implications for infants in the intensive care unit nursery setting. J Pediatr Gastroenterol Nutr 1986; 5: 116–121
25 Widdowson EM, Southgate DAT, Hey EN. Body composition of the fetus and infant. In: Visser HKA ed. Fifth Nutricia Symposium. Nutrition and metabolism of the fetus and infant. The Hague: Martinus Nijhoff, 1979: pp. 169–177
26 Catzeflis C, Schutz Y, Micheli J-L, Welsch C, Arnaud MJ, Jequier E. Whole body protein synthesis and energy expenditure in very low birth weight infants. Pediatr Res 1985; 19: 679–697
27 Jackson AA, Badaloo AV, Forrester T, Hibbert JM, Persaud C. Urinary excretion of 5-oxoproline (pyroglutamic aciduria) as an index of glycine insufficiency in normal man. Br J Nut 1987; 58: 207–214
28 Hamilton CMH, Shaw JCL. Changes in sodium and water balance, renal function and aldosterone excretion during the first seven days of life in very low birth weight infants. Pediatr Res 1984; 18: 91

29 Shaffer SG, Bradt SK, Meade VM, Hall RT. Extracellular fluid changes in very low birthweight infant during first 2 postnatal months. J Pediatr 1987; 111: 124–128
30 Shaw JCL. Absorption and retention of sodium, postassium, magnesium and calcium by preterm infants. In: Proc 2nd Ross Clin Res Conf Meeting Nutritional Goals for Low Birth Weight Infants. Columbus, Ohio: Ross Lab, 1982; 97–103
31 Roy RN, Chance GW, Radde IC, Hill DE, Willis DM, Sheepers J. Late hyponatraemia in very low birth weight infants (<1.3 kg). Pediatr Res 1976; 10: 526–531
32 Gross SJ. Growth and biochemical response of preterm infants fed human milk or modified infant formula. N Engl J Med 1983; 308: 237–241
33 Sulyok E, Nemeth M, Tenyi I, Csaba I, Györy E, Ertle T, Varga F. Postnatal development of Renin-Angiotensin-Aldosterone system, RAAS, in relation to electrolyte balance in premature infants. Pediatr Res 1979; 13: 817–820
34 Lichardus B, Sulyok E, Kovacs L, Michajlovskij N, Lehotska V, Nemethova V, Varga L, Ertl T. Renal salt-wasting increases vasopressin excretion in preterm infants. Monogr Neural Sci 1986; 12: 179–184
35 Tulassay T, Seri I, Rascher W. Atrial natriuretic peptide and extracellular volume contraction after birth. Acta Paediatr Scand 1987; 76: 444–446
36 French TJ, Colbeck M, Burman D, Spiedel BO, Hendy RA. A modified cow's milk formula suitable for low birthweight infants. Arch Dis Child 1982; 57: 507–510
37 Royer P. Growth and development of bony tissues. In: Davies JA, Dobbing J. eds. Scientific Foundations of Paediatrics. 2nd ed. London: William Heineman, 1969
38 Kayshap S, Forsyth M, Zucker C, Ramakrishnan R, Dell RB, Heird WC. Effects of varying protein and energy intakes on growth and metabolic response in low birth weight infants. J Pediatr 1986; 108: 955–963
39 Rowe JC, Goetz CA, Carey DE, Horak E. Achievement of in utero retention of calcium and phosphorus accompanied by high calcium excretion in very low birth weight infants fed a fortified formula. J Pediatr 1987; 110: 581–585
40 Gross SJ. Bone mineralisation in preterm infants fed human milk with and without mineral supplementation. J Pediatr 1987; 111: 450–458
41 Koo WWK, Gupta JM, Nayanar VV, Wilkinson M, Posen S. Skeletal changes in preterm infants. Arch Dis Child 1982; 57: 447–452
42 Rowe JC, Carey DE. Phosphorus deficiency syndrome in very low birth weight infants. Pediatr Clin North Am 1987; 34: 997–1017
43 Senterre J, Putet G, Rigo J. Effects of vitamin D and phosphours supplementation on calcium retention in preterm infants fed banked human milk. J Pediatr 1983; 103: 305–307
44 Carey DE, Cynthia A, Goetz RN, Horak E, Rowe J. Phosphours wasting during phosphorus supplementation of human milk feedings in preterm infants. J Pediatr 1985; 107: 790–796
45 Day GM, Chance GW, Radde IC, Reilly BJ, Park E, Sheepers J. Growth and mineral metabolism in very low birth weight infants: II. Effects of calcium supplementation on growth and divalent cations. Pediatr Res 1975; 9: 568–575
46 Bhatia J, Fomon SJ. Formulas for premature infants: fate of the calcium and phosphorus. Pediatrics 1983; 72: 37–40
47 Kildeberg P. Quantitative Acid-Base Physiology. System Physiology and Pathophysiology of Renal, Gastrointestinal, and Skeletal Acid-Base Metabolism. Odense University Press, 1981
48 Kildeberg P, Winters RW. Balance of Net Acid: Concept, Measurement and Applications. Adv Pediatr 1978; 25: 349–381
49 Kildeberg P. Disturbances of hydrogen ion balance occurring in premature infants. I. Late Metabolic Acidosis. Acta Paediatr Upsala 1964; 53: 517–519

50 Shaw JCL. Trace elements in the fetus and young infant. I Zinc. Am J Dis Child 1979; 133: 1260–1268
51 Dauncey MJ, Shaw JCL, Urman J. The absorption and retention of magnesium, zinc and copper by low birthweight infants fed pasteurised human breast milk. Pediatr Res 1977; 11: 991–997
52 Tyrala EE. Zinc and copper balances in preterm infants. Pediatrics 1986; 77: 513–517
53 Shaw JCL. Trace elements in the fetus and young infant. II. Copper, Manganese, Selenium and Chromium. Am J Dis Child 1980; 134: 74–81
54 Shaw JCL. Copper and non accidental injury. Arch Dis Child 1988; 63: 448–455
55 Knight P, Heer D, Abdenour G. CaxP and Ca/P in the parenteral feeding of preterm infants. J Parenter Enteral Nutr 1983; 7: 110–114

The gastrointestinal tract

P J Milla
W M Bisset
Department of Child Health, Institute of Child Health, London

> The extremely limited energy reserves of the very premature infant dictate an urgent need to establish an adequate nutrient intake very shortly after birth. By 22—28 weeks gestation the fetal intestinal mucosa morphologically resembles the adult in the small intestine, but in the large intestine fetal villi are still present. Functionally the activity of many digestive enzymes associated with villous absorptive cells and the distribution of endocrine cells has almost reached adult values. Other functions are however less well developed, including absorption, motor activity and that of the accessory organs (liver and biliary system, pancreas). As a consequence of such disparate development of function a knowledge of the pattern of development in the human is essential for the provision of optimal nutritional care of the very preterm infant.

Whether the infant who is born extremely prematurely before 28 weeks gestation will survive is dependent on its ability to successfully adapt from intrauterine to extrauterine life. The extremely limited energy reserves, a 600 g infant has less than 6 g of stored fat, dictate an urgent need to establish an adequate nutrient intake. Adequate nutrition is dependent on the degree of maturation of the gastrointestinal tract at this age. In addition to digestion absorption and motor activity, the mucosa must also act as a barrier to lumenal macromolecules and this is a function of many factors which include: the cell types present, the distribution, composition and organisation of the various cells' subcellular organelles and the presence and continuity of the epithelial cell barrier. These proceed at different species specific rates resulting in different function appearing at different times as shown in Figure 1. A sound understanding of the different aspects of the

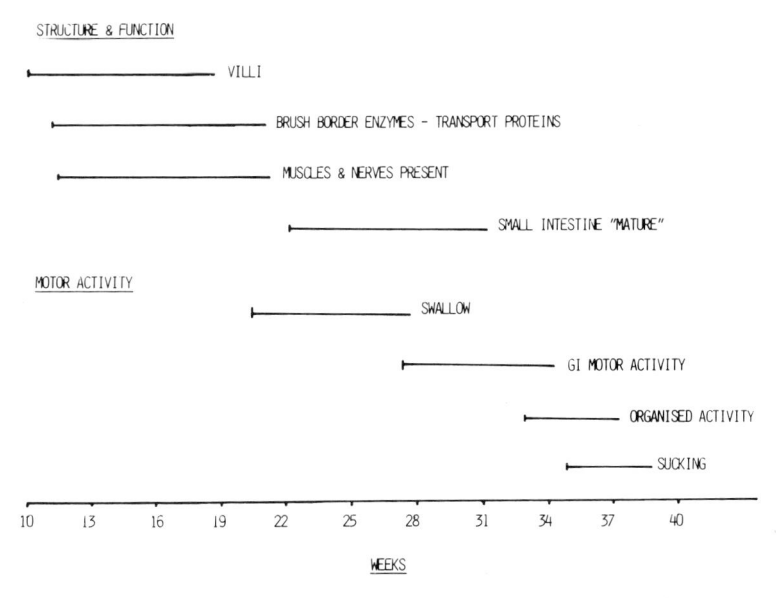

Fig. 1 The general timetable of development of human gastrointestinal structure and function.

developing gastrointestinal tract and especially the state of development between 24 and 28 weeks gestation is essential for the successful nutritional care of infants born at such a time.

DEVELOPMENT OF THE STRUCTURE OF THE GASTROINTESTINAL TRACT

Three major phases of development of the human gastrointestinal tract occur; an early period of proliferation and morphogenesis, an intermediate period of differentiation when many different and distinctive cell types appear and a later period of maturation resulting in a bowel capable of transporting, digesting and absorbing nutrients.

Proliferation and morphogenesis

The gastrointestinal tract first appears at 4 weeks gestation as a tube of stratified epithelium which extends from the mouth to the cloaca and can be divided into three distinct parts; the foregut (oesophagus, stomach, proximal duodenum, liver and pancreas), midgut (small intenstine through to the proximal 2/3 of transverse colon), and hindgut. The most proximal part forms the oesophagus and is separated by the newly formed diaphragm from the fusiform dilatation of the foregut which between 5-7 weeks gestation forms the stomach. The rapidly growing distal intestine herniates through the umbilicus but subsequently by 10 weeks the loop of bowel undergoes a counter-clockwise rotation and returns to the abdominal cavity. By 9 weeks pancreatic and hepatic tissue has clearly appeared and by 12 week bile secretion has started. Thus by 12 weeks the gross abdominal structures are well developed with a similar layout to that found in the newborn infant.[1]

At 5 weeks gestation the epithelium of the oesophagus has a double layer of cells, by 10 weeks the epithelium is ciliated and it is not until after 20 weeks that the stratified squamous epithelium found in the newborn infant develops.

The development of the myenteric plexus by 9 weeks and differentiated ganglion cells by 13 weeks is associated with the appearance of oesophageal muscle.[2] In the stomach circular smooth muscle appears by 9 weeks with glandular pits first forming at 10 weeks with parietal cells visualised by 11 weeks and mucin secreting cells by 16 weeks gestation.[2]

In the small intestine, rudimentary villi appear at 8 weeks with an apical layer of cells with short and irregular microvilli. Coincident with the end of this first phase of development is the formation of crypts and elongation of the primitive villi. The precise nature of the transformation of the simple stratified epithelium to the complex epithelium with well developed crypts and villi which occurs by 14 weeks gestation is not clear.[3] This process like many others proceeds in a craniocaudal direction.

The mucosa of the colon is poorly differentiated at 8 weeks gestation but between 9 and 11 weeks longitudinal folds develops. Between 14 and 16 weeks true villus structure similar to those in the small intestine have developed which continue to develop and elongate up to 28 weeks have developed gestation.[4] The reason for the formation of colonic villi is unknown, as is whether they provide a digestive or absorptive advantage for the infant born extremely prematurely prior to 28 weeks gestation.

The appearance of neural and muscular elements also follows a craniocaudal gradient with Auerbach's plexus appearing at 9 weeks and Meissner's plexus together with smooth muscle at 13 weeks in the small intestine and a week later in the proximal colon. By 24 weeks ganglion cells have migrated to within 1 cm of the anus.

Cellular differentiation

Towards the end of the preceding period of morphogenesis differentiation of different cell types begins to occur. The various tissues of the gastrointestinal tract follow an inherent species dependent pattern of differentiation. Differentiation into ectoderm, mesoderm and endoderm is followed by anatomical specialisation which involves interactions between these three layers.

The epithelium of most of the digestive tract is endodermal in origin but differentiates into squamous epithelium in the oesophagus and into absorptive, secretory, goblet and endocrine cells elsewhere. The earliest cells to appear in stratified epithelium are goblet cells and fetal endocrine cells.[5] These initial endocrine cells (precursor cells) appearing at 9 weeks together with later transitional cells (12 weeks gestation) appear at times of very rapid differentiation, that is stratified to columnar epithelium, formation of villi and crypts and new specialised cell types such as absorptive cells. It seems likely that the fetal endocrine cells play an important part in creating the correct micro-environment for differentiation to occur.

All the fetal endocrine cells have two populations of secretory granules. One has the former function and these later disappear and one is the precursor of those found in adult endocrine cells. Initially, a single layer of undifferentiated stratified epithelial cells is arranged radially towards the lumen. At about 8–10 weeks gestation they undergo a transition to columnar cells followed immediately by the formation of secondary lumina and junctional complexes (Fig. 2a, b). Secondary lumina seem to have a role in remodelling of the mucosa and eventual villus formation[6] (Fig. 2c). Crypt cells consist of undifferentiated columnar epithelial cells and Paneth cells, both are present from 10–11 weeks gestation and are secretory in nature. When crypt cells first appear they differ from mature adult crypt cells in that they contain large aggregates of glycogen and only very small secretory granules. By 16 weeks they resemble adult cells.[6] The villi of fetal intestine are lined by columnar epithelial cells. Interspersed amongst these are a number of other cell types including tuft cells and putative M cells. The role of the former is unknown but the latter are associated later with Peyer's patches and are thought to have a role in macromolecular uptake.[7] The majority of cells are however, absorptive cells which initially are characterised by short microvilli, large infra- and supra nuclear glycogen deposits moderately developed Golgi apparatus and many vesicles and tubules in the apical cytoplasm. The apical tubular system undergoes a dramatic increase in complexity between 14 and 17 weeks gestation as shown in Figure 2d but by 24 weeks is undetectable in proximal small intestine.

Maturation

Between 18 and 22 weeks gestation many of the features distinctive of fetal intestine disappear, such as the apical tubular system and this introduces the final phase of maturation. Apart from the colon which retains villi until 28 weeks gestation the epithelium of the intestine is now adult in type. The limited amount of data regarding brush border digestion and absorption suggests that functional maturation does indeed occur up to and beyond full term and is discussed below.

DEVELOPMENT OF INTESTINAL FUNCTION

The development of function of different regions of the gut correlates with structural development. Data regarding the human fetus and infant prior to 28 weeks gestation is scanty but it is clear that digestion, absorption and secretion are relatively advanced compared to motor function.

Intestinal motor activity

The motor activity of the gut moves the intraluminal contents from one specialised region of the gut to another and in older children the pattern of motility is integrated and related to the physiological function of the particular region of the gut.

Studies of intestinal motor activity in the very preterm infant have however been limited by both technical and ethical constraints and as a result little detailed information is available. An amniographic study has shown that when contrast is injected into the amniotic cavity there is very little transit down the fetal gut before 28 weeks gestation.[8] It is also clear that although the intestine is structurally mature by 24 weeks gestation, in the majority of very preterm infants, immaturity of motor function is a major limiting factor to the introduction of enteral nutrition, and such problems are further compounded in infants with respiratory distress.[9]

Swallowing has been observed in utero as early as 16 weeks

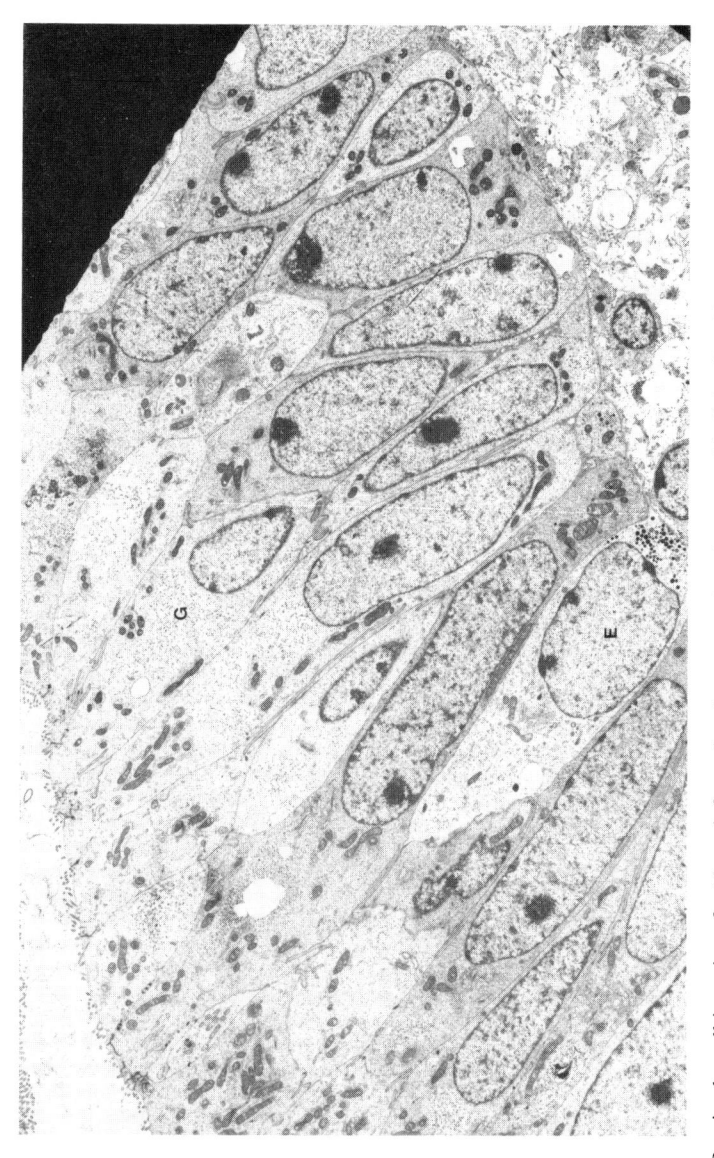

Fig. 2a Proximal small intestine of a 10 week fetus showing very early columnar epithelial cells with short microvilli junctional complexes, infra and supra nuclear glycogen deposits (G). A primitive endocrine cell is shown E (×4000)

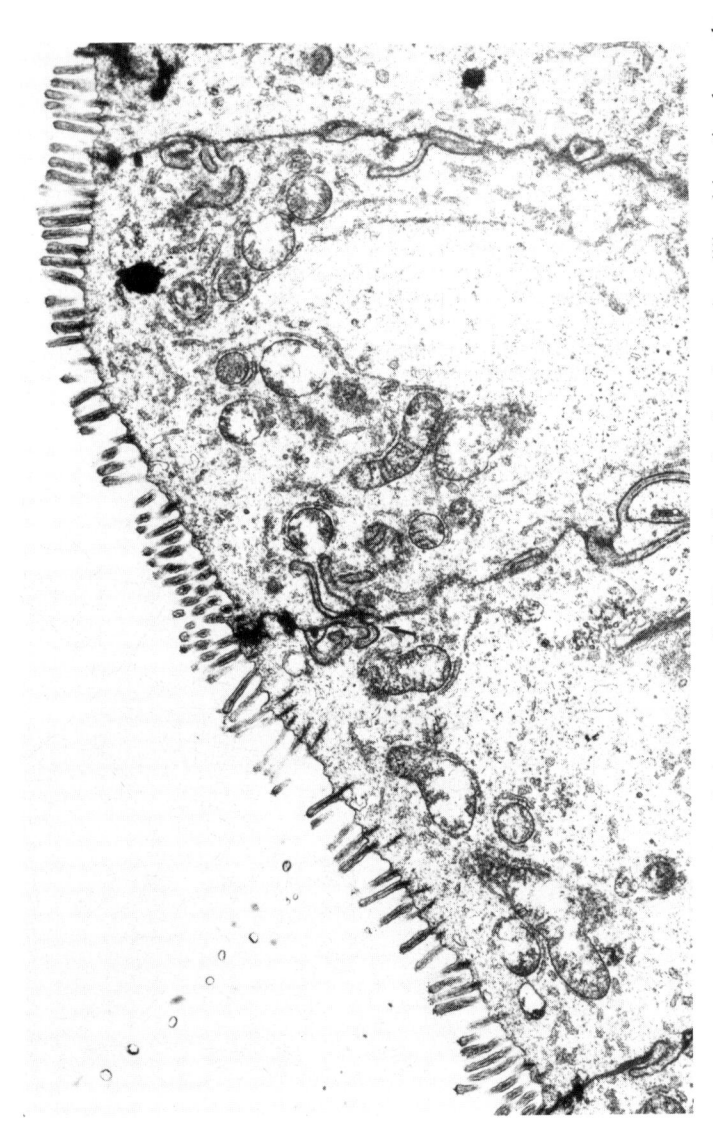

Fig. 2b The apical portion of a small intestinal enterocyte of a 10 week fetus showing short microvilli and junctional complexes (arrow) (×16 400)

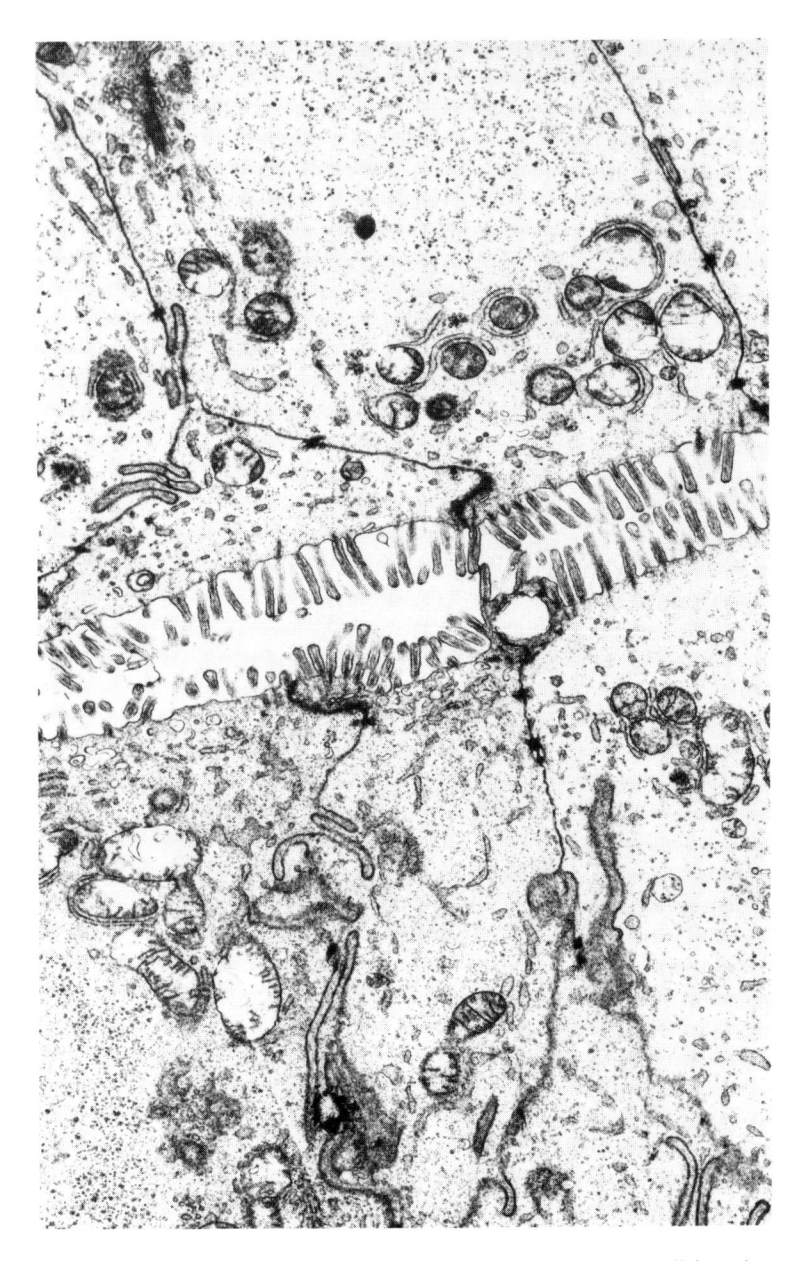

Fig. 2c A well developed secondary lumina in a 10 week fetal small intestine (× 16 400)

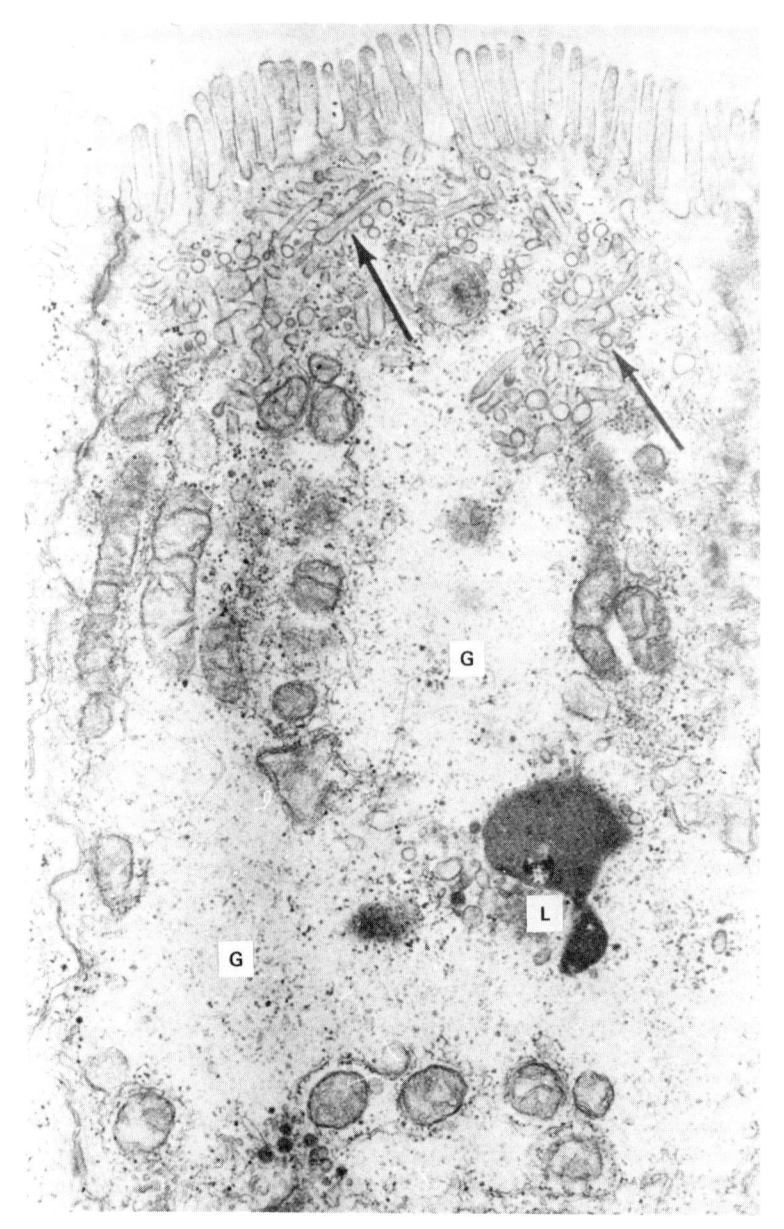

Fig. 2d The apical half of a villous absorptive cell from the small intestine of a 17 week human fetus showing a very abundant apical tubular system (arrows), glycogen (G) and lysosomes (L) (× 16 400). By 22–24 weeks apical tubular system will have disappeared.

Figure 2abc courtesy Professor BD Lake, Institute of Child Health, London gestation and studies using ^{51}Cr-tagged red blood cells have shown that the fetus swallows 13–16 mls/day of amniotic fluid at 20 weeks increasing to 450 ml per day at term.[10] In oesophageal motility studies in preterm infants, broad biphasic poorly propogated contractions are seen and it is likely that in the very preterm infant only very immature activity is present.[11,12] Similarly, lowered oesophageal pressure is markedly reduced in the very preterm infant. Paradoxically the development of effective nutritive sucking lags behind the development of oesophageal motility and is delayed until 33–35 weeks gestation.

Gastric emptying is poor in the very preterm infant and it has been shown that in the fasting state pressure generated in the gastric antrum at 27–28 weeks is low at 5–8 mmHg ($\sim$0.7–1.1 kPa) as compared with levels of 30 mmHg ($\sim$4.0 kPa) by term.[13] In preterm infants from 27–36 weeks gestation motor activity of the small intestine has been clearly defined by the use of multilumen manometric catheters to record both the magnitude and organisation of contractile activity.[13] Before 28 weeks gestation motor activity is of low magnitude (<4 mmHg, $\sim$0.5 kPa) and is apparently random, failing to show the same degree of organisation or propagation as is found in the older infant, where from 30–34 weeks clusters of phasic propagated contractions occur (the fetal pattern) and from 34 weeks to term cyclical phasic contractions (migrating motor complex pattern) develop. Nutritive sucking was noted to occur with the latter. In adults as absence of this activity is frequently associated with bacterial overgrowth and it is quite possible that the hypomotility of the preterm gut is a contributing factor to the development of necrotising enterocolitis. In one study pretreatment of the mother with beta-methasone resulted in an increase in duodenal pressure and contraction frequency which was most marked in infants between 26–29 weeks gestation. In infants with a central nervous system abnormality contractility was reduced by 50%.[14]

Little is known about colonic motility in the very preterm infant although in some a failure to evacuate the colonic contents results in abdominal distension which is only relieved by a rectal examination or glycerine suppository.

Immaturity of enteric neural, humoral and myogenic controls results in the reduced intestinal motility seen in the very preterm infant and in many enteral feeding has to be delayed until the controlling mechanisms develop.

Digestion, absorption, and secretion

Stomach—In one study hydrochloric acid is not found to any great extent in those born before 28 weeks gestation.[15] In others however acid secretion was not related to gestational age and acid secretion was present by 6 hours after birth.[16,17] Other gastric secretions pepsin and mucous are present before 28 weeks gestation.[18]

Pancreas—There is no data regarding pancreatic enzyme secretion in very preterm infant but as even at term pancreatic secretion is very low,[2] it is unlikely that much pancreatic digestion occurs.

Small and large intestine digestive enzymes

The brush border of the intestine possesses an integrated system for the final digestion and absorption of nutrients which is relatively well developed by 22–24 weeks gestation. Brush border disaccharidases develop as the microvillus appears in a craniocaudal direction which extends to the distal colon prior to 28 weeks. Recent studies using improved methods of fetal dating and enzyme activity of a brush border membrane fraction have clearly shown that α-glucosidases (maltase, sucrase–isomaltase are present at 12 weeks and reach 70% of adult values by 14 weeks gestation, whereas β-galactosidase (lactase) is present to 50% of adult values at 14 weeks gestation.[3] These data are at variance with earlier data[19] whereby it was suggested that lactase was only present in trace amounts until 32 weeks gestation, but are in keeping with clinical experience of tolerance to lactose in the very preterm infant. It is of interest, though the function is unknown, that α-glucosidases are present in colonic brush border until such time as colonic villi disappear.

Small peptides are hydrolysed by brush border and cytosolic peptidases. These peptidases seem to follow α-glucosidases in their pattern of development and distribution throughout the gut and like sucrase disappear from the colon in the last trimester.[25]

Small and large intestine—Absorption and secretion

Development of transporting function is closely integrated with morphogenesis and differentiation of crypt and villous columnar epithelial cells.

The appearance of specialised transport systems for aqueous organic solutes in the brush border membrane is associated with the development of junctional complexes, a microvillus as shown in Figure 2, and the transport enzymes Na^+/K^+-ATPase. and adenylate cyclase[26] and the intracellular protein calcium dependent regular protein or calmodulin[27]. Thus at 11–12 weeks gestation the morphological and biochemical development of the epithelium has proceeded in an integrated fashion to the point where specialised physiological function can occur—active Na^+ dependent co-transport of glucose and alanine has been studied in everted sacs constructed from jejunum and ileum of fetuses from 10–18 weeks gestation[28]. The active transport of both substances had increased three-fold by 18 weeks. Glucose kinetics showed a fall in Km to 1.8 mM by 21 weeks gestation and phloridzin sensitivity[29]. D-Xylose D-fructose and D-alanine were all transferred passively.[29] Thus from as early as 10 weeks, specific transport mechanisms are present which by 21 weeks are well developed, exhibiting stereo specificity, Na^+ dependency, electrogenic, active and obey saturation kinetics—all features of Na^+ co-transporting systems found in mature man. Whilst there is very little data between 24 and 28 weeks gestation studies in older preterm infants suggest a later rise in Km and V_{max}[20] which continues to adult life[21] and indicates increasing capacity to absorb substrates. Interestingly, in malnourished premature infants the rise in V_{max} was not as marked.[20]

Little is known regarding other electrolyte transport mechanisms but several facts suggest their presence. Transmural potential difference (p.d.) measurements show the presence of a small endogenous p.d. mucosa negative to serosa which has marked sodium dependence. Reversal of the polarity of the p.d. on lowering the Na^+ concentration of the bathing solution on the mucosal side, which increased in magnitude as the concentration of Na^+ fell, indicates that the pathways through which Na^+ moved down its electrochemical gradient are negatively charged. Increases in endogenous p.d. with gestational age suggests increasing numbers of these transport sites as maturation proceeds. The presence of hydramnios in the second and third trimesters in mothers of infants with both congenital chloridorrhoea[22] and Na^+/H^+ exchange deficiency[23] suggests the presence of Na^+/H^+ and Cl^-/HCO_3^- exchange mechanisms in very preterm infants.

No formal studies of secretion have been carried out in fetal intestine but activation of adenylate cyclase in fetal intestine by cholera toxin[24] clearly indicates the presence of specific receptors and the metabolic processes required for this keystep in secretion.

The colon is an organ of conservation of salt and water. In older preterm infnats (30–34 weeks gestation) electrogenic absorption of Na^+ has been demonstrated but not Cl^-/HCO_3^- exchange.[30] A comparison with renal Na^+ handling and the presence and response to hyperaldosteronism suggests that at this age the colon is the more importaint salt retaining organ.[31] However, there is no data regarding the very preterm infant or the nature of transport in the villi of the colon at this stage of development.

Study over recent years of colonic carcinoma cells lines may provide some insights into the function of early fetal colonic epithelium. Such cells have many of the characteristics of fetal colon with similar glycogen and sucrase-isomaltase content. Ion transport is clearly present and electrogenic Na^+ transfer has been demonstrated.[32]

CONCLUSION

By 22 weeks gestation, the fetal intestinal mucosa resembles the adult and has some of the same functional capabilities. Many of the digestive enzymes associated with villous absorptive cells and the distribution of endocrine cells attain adult levels and patterns towards the end of the second trimester. However, other functions such as absorption and motor activity are less well developed, as is the function of accessory organs the pancreas and biliary system. As a consequence of such disparate development of function a knowledge of the pattern of development is essential for the provision of optimal nutritional care of very preterm infants.

REFERENCES

1 Arey LB. Developmental Anatomy. Philadelphia: Saunders, 1974
2 Grand RJ, Watkins JB, Torti FM. Development of the human gastrointestinal tract. Gastroenterology 1976; 70: 790–810
3 Lacroix B, Kedinger M, Simon-Assmann P, Haffen K. Early organogenesis of human small intestine: Scanning electro microscopy and brush border enzymology. Gut 1984; 25: 925–930
4 Lacroix B, Kedinger M, Simon-Assmann P, Rousset M, Zweibaum A, Haffen K. Developmental pattern of brush border enzymes in the human fetal colon. Correlation with some morphogenic events. Early Hum Dev 1984; 9: 95–103
5 Moxey PC, Trier JS. Endocrine cells in the human fetal small intestine. Cell Tissue Res 1977; 183: 33–50
6 Moxey PC, Trier JS. Specialised cell types in the human fetal small intestine. Anat Rec 1978; 191: 269–286
7 Von Rosen L, Podjaski B, Bettman L, Otto H. Observations on the ultrastructure and function of the so-called microfold or membranous cells (M cells) by means of peroxidase as a tracer. Virchows Arch [Pathol Anat] 1981; 90: 289–312

8 McLain CR. Amniography studies on the gastrointestinal motility of the human fetus. Am J Obstet Gynaecol 1963; 86: 1079–1087
9 Dunn PM. Intestinal obstruction in the newborn with special reference to transient functional ileus associated with respiratory distress syndrome. Arch Dis Child 1963; 38: 459–467
10 Prichard JA. Fetal swallowing and amniotic fluid volume. Obstet Gynaecol 1966; 28: 606–610
11 Gryboski JD. The swallowing mechanism of the neonate 1. Esophageal and gastric motility. Pediatrics 1965; 35: 445–452
12 Diamant NE. Development of esophageal function. Am Rev Respir Dis 1985; 131 (Suppl) :S29–S32
13 Bisset WM, Watt JB, Rivers JPA, Milla PJ. The ontogeny of fasting small intestinal motor activity in the human infant. Gut 1988; 29: 483–488
14 Morriss FH, Moore M, Weisbrodt NW, West MS. Ontogenic development of gastrointestinal motility: IV. Duodenal contractions in preterm infants. Pediatrics 1986; 78: 1106–1113
15 Ahn CI, Kim YJ. Acidity and volume of gastric contents in the first week of life. J Korean Med Assoc 1963; 6: 948–950
16 Harries JT, Fraser AJ. The acidity of the gastric contents of premature babies during the first fourteen days of life. Biol Neonate 1968; 12: 186–193
17 Hyman P, Clarke DD, Everett S, et al. Gastric acid secretory function in preterm infants. J Pediatr 1985; 106: 467–471
18 Werner B. Peptic and tryptic capacity of the digestive glands in newborns. Acta Paediatr Scand 1948; 35 (Suppl 70): 1
19 Lebenthal E, Lee PC. Glucoamylase and disaccharidase activities in normal subjects and in patients with mucosal injury of the small intestine. J Pediatr 1980; 97: 389–393
20 McNeish AS, Ducker DA, Warren IF, Davies DP, Harran MJ, Hughes CA. The influence of gestational age and size on the absorption of D-xylase and D-glucose from the small intestine of the human neonate. In: Development of Mammalian Absorptive Processes: Ciba Foundation Symposium. Amsterdam: Excerpta Media, 1979: pp. 267–275
21 Milla PJ. Aspects of fluid and electrolyte absorption in the newborn. J Pediatr Gastroenterol Nutr 1983; 2: 272–276
22 Holmberg C, Perheentupa J, Launiala K, Hallman N. Congenital chloride diarrhoea. Arch Dis Child 1977; 52: 255–267
23 Booth IW, Stange G, Murer H, Fenton TR, Milla PJ. Defective jejunal brush border Na^+/H^+ exchange: a cause of congenital secretory diarrhoea. Lancet 1985; i: 1066–1069
24 Grand RJ, Torti FM, Jaksina S. Development of intestinal adenyl cyclase and its response to cholera enterotoxin. J Clin Invest 1973; 52: 5053–2059
25 Lindberg T. Intestinal dipeptidases; characteristics development and distribution of intestinal dipeptidases in the human foetus. Clin Sci 1966; 30: 505–515
26 Rosenberg IH. Development of fetal guinea pig small intestine amino acid transport and Na K ATPase. Fed Proc 1966; 25: 456–859
27 Rochette-Egly C, Lacroix B, Pflieger H, Doffoel M, Kedinger M, Haffen K. Calmodulin in normal and cystic fibrosis human intestine at different development stages. Gut 1988 29: 571–579
28 Koldovsky O, Heringova A, Jirsova V, Jivasek JE, Uher J. Transport of glucose against a concentration gradient in everted sacs of jejunum and ileum of human fetuses. Gastroenterology 1965; 48: 185–187
29 Levin RJ, Koldovsky O, Hoskova J, Jirsova V. Electrical activity across human foetal small intestine associated with absorption processes. Gut 1968; 9: 206–213
30 Jenkins HR, Fenton TR, McIntosh NI, Dillon MJ, Milla PJ. Development of epithelial electrolyte transport processes in early childhood. Pediatr Res 1987; 22 Abstract No. 6: 97

31 Jenkins HR, Fenton TR, Savage MO, Dillon MJ, Milla PJ. Development of colonic transport processes: the influence of aldosterone. Gut 1986; 27: Abstract A 1283–1284

32 Grasset E, Pinto M, Dussaulx E, Zweibaum A, Desjeux JF. Epithelial properties of human colonic carcinoma cell line CaCo–2: electrical parameters. Am J Physiol 1984; 242: C260–267

Cardiovascular adaptation in the very immature infant

Andrew R Wilkinson
Neonatal Unit, Department of Paediatrics John Radcliffe Hospital, Oxford, UK

> At term the fetus has developed the biochemical, anatomical and physiological means whereby critical adjustments in the circulation can be made smoothly. When birth takes place two thirds of the way through gestation, or earlier, the baby must attempt to adapt to an extra-uterine existence without the benefit of these mechanisms. Some can be triggered effectively but many are labile and the clinical condition fluctuates between a fetal and neonatal state.
>
> Little is known about the human at this early stage of life and until recently much of our knowledge has been inferred from experiments in animals. Non-invasive techniques of investigation are revealing more information about the circulation and clinical management has been successful in improving the outlook for these babies enormously. However, much more remains to be understood in order to suggest safe and effective ways of intervening to support the newborn with a compromised circulation postnatally.

The major changes that occur in the circulation at birth, particularly the increase in blood flow to the lungs, must be initiated even though the control mechanisms are not fully developed. It is not surprising therefore that the very immature infant often shows signs of difficulty in adapting to extra-uterine life. Very little is known about the human myocardium and cardiovascular control at this stage of gestation. Most of our information about the physiology of the fetal circulation has been derived from experiments in animals, though recent 2-dimensional ultrasound and Doppler studies have begun to give more direct information about the circulation in the human fetus. Nevertheless, most of the information relates to mature babies which should not be applied to the very immature without some qualification.

The circulation adapts throughout pregnancy to the vital role of transporting oxygen, heat and hormones, to the cells and of removing carbon dioxide and other waste products. Changes in the proportion of the ventricular output distributed to various organs, the body, limbs and placenta, in relation to fetal growth occurs but the predominant changes are thought to take place during the third trimester.[1] We still know very little about the mechanisms responsible for these changes and how, if at all, they could be harnessed and manipulated in ways that might lead to improvements in postnatal life. When development is interrupted less than two thirds of the way through gestation the whole timetable of ontogeny is disrupted.

This chapter describes the physiology of the fetal circulation and outlines the major changes that occur after birth and the clinical problems that arise in the immature newborn when the adaptation is less than complete.

FETAL CIRCULATION

Distribution of blood flow

Oxygenation of the fetal blood takes place in the placenta and the partial pressure is 4.0–4.7 kPa (30–35 mmHg) in the umbilical venous blood. Recent studies in fetal lambs have shown that about 55% of umbilical venous blood passes through the ductus venosus, the remainder being distributed to both right and left lobes of the liver.[2] When umbilical blood flow is reduced, flow through the ductus venosus is increased proportionately—probably as the result of active dilatation of the ductus venosus or alternatively vaso-constriction in the hepatic circulation, or both.[3] At the junction of the ductus venosus and the left hepatic vein with the inferior vena cava there is a thin membrane protruding from the lower edge of the orifice which directs the well oxygenated blood towards the left and posteriorly.[4] This blood with a high oxygen content, streams within the inferior vena cava preferentially towards the foramen ovale. After mixing with a small fraction of superior vena caval blood it passes through the foramen ovale to the left atrium and hence to the left ventricle. The foramen ovale is maintained in the fetus by the considerable flow of blood through it. Blood leaving the left ventricle has a higher Po_2, approximately 3.3 kPa (25 mmHg) than the right ventricle, 2.4 kPa (18 mmHg). The left ventricle ejects about 35% of the combined ventricular output.[5] Of this 85% supplies the coronary arteries, brain, head, neck, and arms. The remainder passes through the aortic isthmus to mix with blood from the ductus arteriosus. Blood returning from the head, brain and upper body in the superior vena cava is desaturated, Po_2 1.6–1.9 kPa (12–14 mmHg) and passes into the right atrium where it mixes with the inferior vena caval blood that has not passed through the foramen ovale. After passing through the tricuspid valve to the right ventricle this mixed blood has a Po_2 of 2.4–2.5 kPa (18–19 mmHg). In fetal life the majority of blood leaving the right ventricle is directed through the widely patent ductus arteriosus to the aorta. Only 7% passes to the lungs. About 35% of the mixed blood in the descending aorta is distributed to the lower body and legs but the majority flows to the placental circulation with its low vascular resistance through the two umbilical arteries which arise from the internal iliac arteries. Blood is then distributed to the intervillus spaces of the placenta to be re-oxygenated.

The fetal myocardium and cardiac output

Growth and development of the heart continues throughout pregnancy and after birth but little is known about the structure and function *in-utero* in humans. Most data are available from experiments in fetal sheep with chronically implanted catheters, but the majority of studies have been carried out late in pregnancy. The contractility of the isolated fetal myocaridal tissue has been found to be less than in adults.[6,7] Biochemical investigations show fewer contractile elements, the sarcomeres, and the calcium, which regulates the tension during contraction, is accumulated relatively slowly.[8] Ultrastructural studies show that the ratio of contractile to noncontractile tissue in the newborn myocardium is noticeably less than in adults.[6,9] Despite these findings of immaturity in the fetal myocardium, the pumping performance is impressive.[10] The stroke volume of the newborn heart, expressed as ml/kg body weight, is twice that of the adult.[11] As the heart rate is also approximately double the rate in the adult, the cardiac output is four times greater in the newborn, approximately 180–240 mg/min/kg. Experimental evidence that there is little ability to increase stroke volume suggesting that the fetal heart is functioning maximally must be balanced against the immediate postnatal increase in myocardial contractility which can lead to a doubling of left ventricular output. Sympathetic stimulation does not seem to be responsible[10] though it has been suggested that cooling may stimulate neurohormonal responses.[12] Recent studies suggest that triiodothyronine (T3) may be important, particularly during late gestation, in the maturation of the fetal myocardium.[13] Whether the T3 effect alters cardiac myosin adenosine triphosphate activity[14] or is responsible for the development of a new type of myosin is not known.[15] The extremely preterm infant will not have benefited from the changes that T3 brings about in the myocardium. Further study is needed of this hormonal effect.

Refinement of the non-invasive range-gated, pulsed Doppler and echocardiographic techniques has enabled some measurements to be made in the human newborn. These suggest that cardiac output in babies less than 1000g is as high as 260 ml min^{-1} kg^{-1} [16,17] Providing the limitations and potential errors are taken into account this direct information, hitherto unobtainable, about the human newborn is going to assist in managing babies with disturbed cardiovascular adaptation to extra-uterine life.

Autonomic control

The fetal myocardium has been studied by histochemical, biochemical and pharmacological methods to determine the ontogony of autonomic control. Considerable species differences have been found making it difficult to speculate about the human heart. Limited studies have shown that although acetylcholine release can be stimulated from as early as 13 weeks, the ganglia are immature suggesting that vagal transmission begins later.[18] Parasympathetic neurotransmission tends to develop before sympathetic and has been shown in fetal lambs at 60% of gestation.[19] Circulating catecholamines may influence sympathetic tone and modulate myocardial control in the fetus.[6,20] However, even at term innervation is incomplete and continues postnatally, so at the beginning of the third trimester the potential for an imbalance between sympathetic and parasympathetic stimulation exists.

Baroreceptor control

It is not clear to what extent baroreceptor reflexes play any part in the control of the fetal and neonatal circulation though postnatally sensitivity increases and in the adult baroreceptors plays a major role. Developmental changes have been clearly shown in fetal lambs from 50% of gestation to term but immaturity of neuronal development and neurotransmission at any point in the reflex may be responsible for an inadequate response. Some experimental work suggests wide variation in responses with a gradual maturation *in utero* but other workers have not been able to confirm this.[21,22] Other studies show that the change in heart rate that results from changes in blood pressure may be masked by increased vagal tone.[23,24] These findings may be relevant to the interpretation of heart rate and blood pressure changes in the extremely preterm infant.

Chemoreceptor function

The aortic chemoreceptors respond to hypoxaemia and acidosis giving rise to bradycardia whilst cardiac output and umbilical blood flow is preserved in the fetus.[25] On the other hand, the carotid chemoreceptors were, until recently, thought to be inactive *in utero* and to respond only to extreme hypoxaemia. However, recent studies have shown that in intact unanaesthetised fetuses at 80% of gestation, acute hypoxaemia induced by injection of sodium cyanide, causes bradycardia, respiratory effort but no consistent change in blood pressure.[26] After birth hypoxia leads to a tachycardia and increase in cardiac output associated with respiratory effort.

PERINATAL CHANGES IN THE CIRCULATION

As soon as the umbilical cord is clamped there is an increase in peripheral resistance and a decrease in venous return to the right atrium. The ductus venosus closes, though the factors which initiate this are not known. Patency may be demonstrated up to 7 days after birth but little if any blood is thought to pass through this channel after birth. Immediately after birth the simultaneous decrease in pulmonary resistance, which facilitates an increase in pulmonary blood flow and rise in left atrial pressure, and the decrease in inferior vena caval pressure, leads to closure of the foramen ovale. The pressure in the left atrium normally exceeds that in the right atrium by 1–2 mmHg. Only if pressure in the right atrium exceeds that in the left atrium will blood again flow through the foramen ovale. Nevertheless permanent closure of the foramen ovale occurs only after some months.

Right-to-left shunting will occur whenever this gradient is reversed and right atrial pressure exceeds that in the left atrium. In the very immature this is usually related to severe surfactant deficiency when the pulmonary disease leads to hypoxaemia and acidosis. Both are factors which maintain pulmonary vasoconstriction thus maintaining elevated pulmonary arterial and right ventricular pressure. The high right atrial pressure that results may lead to a right-to-left shunt through the foramen ovale of up to 50% of venous return. Other pulmonary disease in the immature, particularly infection, will have similar effects. Thus the distribution of blood may be maintained through the fetal channels, the foramen ovale and the ductus arteriosus, when pulmonary hypertension is persistent. This state may mimic congenital heart disease but in the immature is much more commonly associated with severe lung disease.

Heart rate and blood pressure

It is still impossible to define exactly what heart rate and blood pressure should be regarded as 'normal' in such an abnormal situation as a baby born three months before term. Some studies have given details of the expected values in babies without apparent cardiopulmonary disease but some of the reports have not distinguished between appropriately grown and growth-retarded babies. The latter are likely to have a more mature autonomic nervous system and the heart rate is correspondingly lower.

At birth heart rate in the extremely preterm is approximately 160 beats per minute and no difference has been found with changes in sleep state.[27] Variability in heart rate reflecting autonomic development has been studied in babies with birthweights less than 1000g and correlations made with disease states.[28] Blood pressure has been measured directly through umbilical arterial catheters[29] or noninvasively by Doppler ultrasound and oscillometric methods.[30] The latter is unreliable in very low birthweight infants as it tends to over-estimate pressure in hypotensive infants.[31] Values reported for infants with birth weights less than 1000g suggest a mean value of approximately 30 mmHg during the first day after birth.[28,29] Perinatal asphyxia and severe hyaline membrane disease are frequently associated with hypotension and clinical signs of shock. Myocardial function may be improved by an infusion of an inotropic drug such as dopamine. A dose of 2–8 μg kg^{-1} min^{-1} is usually sufficient. Drugs used in the intensive care nursery may have marked effects on blood pressure. Mydriatics lead to a significant and sustained rise in blood pressure.[32] Paralysis with pancuronium leads to increased catecholamine secretion and may elevate heart rate and blood pressure[33] though other reports describe unpredictable effects on blood pressure.[34] The relationship between arterial blood pressure and cerebral blood flow is complex. Initial reports that fluctuations in arterial pressure are associated with an increased incidence of intracranial haemorrhage in preterm infants[35] have been followed by the suggestion that ischaemia after hypotension is potentially far more damaging to the developing brain.[36,37] Some reports suggest an increased incidence of episodes of hypertension in very low birth weight infants with intracranial haemorrhage but others have not found this.[38,39]

THE DUCTUS ARTERIOSUS

Patency of the ductus arteriosus is actively maintained *in utero* by the influence of prostaglandins, particularly PGE$_1$ and PGE$_2$ but the sensitivity of the ductal tissue to the effects of prostaglandins decreases throughout gestation. Although produced in relatively small quantities, when compared with other prostaglandins, PGE$_2$ is the most potent dilator of the ductus arteriosus. The precise source of circulating PGE$_2$ is not known. Although the ductus is able to synthesize and catabolize PGE$_2$ very little is produced at the low oxygen tension prevailing in the fetus.[40] Significant amounts probably come from the placenta. Pulmonary metabolism and plasma clearance rates are lower in early gestation when compared with term. Thus the levels of PGE$_2$ are higher in the preterm than later in gestation.[41] This has been found prenatally in preterm fetal lambs and the levels are maintained postnatally for a number of hours.[42] After birth at term the ductus arteriosus constricts and functional closure has occurred in 50% by 24 hours, 90% by 48 hours and all by 96 hours.[43] The ductus closes first by contraction of smooth muscle and then by breakdown of the endothelium with proliferative connective tissue changes leading to a permanent closure. The rise in oxygen tension in arterial blood is the most important factor responsible for ductal constriction. Hence after inflation of the lungs the mechanisms which initiate pulmonary vascular dilatation and the increase in pulmonary blood flow are intimately related to ductal closure.

The vasoconstrictor substances, leukotrienes C4 and D4, products of 5'lipoxygenase metabolism of arachidonic acid may control pulmonary vascular tone *in utero*.[44] Inhibition of leukotrienes may be vital to normal postnatal adaptation but the mechanisms will not be developed in the extremely preterm infant. In the future specific inhibitors of leukotrienes may have a therapeutic role.[45]

The mechanisms whereby oxygen produces constriction of the ductus is not fully understood. Oxygenation of cytochrome a_3 and the production of adenosine triphosphate may be responsible by leading to alterations in intracellular calcium concentrations. Thromboxane (TxA_2) produced in the lungs is a vasoconstrictor and although levels increase perinatally it is very labile and unlikely to have a specific effect on the ductus arteriosus.[46] The role of sympathetic and parasympathetic innervation of the ductus is controversial. Acetylcholine can produce constriction and noradrenaline nerve terminals have been described in the media. These penetrate further in the more mature fetuses but the concentration of catecholamines necessary to produce constriction is far greater than physiological levels.[47] The vasoactive peptide bradykinin and other factors such as histamine and 5-hydroxytryptamine do produce constriction of the mature ductus in vitro but the effect of the preterm ductus is minimal.[48]

In the very immature persistent patency of the ductus arteriosus (PDA) is common. A large haemodynamically significant PDA has been reported in 42% of infants with a birth weight less than 1000g.[49] Surfactant deficiency predisposes to this condition. Initially persistence of high pulmonary pressure may maintain the right-to-left flow through the ductus arteriosus and in these babies the ductus does not constrict. Later PDA leads to the development of a left-to-right shunt and a large recirculation of blood through the lungs. Perinatal asphyxia and excessive fluid therapy may lead to PDA independent of lung disease. Intrauterine growth retardation and maternal steroid therapy reduce the incidence, possibly by a direct effect stimulating the ductal response to oxygen and decreasing sensitivity to PGE_2.[50] Endogenous glucocorticoids may reduce the sensitivity of the ductus to PGE_2 and play a role in triggering the biochemical changes that determine ductal constriction. An infusion of hydrocortisone into preterm fetal lambs leads to a reduced calibre of the ductus postnatally and prenatal maternal steroid therapy reduces the incidence of PDA in preterm infants at all gestations.[50] This effect appears to be independent of the effect of steroids on lung function. In term infants responsiveness of the ductus arteriosus both to hypoxia and to PGE_2 decreases rapidly after birth and seems to be due to the reduced luminal blood flow. Once constricted ischaemic change in the wall occurs and permanent closure ensues. However, in as many as a third of preterm infants the ductus may re-open after initial closure. Continued responsiveness to PGE_2 and the higher circulating concentration may be responsible. This in turn may be the result of low circulating levels of thyroid hormone in the extremely preterm.[46]

Diagnosis

Signs of a significant PDA usually develop after 3–7 days of life. A murmur, usually confined to systole, may be present though is commonly intermittent. Ventilatory support may need to be increased. A widened pulse pressure with tachycardia and bounding pulses develops. The heart size may be increased on chest radiograph but this is not invariable. Echocardiography is useful, first in excluding other congenital heart disease, and then M mode may show an increased ratio between the diameter of the left atrium and the aortic route. Usually less than 1.0, this ratio may be in excess of 1:1.5. The patent ductus may be visualized by 2-dimensional echocardiography and the shunt of blood documented by contrast or Doppler studies.

Management

Fluid intake should be restricted to about 100–120 ml kg^{-1} d^{-1} and then gradually liberalized providing the signs do not progress. If florid signs of cardiac failure are present at the time of diagnosis a diuretic should be given. Chlorothiazide, 20–40 mg/kg 12 hourly is effective. Although commonly used, frusemide should be reserved for emergency intravenous therapy as there is work showing that this drug can promote prostaglandin synthesis thereby possibly prolonging patency of the ductus.[52] Ventilation should be adjusted to avoid hypoxia and optimal oxygen carrying capacity maintained by correcting anaemia. Serum electrolytes must be measured 12 hourly and supplementation adjusted appropriately.

Agents such as indomethacin that inhibit the synthesis of prostaglandins are effective in promoting ductal closure. In a large multicentre randomised trial, the very immature infants of less than 28 weeks gestation with a haemodynamically significant shunt who were given indomethacin were 3 times more likely to have effective closure of the duct than those who only received fluid restriction.[53] The most common regime is to give 3 doses of indomethacin 0.2 mg kg^{-1} at intervals of 12 hours. However, because indomethacin is metabolized more rapidly as postnatal age increases some have recommended reducing the dose if the drug is given at less than 48 hours of age and increasing to 0.25 mg kg^{-1} after 8 days. There does not appear to be merit to giving 'early' prophylactic indomethacin into *all* low birth weight babies. One study showed a high incidence of side effects particularly when serum indomethacin concentrations exceeded 1.0 µg/ml.[54] To prevent relapse repeated doses for as long as a week has been suggested but considering the effect that indomethacin has of reducing cerebral blood flow more studies are needed before this approach can be regarded as safe.[55,56]

REFERENCES

1. Rudolph AM, Heymann MA. The circulation of the fetus in utero. Circ Res 1967; 21: 163–184
2. Edelstone DI, Rudolph AM, Heymann MA. Liver and ductus venosus blood flows in fetal lambs in utero. Circ Res 1978; 42: 426–433
3. Edelstone DI, Rudolph AM, Heymann MA. Effects of hypoxemia and decreasing umbilical flow on liver and ductus venosus blood flows in fetal lambs. Am J Physiol 1980; 238: H656–H663
4. Bristow J, Rudolph AM, Itskovitz J. A preparation for studying liver blood flow, oxygen consumption, and metabolism in the fetal lamb in utero. J Dev Physiol 1981; 3: 255–266
5. Heymann MA, Creasy RK, Rudolph AM. Quantitation of blood flow pattern in the foetal lamb in utero. In: Foetal and Neonatal Physiology (Proceedings of the Sir Joseph Barcroft Centenary Symposium). Cambridge: Cambridge University Press, 1973: pp. 129–135
6. Friedman WF. The intrinsic properties of the developing heart. In: Friedman WF, Lesch M, Sonnenblick EH, eds. Neonatal Heart Disease. New York: Grune and Stratton, 1973: pp. 21–49
7. Davies P, Dewar J, Tynan M, Ward R. Postnatal developmental changes in the length-tension relationship of cat papillary muscles. J Physiol (London) 1975; 253: 95–102
8. Nayler WG, Fassold E. Calcium accumulating and ATPase activity of cardiac sacoplasmic reticulum before and after birth. Cardiovasc Res 1977; 11: 231–237
9. Olivetti G, Anversa P, Loud AV. Morphometric study of early postnatal development in the left and right ventricular myocardium of the rat. II. Tissue growth, capillary growth and sacroplasmic alterations. Circ Res 1980; 46: 503–512
10. Klopfenstein HS, Rudolph AM. Postnatal changes in the circulation, and responses to volume loading in sheep. Circ Res 1978; 42: 839–845
11. Berman W, Musselman J. Myocardial performance in the newborn lamb. Am J Physiol 1979; 237: H66–H70
12. Rudolph AM, Iwamoto HS, Teitel DF. Perinatal cardiovascular adjustments. In: Jones CT, ed. Fetal and Neonatal Development. Perinatology Press, 1988: 598–604

13 Breall JA, Rudolph AM, Heymann MA. Role of thyroid hormone in postnatal circulatory and metabolic adjustments. J Clin Invest 1984; 73: 1418–1424
14 Morkin E. Stimulation of cardiac myosin adenosine triphosphatase in thyrotoxicosis. Circ Res 1979; 44: 1–7
15 Fink IL, Morkin E. Evidence for a new cardiac myosin species in thyrotoxic rabbits. FEBS Lett 1977; 81: 391–394
16 Alverson DC, Eldridge M, Dillon T, Yabek SM, Berman W Jr. Noninvasive pulsed Doppler determination of cardiac output in neonates and children. J Pediatr 1982; 101: 46–50
17 Walther FJ, Siassi B, Ramadan NA, Ananda AK, Wu PYK. Pulsed Doppler determinations of cardiac output in neonates: normal standards for clinical use. Pediatrics 1985; 76: 829–833
18 Walker D. Functional development of the autonomic innervation of the human fetal heart. Biol Neonate 1975; 25: 31–43
19 Lebowitz EA, Novick JS, Rudolph AM. Development of myocardial sympathetic innervation in the fetal lamb. Pediatr Res 1972; 6: 887–893
20 Tynan M, Davies P, Sheridan D. Postnatal maturation of noradrenaline uptake and release in cat papillary muscles. Cardiovasc Res 1977; 11: 206–209
21 Shinebourne EA, Vapaavouri EK, Williams RL, Heymann MA, Rudolph AM. Development of baroreflex activity in unanaesthetised foetal and newborn lambs. Circ Res 1972; 31: 710–718
22 Dawes GS, Johnston BM, Walker DW. Relationship of arterial pressure and heart rate in fetal newborn and adult sheep. J Physiol (London) 1980; 309; 405–417
23 Macdonald AA, Rose J, Heymann MA, Rudolph AM. Heart rate response of fetal and adult sheep to hemorrhage stress. Am J Physiol 1980; 239: H789–H793
24 Wood C, Walker AM, Yardley R. Acceleration of the fetal heart rate. Am J Obstet Gynecol 1979; 134: 523–527
25 Dawes GS, Duncan SL, Lewis BV, Merlet CL, Owen-Thomas JB, Reeves JT. Cyanide stimulation of the systematic arterial chemoreceptors in foetal lambs. J Physiol (London) 1969; 201: 117–128
26 Itskovitz J, Rudolph AM. Cardiorespiratory response to cyanide of arterial chemoreceptors in fetal lambs. Am J Physiol 1987; 252: H916–H922
27 Siassi B, Hodgman J, Cabal L, Hon EH. Cardiac and respiratory activity in relation to gestation and sleep states in newborn infants. Pediatr Res 1979; 13: 1163–1166
28 Cabal LA, Larrazabal C, Siassi B. Hemodynamic variables in infants weighing less than 1000 grams. Clin Perinatol 1986; 13: 327–338
29 Versmold HT, Kitterman JA, Phibbs RH, Gregory GA, Tooley WH. Aortic blood pressure during the first 12 hours of life in infants with birth weight 610 to 4220 grams. Pediatrics 1981; 67: 607–613
30 Dweck H, Reynolds DW, Cassady G. Indirect blood pressure measurements in newborns. Am J Dis Child 1974; 127: 492–494
31 Diprose GK, Evans DH, Archer LNJ, Levene MI. Dinamap fails to detect hypotension in very low birthweight infants. Arch Dis Child 1986; 61: 771–773
32 Lees BJ, Cabal LA. Increased blood pressure following pupillary dilatation with 2.5% phenylephrine hydrochloride in preterm infants. Pediatrics 1981; 68: 231–234
33 Cabal LA, Siassi B, Artal R, Gonzalez F, Hodgman J, Plajstek C. Cardiovascular and catecholamine changes after administration of pancuronium in distressed neonates. Pediatrics 1985; 75: 284–287
34 Reynolds EOR, Hope PL, Whitehead MD. Muscle relaxation and periventricular hemorrhage. N Engl J Med 1985; 313: 955–956
35 Perlman JM, McMenamin JB, Volpe JJ. Fluctuating cerebral bloodflow velocity in respiratory-distress syndrome. N Engl J Med 1983; 309: 204–209

36 Young RSK, Hernandez MJ, Yagel SK. Selective reduction of blood flow to white matter during hypotension in newborn dogs: A possible mechanism of periventricular leukomalacia. Ann Neurol 1982; 12: 445–448
37 Weindling AM, Rochefort MJ, Calvert SA, Fok T-F, Wilkinson AR. Development of cerebral palsy after ultrasonographic detection of periventricular cysts in the newborn. Dev Med Child Neurol 1985; 27: 800–806
38 Bancalari E, Gerhardt T, Feller R, Gannon J, Melnick G, Abdenour G. Muscle relaxation during IPPV in prematures with RDS. Pediatr Res 1980; 14: 590
39 Weindling AM, Wilkinson AR, Cook J, Calvert SA, Fok T-F, Rochefort MJ. Perinatal events which precede periventricular haemorrhage and leukomalacia in the newborn. Br J Obstet Gynaecol 1985; 92: 1218–1223
40 Clyman RI, Mauray F, Demers LM et al. Does oxygen regulate prostaglandin induced relaxation in the lamb ductus arteriosus? Prostaglandins 1980; 19: 489–498
41 Clyman RI, Mauray F, Heymann MA et al. Effect of gestation age on pulmonary metabolism of prostaglandin E_1 and E_2. Prostaglandins 1981; 21: 505–513
42 Clyman RI, Mauray F, Roman C et al. Effect of gestational age on ductus arteriosus response to circulating prostaglandin E_2. J Pediatr 1983; 102: 907–911
43 Gentile R, Stevenson JG, Dooley T, Franklin D, Kawabori I, Pearlman A. Pulsed Doppler echocardiographic determination of time of ductal closure in normal newborn infants. J Pediatr 1981; 98: 443–448
44 Schreiber MD, Heymann MA, Soifer SJ. The differential effects of leukotriene C_4 and D_4 on the pulmonary and systemic circulations in newborn lambs. Pediatr Res 1987; 21: 176–182
45 Lebidois J, Soifer SJ, Clyman RI, Heymann MA. Piriprost: A putative leukotriene synthesis inhibitor increases pulmonary blood flow in fetal lambs. Pediatr Res 1987; 22: 350–354
46 Clyman RI. Ductus arteriosus: Current theories of prenatal and postnatal regulation. Sem Perinatol 1987; 11: 64–71
47 Aronson SG, Gennser G, Owman C et al. Innervation and contractile response of the human ductus arteriosus. Eur J Pharmacol 1970; 11: 178–186
48 Friedman WF, Printz MP, Kirkpatrick SE, Hoskins EJ. The vasoactivity of the fetal lamb ductus arteriosus studied in utero. Pediatr Res 1983; 17: 331–337
49 Ellison MD, Peckham GJ, Lang P et al. Evaluation of the preterm infant for patent ductus arteriosus. Pediatrics 1983; 71: 364–372
50 Clyman RI, Ballard PL, Sniderman S, Ballard RA, Roth R, Heymann MA, Granberg JP. Prenatal administration of betamethasone for prevention of patent ductus arteriosus. J Pediatr 1981; 98: 123–126
51 Clyman RI, Mauray F, Roman C, Rudolph MD, Heymann MA. Effects of an antenatal glucocorticoid administration on ductus arteriosus of preterm lambs. Am J Physiol 1981; 241: H415–H420
52 Green TP, Thompson TR, Johnson DE, Lock JE. Furosemide promotes patent ductus arteriosus in premature infants with respiratory distress syndrome. N Engl J Med 1983; 308: 743–748
53 Gersony WM, Peckham GJ, Ellison RC, Miettinen OS, Nadas AS. Effects of indomethacin in premature infants with patent ductus arteriosus: Results of a national collaborative study. J Pediatr 1983; 102: 895–906
54 Rennie JM, Doyle J, Cooke RWI. Early administration of indomethacin to preterm infants. Arch Dis Child 1986; 61: 233–238
55 Evans DH, Levene MI, Archer LNJ. The effect of indomethacin on cerebral blood-flow velocity in premature infants. Dev Med Child Neurol 1987; 29: 776–782
56 Colditz P, Murphy D, Rolfe P, Wilkinson AR. Effect of infusion rate of indomethacin on cerebrovascular measurements in the preterm infant. Arch Dis Child 1988 (in press)

Development of immunity

Andrew Whitelaw
Department of Paediatrics and Neonatal Medicine, Royal Postgraduate Medical School, Hammersmith Hospital, London

Jacqueline Parkin
Department of Immunology, St Mary's Hospital Medical School, London

> Infants born before 28 weeks gestation have low IgG levels which then fall further. Newborn infants have less effective polymorphonuclear chemotactic movement than adult cells. These defects are more marked in preterm infants and persist for longer. C3, C4 and complement factor B are signficantly lower before 32 weeks than at term and in infants born at 27 weeks C3 and C4 are persistently low. Opsonic activity against *Staphylococcus epidermidis* decreases with decreasing gestational age. Septicaemic very immature infants are liable to develop neutrophil storage pool exhaustion.
>
> The multiple immune deficiencies in infants born before 28 weeks render them extremely vulnerable to bacterial invasion. Replacement therapy with immunoglobulin is now of proven value. Granulocyte transfusion or exchange transfusion are both logical but lack consistent confirmation as therapies. Active immunisation can be carried out as usual even in the most immature infants.

An immune response is not essential for normal fetal growth and development but becomes absolutely necessary for survival after birth. For infants born before 28 weeks, infection is a major problem. This is because:

1. Infection in the mother's cervix may have brought about preterm labour or premature rupture of the membranes
2. Such very immature infants are less immunologically competent than full term infants, older children and adults
3. They often require intensive care support with invasive

procedures such as endotracheal intubation and intravenous nutrition
4. They are cared for and handled by considerable numbers of staff with the possibility of cross-infection.

This chapter describes the development of immunity in the fetus, how this is modified by birth, and how the immature infant responds to infection. The roles of maternal immunity, mother's milk, immunological support therapy and active immunisation are also discussed.

B LYMPHOCYTE DEVELOPMENT

Stem cells arise from the yolk sac and by 8 weeks of gestation, pre B cells and pre T cells arise, predominantly in the fetal liver. Pre B cells are characterised by small amounts of μ chain in the cytoplasm, but initially lack surface antigen receptors and their development is not dependent on antigen or T cells. At this stage, clonal diversity develops. By 9 weeks, immature B lymphocytes develop the first surface immunoglobulin which is surface IgM. It is during the short period of time around 10–12 weeks when B cells have IgM, Fc and antigen receptors, but lack IgD, that tolerance can be induced by exposure to antigen. This may be because surface IgD is necessary for B cells to proliferate in response to certain antigens.[1] After 10 weeks gestation, mature B cells appear with surface IgG, IgD, IgA or IgM. A characteristic feature of fetal and newborn B cells is the presence of multiple surface immunoglobulin isotypes.[2] After 15 weeks, the complete variety of mature B cells exist, including the presence of multiple immunoglobulin IgG classes with the same antibody specificity.[3] Mature B cells, in cooperation with T cells may differentiate into memory cells, self-antigen memory cells, circulating antigen sensitive cells or plasma cell blasts.

IMMUNOGLOBULIN SYNTHESIS

Other immunoglobulin classes are not produced in significant amounts until many weeks after birth. Initial immunoglobulin synthesis is mainly IgM from 30 weeks gestation. However, in vitro studies have shown fetal cells to be capable of IgM and IgG synthesis from mid-gestation.[4]

IgM

IgM is not transfered across the placenta, and cord levels are normally less than 20 mg/dl at term. Evans et al.[5] found cord IgM levels below 28 weeks gestation to have a mean of 3.0 mg/dl with a range of 0–17 mg/dl and 75% of samples having undetectable IgM whereas at full term mean IgM was 17 mg/dl. IgM production increases significantly by the end of the first week after birth, regardless of gestational age, being stimulated by antigens from the neonatal gastrointestinal tract.

IgG

IgG is transfered across the placenta from as early as 8 weeks gestation. There is passive transfer of IgG which is proportional to the mother's IgG level. There is also evidence of an active transfer, probably via Fc receptors in the placenta, which is inhibited by high maternal IgG levels.[6] Fetal IgG levels are very low until after 17 weeks and then begin to increase until at term cord IgG is slightly higher than that of the mother. Both Evans et al.[5] and Hyvarinen et al.[7] found cord IgG at 28 weeks to be less than 50% of cord IgG at term. After birth, IgG levels fall as none is being synthesised, with a half-life of 25 days. Thus infants born before 28 weeks gestation are born with much lower IgG levels which then progressively fall only increasing after 4–6 months.

IgG subclasses

IgG subclasses in cord blood are similar to those of the mother, 70% IgG1, 20% IgG2, 7% IgG3, 3% IgG4, indicating no selectivity in placental transfer.[3] Oxelius and Svenningsen[8] studied IgG subclasses sequentially in infants as immature as 27 weeks and found that all four subclasses fell from 30–40% of adult level at birth to 20% of adult level at 6–8 weeks.

IgA

IgA does not cross the placenta and is synthesised to a negligible extent in fetal life. Mean serum IgA is 10 mg/dl below 28 weeks.[5] Secretory IgA is the chief immunoglobulin of exocrine gland secretions and first appears in the intestine about 4 weeks after birth.[9] Secretory IgA can be acquired from breast milk.

Infants of less than 28 weeks are particularly susceptible to septicaemia, lacking IgM and having diminished levels of IgG, while their blood stream is frequently invaded by foreign bodies such as indwelling catheters. After the first few weeks, the serum levels of IgG are even lower than at birth.

T LYMPHOCYTE DEVELOPMENT

The thymus develops from the third and fourth pharyngeal pouches at about six weeks of gestation. Thymocytes begin to develop by 8 or 9 weeks gestation, proliferating in the thymic cortex and then moving to the medulla to mature into T lymphocytes. The thymic epithelium is the origin of inducer hormones such as thymosin, thymopoietin. The thymic epithelium and specialised 'nurse cells' induce precursor cells to develop surface receptors — and acquire suppressor and helper functions. It is at this stage that the gene re-arrangement of the α and β chains of the T cell receptor occurs and acquisition of the interleukin-2 receptor plays a vital role in the induction of proliferative responses. 70% of developing thymocytes die within the thymus, perhaps because cells capable of reacting against the body's own antigens are removed.[3]

T lymphocyte function

A mixed lymphocyte response has been demonstrated using fetal liver cells as early as 8 weeks gestation. Phytohaemagglutinin responses have been shown at 10 weeks using thymus cells and at 13–14 weeks using spleen cells. Mixed lymphocyte responses occur in the thymus by 12 weeks and in blood by 14 weeks.[10] By 24 weeks T lymphocyte function in the fetus is sufficient to prevent graft-versus-host disease when viable adult lymphocytes are given to the fetus for treatment of rhesus iso-immunisation. Furthermore, fetal lambs can reject skin grafts in mid-trimester.[11] However, there is also evidence of diminished T lymphocyte function in newborns. Neonates are usually non-reactive to skin tests with *Candida*, streptokinase-streptodornase or purified protein derivative[12] and show diminished skin reactivity when previously sensitised with BCG vaccine or dinitrochlorobenzene.[13] Cytotoxic T cell responses have also been shown to be markedly reduced in a study of fetuses of 16–26 weeks gestation. In some cases this function could be restored by the addition of T cell growth factor (TCGF) suggesting a deficiency in helper cells. In others, TCGF had no effect implying that cytotoxic percursor cells may also be deficient at this stage in development.[14] Defects in cytotoxic T cell function are potentially of clinical relevence as they are directly involved in the control of many viral infections. Increased suppressor cell activity and suppression of B cell differentiation have been demonstrated by several workers.[16] Despite the in vitro evidence of defects in cell mediated immunity, some in vivo studies have shown normal delayed hypersensitivity reactions even in preterm infants. Dawodo[15] administered BCG vaccine to 12 preterm infants of 32–36 weeks gestation and found that 10 developed a definite Mantoux reaction subsequently. However, we do not know whether these processes are significantly different in infants of less than 28 weeks compared to those at term.

PHAGOCYTE FUNCTION

Movement

Newborn polymorph cells show impaired movement towards a chemical stimulus when compared to adults cells.[17] The binding of chemotactic peptides to polymorphs appears to be normal so the defect may lie in decreased cell deformability or events subsequent to receptor peptide binding.[18] In addition, newborn polymorph cells have less effective adherence to surfaces than do adult cells. Christensen and Rothstein showed that migration of polymorph cells into a subcutaneous sponge was less in newborn rats than in 4 week old rats.[19] Although there are no data relating specifically to infants under 28 weeks, a study by Sacchi[20] demonstrated that the postnatal development of chemotactic ability is delayed in preterm infants, and that the degree of delay is proportional to the gestational age. Despite all infants showing a marked impairment in chemotaxis at birth, this was no longer present in term infants by the time of regaining their birth weight (15–17 days). In contrast, in 18 preterm infants the defect remained unchanged. On longer term follow-up of 9 preterm infants, four infants of 34 weeks gestation or more developed normal chemotaxis by 43 weeks postmenstrual age. None of the infants with gestation less than 34 weeks had become normal by term.

Phagocytosis

Despite many studies being performed there is controversy concerning neutrophil function in the neonate, and very little information available on the development of function in utero. The discrepancies may be due to the varying assay systems and target organisms used, the time of investigation in relation to birth, the clinical state of the patients and even the mode of delivery.[21] In general, healthy term neonates have been found to have normal phagocytic ability. However, under conditions of 'stress' such as low concentrations of serum for opsonisation of the target organism, defects have been found.[22] This suggests that, in sub-optimal conditions, neutrophil function is deficient and this may be reflected in vivo by the abnormalities in phagocytic and bactericidal ability observed in sick neonates.[23,24] In contrast, defects in polymorph phagocytic function have been noted more consistently in both healthy and sick preterm infants. One longitudinal study of infants of 27–34 weeks gestation showed phagocytosis to be reduced particularly in the first week of life and this period was prolonged in sick patients.[25]

Bactericidal activity

The results with neonatal polymorphs have been conflicting. Forman and Steihm,[23] Park et al.[24] and McCracken and Eichenwald[26] found no difference between neonatal and adult cells in the killing of bacteria such as *Staphylococcus aureus*, *Escherichia coli* and *Pseudomonas aeruginosa*. However, Cocchi and Marianelli[27] and Mills et al.[28] found evidence of reduced killing of *P. aeruginosa* and *E. coli*. Ambruso et al.[29] studied oxidative metabolism in polymorphs in the resting state and following stimulation. Cord blood polymorphs produced relatively less hydroxyl radical than superoxide when compared to adult controls. Hydroxyl radical is an important means of killing ingested bacteria.

COMPLEMENT

Neutrophil phagocytosis and killing is not only dependent on cellular function but also on serum opsonisation. The levels of two major opsonins, complement and immunoglobulin, are related to gestational age and preterm infants are therefore particularly deficient. Kovar et al.[30] showed that infants under 32 weeks gestation have significantly lower levels of C4 (classical pathway), factor B (alternative pathway) and C3 (common pathway) than do infants at term.

Our own studies on small numbers of very preterm infants (27–29 weeks) have demonstrated that C3 and C4 are substantially reduced in the first week. Even after four weeks C3 and C4 was reduced in the 27 week gestation infants (Figs. 1 and 2).

Changes in Complement Levels with Time

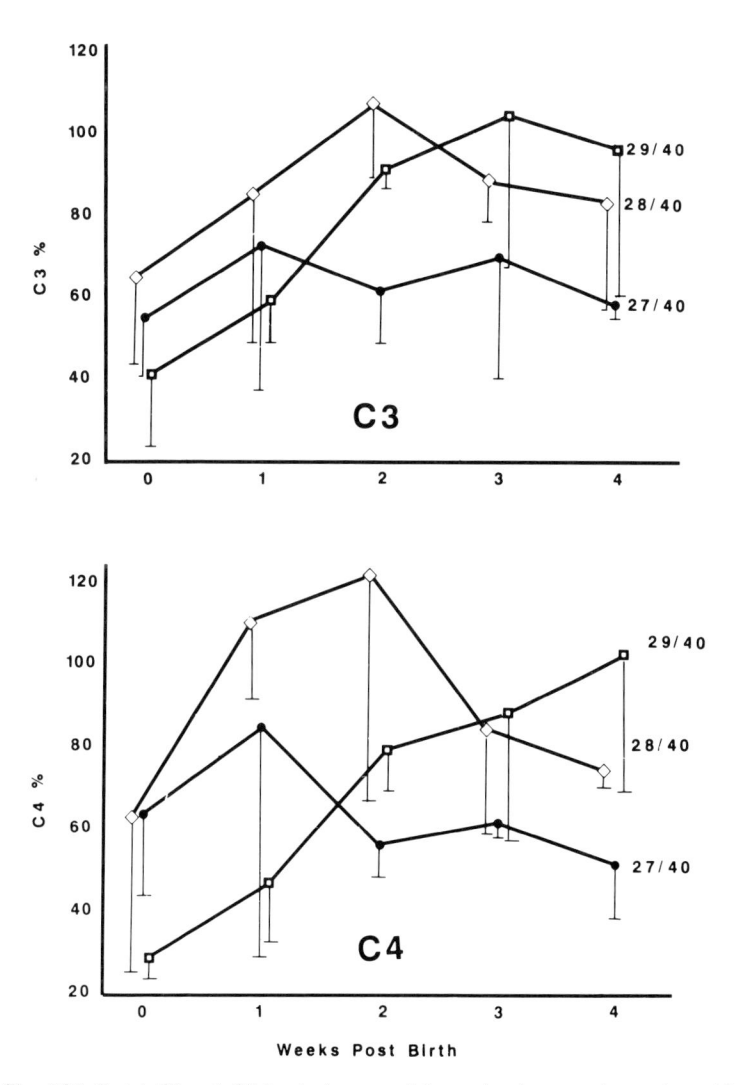

Figs 1&2 Serial C3 and C4 levels (measured by rocket immunoelectrophoresis) expressed as a percentage of pooled adult sera in preterm infants of 27 weeks (N=4), 28 weeks (N=4), and 29 weeks (N=3) gestation.

Opsonisation

Dossett et al.[31] found opsonic activity against *E. coli* and *Serratia marcescens* (*Chromobacterium prodigiosum*) by newborn sera to be less than maternal sera. However, there was no difference when *S. aureus* and group B (β-haemolytic) streptococci were examined. Forman and Steihm[23] found that sera from infants with birth weights below 2000 g showed deficient opsonisation against *S. aureus* and *Serratia*. McCracken and Eichenwald[26] found that infants weighing less than 3000 g showed diminished opsonisation against *S. aureus, E. coli* and *P. aeruginosa*. No data exist for infants under 28 weeks. Very immature infants are particularly prone to invasion by *Staphylococcus epidermidis*, this organism being the commonest found in late neonatal septicaemia.[32] Fleer et al.[33] reported that opsonic activity against *S. epidermidis* decreased with decreasing gestational age. Opsonisation was abolished by heating to 56°C, or the presence of EDTA but was not blocked by MgEGTA, indicating that the alternative complement pathway was involved. Although these preterm infants' sera had detectable antibody to *Staphylococcal* peptidoglycan, these IgG antibodies appeared to have no heat stable opsonising activity.

In our own studies using *Candida albicans* as a target, serum opsonic activity was lower at 27 weeks gestation than at 28 or 29 weeks. However, opsonic activity[34] matured in the first two to three weeks attaining adult control levels (Fig. 3). In contrast, the serum factors involved in stimulating intracellular killing of the same target *Candida*, 'procidins',[34] were similarly reduced at 27, 28 and 29 weeks gestation and increased at similar rates (Fig. 4).

NEUTROPHIL NUMBERS

During mid-trimester, total white cell, neutrophil and lymphocyte counts increase but the increase is greater for neutrophils.[35] Total neutrophil count tends to be lower in infants of 23–27 weeks than at term. However, McIntosh[36] has made the important observation that infants weighing less than 1000 g who are small for gestational age have significantly lower neutrophil counts compared with those infants who are appropriate for their dates and, of the same weight. We have also observed this. Such 'small-for-dates' infants may have neutrophil counts below 1000 mm^{-3} or even below 500 mm^{-3} in the absence of infection. Such neutropenia is clinically significant because secondary invasion and septicaemia may occur in such infants even if sepsis was absent initially. It has been suggested that the phenomenon might be due to chronic hypoxia stimulating the marrow to such an extent that neutrophil precursors were crowded out by red cell precursors.

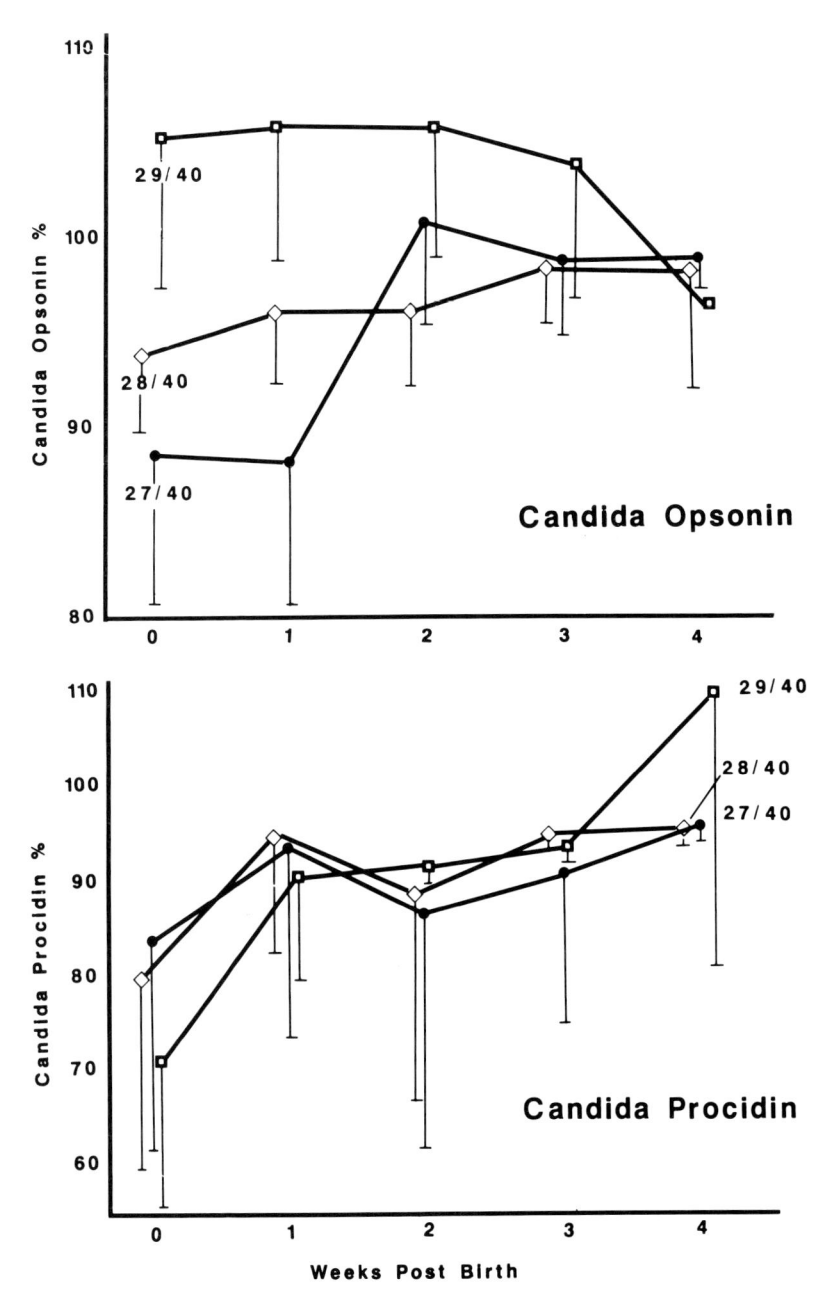

Figs 3&4 Serum opsonin and procidin function against a *Candida* target in preterm infants of 27 weeks (N=4), 28 weeks (N=4) and 29 weeks (N=3) gestation.

Another possibility might be that placental insufficiency has resulted in a deficiency of some nutrient which is required for neutrophil division.

Conversely, very immature infants may have an extremely high neutrophil count in the absence of infection, a leukaemoid reaction. This phenomenon does not seem to render the infant even more vulnerable to infection. It may be linked to high levels of stress hormones such as glucocorticoids and catecholamines which mobilise neutrophils.

Acute phase proteins

A number of proteins are synthesised and released into the bloodstream within hours of acute infection, tissue necrosis and other stresses such as surgery. Philip[37] has examined the role of C reactive protein (CRP), fibrinogen, peptidaminoglycan and fibronectin in the rapid diagnosis of neonatal sepsis. We have recently examined CRP using a highly sensitive solid phase ligand binding radioassay. The normal range of non-infected neonates is below the threshold of commercially available CRP assays. The 95% confidence limit for cord blood is 1.5 mg/l for preterm infants including those below 28 weeks. Such very immature infants are quite capable of responding to infection by increasing CRP. For example, a 26 week infant with proven septicaemia, had a cord CRP level of 1 mg/l and increased it to 15 mg/l by 24 hours. There is inevitably a delay between the infant's liver beginning to increase synthesis and the finding of a serum CRP level over the 95% confidence limit. If the infant is profoundly neutropenic, and deficient in IgG and complement factors, the septicaemia may become overwhelming within 12 hours. Thus one CRP measurement cannot definitely exclude early sepsis.

IMMUNITY AND BREAST MILK

The protective properties of breast milk include secretory IgA, lysozyme, lactoferrin, leukocytes and small amounts of IgG, IgM and IgD. Although mother's milk usually contains high titres of antibodies against *E. coli* O and K antigens, they do not prevent the breast fed infant's gut from being colonised with *E. coli* with the corresponding O and K antigens.[38] Gothefors[39] showed that such strains of organisms from breast fed infants were more sensitive to the bactericidal effect of human serum than were the gut organisms from formula fed infants. This effect probably indicates reduced virulence and is thought to be due to local secretory IgA. Secretory IgA levels are very high, e.g. 1200 mg/dl in colostrum falling to 50–100 mg/dl in mature breast milk.[3]

Although B and T lymphocytes, monocytes and polymorph cells are present in breast milk, it is not clear what their protective role is. The phagocytes may be active in killing bacteria within the pharynx and lumen of the gut. There is a report of transfer of cellular immunity to tuberculin via breast milk[40] but maternal breast milk T lymphocytes have not established a graft even in immunodeficient infants. It has been suggested that breast milk gives protection against necrotising enterocolitis[41] but this protection is certainly not complete. Two large studies from developing countries[42,43] showed a clear protective effect from breast milk against bacterial infection. Although these studies did not concern infants below 28 weeks gestation, it would be very surprising if the feeding of fresh mother's milk did not improve host defences in such infants.

IMMUNISATION

In the past it was a widespread practice to delay active immunisation of preterm infants for several months so that an infant born at 26 weeks might start immunisation at 6 months of age instead of the customary 3 months. This was done in the mistaken belief that such an infant would not respond to the vaccines at an earlier age and would also be at the higher risk of an adverse reaction. We have recently found that infants as immature as 26 weeks gestation can achieve adequate levels of immunity if vaccinated against diphtheria, tetanus, pertussis and polio three months after birth. This is important as parental acceptance of vaccination is likely to be increased by the first dose being given before the infant leaves hospital and because pertussis is extremely dangerous in such infants.

IMMUNOLOGICAL THERAPY

There is ample evidence that infants of 23–27 weeks gestation are at serious risk of infection because of a relative deficiency of immunoglobulins, complement factors and some neutrophil functions. In addition the neutrophil storage pool is likely to become exhausted during sepsis. Thus replacement therapy could be used either prophylactically or as 'rescue'.

Intravenous immunoglobulin

Purified intravenous immunoglubulin has been available in recent years and several studies have concluded that there is benefit. Sidiropoulos et al.[44] gave IV immunoglobulin as rescue therapy to 15 infants with sepsis in a randomised study with 20 infants in a control group receiving only antibiotics. Survival was better in the immunoglobulin treated group. Two trials of prophylactic immunoglobulin in low birth weight infants have both shown significant reductions in sepsis.[45,46]

Fresh frozen plasma

Complement factors can be replaced by giving fresh frozen plasma. However, to substantially raise complement levels would require large volumes of plasma. In a shocked septicaemic infant large volumes of plasma may be needed to restore blood volume and to correct coagulation disturbances, but circulatory overload may occur if more than 20 ml/kg is given.

Exchange transfusion

An alternative therapy in septicaemia is exchange transfusion by which adequate volumes of fresh frozen plasma can be given, replacing complement and immunoglobulins and clotting factors whilst also removing some of the bacterial toxin circulating. While there are plenty of anecdotes on the benefits of exchange transfusion in septicaemia, good controlled studies are lacking.

Granulocyte replacement

Granulocyte replacement can be given as granulocyte concentrate or as buffy coat. Preparation of granulocyte concentrate requires a cell separator (not widely available 24 hours a day) and takes time. Buffy coat is available from most blood transfusion centres and does not require expensive equipment. Christensen has described how neutrophil storage pool (NSP) exhaustion is a peculiarly neonatal problem and has a very high mortality. In his randomised trial, administration of granulocytes significantly improved survival in septicaemic infants with NSP exhaustion.[47] Other trials have not found benefit from granulocyte transfusion. It is not clear whether the later trials may have studied infants at a later stage of septicaemia or whether there may have been more delay in obtaining granulocyte preparations. At present, it cannot be recommended as routine therapy. Christensen has recently shown that intravenous immunoglobulin alters neutrophil kinetics in newborns and facilitates mobilisation of neutrophils and migration into infected tissue.[48]

ACKNOWLEDGEMENT

We thank Dr. M. Rutherford and Professor M. Pepys for their collaboration.

REFERENCES

1 Vitetta E, Uhr JW. IgD and B cell differentiation. Immunol Rev 1977; 37: 50–88
2 Gathings WE, Lawton AR, Cooper MD. Immunofluoresecent studies on the development of pre B cells, B lymphocytes and immunoglobulin isotype diversity in humans. Eur J Immunol 1977; 7: 804–810
3 Miller ME, Stiehm ER. Immunology and resistance to infection. In: Remington JS, Klein JO, eds. Infectious Diseases of the Fetus and Newborn Infant, 2nd edn. Philadelphia: Saunders, 1983: pp. 27–68
4 Lawton AR, Self KS, Royal SA, Cooper MD. Ontogeny of B lymphocytes in the human fetus. Clin Immunol Immunopathol 1972; 1: 84–93
5 Evans HE, Alpata SO, Glass L. Serum immunoglobulin levels in premature and full term infants. Am J Clin Pathol 1971; 56: 416–418
6 Gitlin D, Kumate J, Urrusti J, Morales C. The selectivity of the human placenta in the transfer of plasma proteins from mother to fetus. J Clin Invest 1964; 43: 1938–1951
7 Hyvarinen M, Zeltzer P, Oh W, Stiehm ER. Influence of gestational age on the newborn serum levels of alpha-1-fetoglobulin, IgG globulin and albumin. J Pediatr 1973; 82: 430–437
8 Oxelius VA, Svenningsen NW. IgG subclass concentrations in preterm neonates. Acta Paediatr Scand 1984; 73: 626–630
9 Perkkio M, Savilahti E. Time of appearance of immunoglobulin-containing cells in the mucosa of the neonatal intestine. Pediatr Res 1980; 14: 953–955
10 Stites DP, Pavia CS. Ontogeny of human T cells. Pediatrics 1979; 64 (supplement): 795–802
11 Silverstein AM, Prendergast RA. Fetal Response to antigenic stimulus IV. Rejection of skin homografts by the fetal lamb. J Exp Med 1986; 119: 955–964
12 Miller ME. The immunodeficiencies of immaturity. In: Stiehm ER, Fulginiti VA, eds. Immunologic Disease in Infants and Children, 2nd edn. Philadelphia: Saunders, 1980: 219–238
13 Uhr JW, Dancis J, Neuman CG. Delayed-type hyerpsensitivity in the premature neonatal human. Nature 1960; 187: 1130–1131
14 Rayfield LS, Brent L, Boylston A et al. Human lymphocytes require T cell growth factors for cytotoxic response. Clin Exp Immnol 1987; 69: 451–458
15 Dawodu AH. Tuberculin conversion following BCG vaccination in preterm infants. Acta Paediatr Scand 1985; 74: 564–567
16 Hayward AR, Lawton AR. Induction of plasma cell differentiation of human fetal lymphocytes. Evidence for functional immunity of T and B cells. J Immunol 1977; 119: 1213–1217

17 Miller ME. Phagocyte function in the neonate. Selected aspects. Pediatrics 1979; 64 (suppl): 709–712
18 Strauss RG, Snyder EL. Chemotactic peptide binding by intact neutrophils from human neonates. Pediatric Research 1984; 18: 63–66
19 Christensen RD, Rothstein G. Efficiency of neutrophil migration in the neonate. Pediatrics 1980; 14: 1147–1149
20 Sacchi F, Rondini G, Mingrat G et al. Different maturation of neutrophil chemotaxis in term and preterm newborn infants. J Pediatr 1982; 101: 273–274
21 Frazier JP, Clearly TG, Pickering LK et al. Leukocyte function in healthy neonates following vaginal and Caesarean deliveries. J Pediatr 1982; 101: 269–272
22 Miller ME. Phagocytosis in the newborn infant. J Pediatr 1969; 74: 255–259
23 Forman ML, Stiehm ER. Impaired opsonic activity but normal phagocytosis in low birth weight infants. N Engl J Med 1969; 281: 926–931
24 Park BH, Holmes B, Good RA. Metabolic activities in leukocytes of newborn infants. J Pediatr 1970; 76: 237–241
25 Al-Hadithy H, Addison IE, Gladstone AG et al. Defective neutrophil function in low birth weight premature infants. J Clin Pathol 1981; 34: 366–370
26 McCracken GH, Eichenwald HF. Leukocyte function and the development of opsonic and complement activity in the neonate. Am J Dis Child 1971; 121: 120–126
27 Cocchi P, Marianelli L. Phagocytosis and intracellular killing of *Pseudomonas aeruginosa* in premature infants. Helv Paediatr Acta 1967; 22: 110–118
28 Mills EL, Thompson T, Bjorksten B, Filipovitch D, Quie P. The chemiluminescence and responses and bactericidal activity of neutrophils from newborns and their mothers. Pediatrics 1979; 63: 429–434
29 Ambruso DR, Altenburger KM, Johnston RB. Defective oxidative metabolism in newborn neutrophils: descrepancy between superoxide anion and hydroxyl radical generation. Pediatrics 1979; 64: 722–725
30 Kovar I, Ajina NS, Hurley R. Serum complement and gestational age. J Obstet Gynecol 1983; 3: 182–186
31 Dossett JH, Williams RC, Quie PG. Studies on interaction of bacteria, serum factors and polymorphonuclear leukocytes in mothers and newborns. Pediatrics 1969; 44: 49–57
32 Placzek M, Whitelaw A. Early and late neonatal septicaemia. Arch Dis Child 1983; 58: 728–731
33 Fleer A, Gerrards LJ, Aerts P, Westerdaal NAC, Senders RC, van Dijk H, Verhoef J. Opsonic defence to *Staphylococcus epidermidis* in the premature neonate. J Infect Dis 1985; 152: 930–937
34 Bridges CG, DaSilva GL, Yamamura M, Valdimarsson H. A radiometric assay for the combined measurement of phagocytosis and intracellular killing of candida albicans. Clin Exp Immunol 1980; 42: 226–233
35 Playfair JHL, Wolfendale MR, Kay HEM. The leukocytes of peripheral blood in the human fetus. Br J Haematol 1963; 336–344
36 McIntosh N, Kempson C, Tyler RM. Blood counts in extremely low birth weight infants. Arch Dis Child 1988; 63: 74–76
37 Philip A. Neonatal Sepsis and Meningitis. Boston: Hall, 1985
38 Carlsson B, Kaijser B, Ahlsted S, Gothefors L, Hanson LA. Antibodies against *Escherichia coli* capsular (K) antigens in human milk and serum. Their relation to the *E. coli* gut flora of the mother and neonate. Acta Paediatr Scand 1982; 71: 313–318
39 Gothefors L, Olling S, Winberg J. Breast feeding and biological properties of faecal *E. coli* strains. Acta Paediatr Scand 1975; 64: 807–812
40 Ogra SS, Weintraub D, Ogra PL. Immunological aspects of human colostrum and milk. III Fate and absorption of cellular and soluble components in the gastrointestinal tract of the newborn. J Immunol 1977; 119: 245–248

41 Barlow B, Santulli TV, Heird WC, Pitt J, Blanc WA, Schullinger JN. An experimental study of acute neonatal enterocolitis—the importance of breast milk. J Pediatr Surg 1974; 9: 587–595
42 Narayanan I, Prakash K, Murthy NS, Gujral VV. Randomised controlled trial of the effect of raw and holder pasteurised human milk and of formula supplements on the incidence of neonatal infection. Lancet 1984; 2: 1111–1113
43 Victoria C, Smith P, Vaughan J, et al. Evidence for protection by breast feeding against infant deaths from infectious diseases in Brazil. Lancet 1987; 2: 319–321
44 Sidiropoulos D, Boehme U, von Muralt G, Morell A, Barandan S. Immunoglobulin supplementation in the management of neonatal sepsis. Schweiz Med Wochenschr 1981; 111: 1649–1655
45 Haque K, Zaidi M, Haque S, Bahakim H, El-Hazmi M, El Swailam M. Intravenous immunoglobulin for prevention of sepsis in preterm and low birth weight infants. Pediatr Infect Dis 1986; 5: 622–625
46 Chirico G, Rondini G, Plebani A, Chiara A, Massa M, Ugazio A. Intravenous gammaglobulin therapy for prophylaxis of infection in high risk neonates. J Pediatr 1987; 110: 437–442
47 Christensen RD, Rothstein G, Anstall HB, Bybee B. Granulocyte transfusion in neonates with bacterial infection, neutropenia and depletion of marrow neutrophils. Pediatrics 1982; 70: 1–6
48 Christensen RD. Intravenous immunoglobulin for prophylaxis or treatment of bacterial infection in neonates. J Perinat 1987; 7: 58–61

New non-invasive methods for assessing brain oxygenation and haemodynamics

E O R Reynolds, J S Wyatt, D Azzopardi, D T Delpy, E B Cady, M Cope, S Wray
Departments of Paediatrics, Medical Physics & Bioengineering, and Physiology, University College and Middlesex School of Medicine, The Rayne Institute, London

> Hypoxic-ischaemic injury to the brain is the commonest cause of permanent neurodevelopmental disability in very preterm and other infants who survive after neonatal intensive care.
>
> Two new methods allow normal and abnormal oxidative metabolism to be investigated non-invasively in brain tissue. **Magnetic resonance spectroscopy** is used to measure the concentrations of important phosphorus compounds that are involved in energy metabolism—adenosine triphosphate, phosphocreatine and inorganic orthophosphate—and also to measure intracellular pH. Normal developmental changes with gestation have been defined and abnormalities indicating impaired oxidative phosphorylation detected in a range of conditions of suspected or proven hypoxic-ischaemic injury. **Near infrared spectroscopy** provides continuous cot-side information about cerebral oxygenation and haemodynamics. Quantitative measurements can be made of oxyhaemoglobin, deoxyhaemoglobin, oxidized cytochrome aa3 and various haemodynamic indices.
>
> These two complementary techniques are likely to prove increasingly valuable for: monitoring brain-oxygenation and haemodynamics in babies; investigating the mechanisms of damage to the brain; assessing the results of treatment; and assigning long-term prognosis.

NON-INVASIVE INVESTIGATION OF THE BRAIN

Cerebral periventricular haemorrhage and hypoxic-ischaemic injury are very common in infants born well before term.[1] The introduction of portable ultrasound apparatus for scanning the brain repeatedly in the intensive care nursery has been followed by the publication of a large number of studies of the prevalence, pathogenesis and prognostic significance of these cerebral lesions.[2] The initial studies concentrated on periventricular haemorrhage, which was easy to visualize, even with early linear-array scanners, and it soon became clear that the prevalence of haemorrhage increased sharply with decreasing maturity, so that in infants born before 28 weeks of gestation it was about 80%. More recently attention has shifted towards the role of hypoxic-ischaemic brain injury as a cause of death and long-term disability in very preterm infants. This change of direction arose for two reasons. Firstly follow-up studies of cohorts of infants whose brains had been prospectively scanned with ultrasound showed that periventricular haemorrhage, though extremely common, was responsible for disability only in a minority of disabled very preterm survivors: the haemorrhages appeared innocuous, or almost so, unless they led to post-haemorrhagic hydrocephalus or intraparenchymal haemorrhage (often due to venous infarction associated with disrupted venous drainage.[3]) Secondly the improving quality of ultrasound imaging, especially following the introduction of modern mechanical sector scanners has allowed hypoxic-ischaemic injury to be diagnosed from the development of cystic periventricular leucomalacia, or inferred from the presence of ventricular dilatation in the absence of evidence of obstruction to the drainage of cerebrospinal fluid.[2,4–9] It is now clear that hypoxic-ischaemic injury such as periventricular leucomalacia is a more frequent cause than haemorrhage of permanent damage to the brain in surviving very preterm infants.[4–6,10] The presence of hypoxic-ischaemic injury may be suspected before frank loss of brain tissue occurs from the appearance of increased echodensities on ultrasound scan.[2,7,8] However, studies in which the ultrasound-appearance of the brain has been compared with autopsy findings show that increased echodensities are poor indicators of hypoxic-ischaemic injury[9]—unless they are extremely obvious and persistent.[7,8] It must be concluded that, unlike the situation for cerebral haemorrhage, ultrasound scanning does not provide useful information about early events in this type of injury.

If periventricular leucomalacia and other forms of hypoxic-ischaemic injury to the brain (such as birth asphyxia in term infants) are to be rigorously investigated, new methods are required for identifying them as they occur, and for exploring the mechanisms involved, particularly so that therapeutic interventions can be tested objectively and the prognosis for the infants determined. It was the realization that hypoxic-ischaemic brain injury was the major cause of long-term neurodevelopmental disability in very immature, and other, infants who survive after intensive care that provided the impetus for the introduction of new techniques for investigating this type of injury. The aim of this review is to describe the use of two such techniques—magnetic resonance spectroscopy and near infrared spectroscopy—which show great promise, particularly when used in combination.

MAGNETIC RESONANCE SPECTROSCOPY

Background and theory

Magnetic resonance spectroscopy has been used for many years in analytical chemistry, but has only recently become applicable to studies of animals and human subjects.[11] This development depended on the production of the large, usually superconducting, magnets that are necessary for the provision of a sufficiently strong uniform magnetic field. The principle of the technique depends on the tendency of certain atomic nuclei, notably phosphorus (^{31}P), hydrogen (^{1}H), an isotope of carbon with 1.1% abundance (^{13}C), sodium (^{23}Na) and fluorine (^{19}F), to line up along a magnetic field. This alignment can be disturbed by applying a suitable radiofrequency pulse at right angles to the field. When the pulse ceases, the nuclei return to their previous alignment and in so doing generate a magnetic resonance signal which can be detected. The exact frequency of the signal depends on the chemical compound in which the nuclei reside, and the signal-intensity is proportional to concentration. In practice, the part of the body to be examined is placed within the horizontal bore of the magnet, and a succession of radiofrequency pulses is transmitted by a surface coil, which also acts as an aerial to detect the magnetic resonance signals returning from the tissue. These signals are summed and processed by Fourier transformation to generate a spectrum.

The technique is particularly suited to the investigation of hypoxic-ischaemic injury because it can be used to measure, noninvasively in brain tissue, the relative intracellular concentrations of phosphorus metabolites that are important in energy metabolism, notably adenosine triphosphate (ATP), phosphocreatine (PCr) and inorganic orthophosphate (Pi). Intracellular pH (pH_i) can also be estimated. ATP is the major energy source for the metabolism of the body and is dependent for its synthesis on the processes of oxidative phosphorylation and glycolysis. In conditions of inadequate oxygen supply or when the mechanisms involved in the utilization of oxygen are disrupted, the concentration of ATP will tend to fall. This tendency is however, counteracted by the creatine kinase reaction (Fig. 1). Because of the very high equilibrium constant of this reaction, phosphocreatine acts as a buffer for ATP, so that any impairment of oxidative phosphorylation will result initially in a fall in the concentration of PCr and an approximately equal rise in that of Pi, in other words a fall in the ratio of PCr to Pi. This ratio is a sensitive indicator of the efficacy of oxidative phosphorylation, because it is related directly to the phosphorylation potential [ATP]/([ADP][Pi]) and to the free energy change of hydrolysis of ATP. Only when PCr/Pi has fallen to a low level will the concentration of ATP begin to fall.

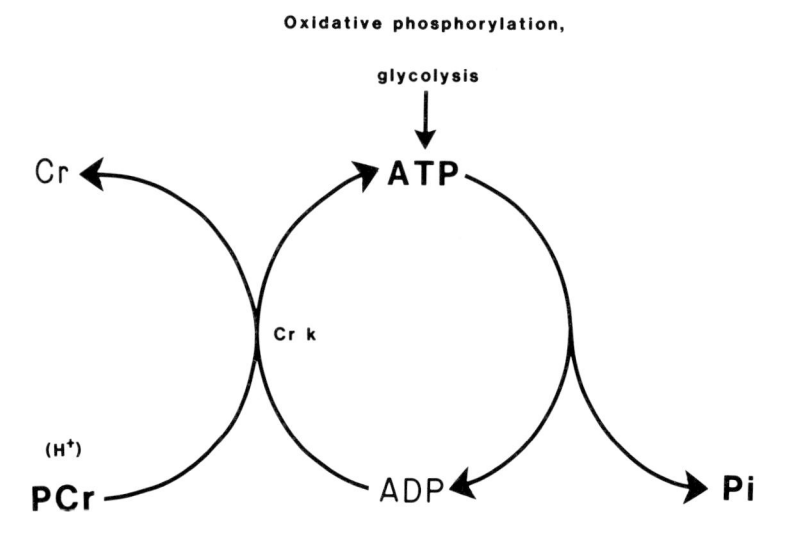

Fig. 1 Creatine kinase reaction. Any tendency for the concentration of adenosine triphosphate (ATP) to fall due to inadequate oxidative phosphorylation is buffered by the creatine kinase reaction. The net effect is a fall in the concentration of phosphocreatine (PCr) and a rise in that of inorganic phosphate (Pi).

Equipment and methods for studying the brain in newborn infants

We have used an Oxford Research Systems TMR 32–200 spectrometer operating at a field strength of 1.89 T. The diameter of the bore of the magnet was initially 20 cm and more recently 27 cm. For transporting and studying infants safely in a strong magnetic field, a special transport system is necessary, especially since ferromagnetic metal cannot, for reasons of safety, be allowed within 3 m of the magnet.[12] The system is based on a transport incubator with the baby carried in a perspex cylinder mounted on the top. This cylinder can be detached and inserted within the bore of the magnet while monitoring and mechanical ventilation, if necessary, are continued. Inside the cylinder, the baby's head lies on a surface coil 5 cm or 7.4 cm in diameter, which transmits the exciting radiofrequency pulses into the brain and also receives the returning magnetic resonance signals. The baby's head is positioned so that signals are obtained from the adjacent cerebral hemisphere, mainly from the temporoparietal cortex.[13] The surface coil can be tuned to the resonance frequencies of both ^{31}P (32.5 MHz) and ^1H (80.3 MHz). The ^{31}P spectra are usually obtained by Fourier transformation of 256 summed free induction decays following radiofrequency pulses repeated at intervals of 2.256 s. The pulse length is chosen to produce a flip angle of 90° at the centre of the coil. The effects of saturation (atomic nuclei not returning fully to their resting state between pulses) caused by the rapid pulse repetition rate have been measured for each metabolite and correction factors derived, so that the values for the gated spectral peak areas can be corrected and made proportional to concentration.[14,15] The resonance frequency of the Pi peak changes with pH_i, which can therefore be calculated from the difference in frequency between the PCr and Pi peaks, using a version of the Henderson-Hasselbach equation.[16]

Studies have been performed at University College Hospital on over 180 infants, often on several occasions, usually because of suspicion of hypoxic-ischaemic brain injury, but also including normal infants.[14,17–21] Similar studies have been done in Philadelphia.[22,23] Few data are available so far from infants born at less than 28 weeks of gestation, but it is nevertheless possible to draw inferences about maturational events in the brain, and about the general effects of hypoxic-ischaemic injury on the ^{31}P metabolites and pH_i, which are not likely to differ greatly with maturity.

Normal changes with brain maturation

Figure 2 shows ^{31}P spectra from two healthy infants without evidence of cerebral abnormalities, one born at 28 weeks of gestation (A) and the other born at term (B). Seven spectral peaks can be seen which are attributable, from left to right, to phosphomonoesters, Pi, phosphodiesters, PCr, and the γ, α and β ^{31}P nuclei of nucleotide triphosphates, mainly ATP.[11] The γ and α peaks include undetectably small contributions from adenosine diphosphate (ADP) and the α peak, a contribution from nicotinamide adenine dinucleotide (NAD). The PCr and Pi peaks are of particular importance for the consideration of oxidative metabolism, for reasons that have been given above. In the immature infant, the area of the PCr peak appears relatively smaller, and that of the Pi peak larger, than in the term one. Data from 30 normal preterm and term infants, born between 24 and 42 weeks of gestation and studied at a median age of 5 days after birth show that PCr/Pi increases in a systematic way with gestation (Fig. 3).[15] It appears, therefore, that the phosphorylation potential of brain

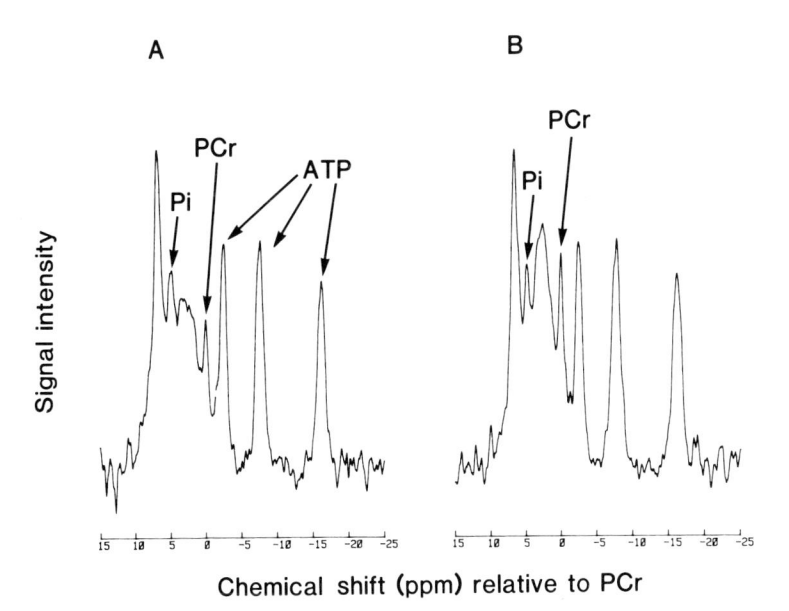

Fig. 2 ^{31}P spectra from two infants with normal brains.
A: Born at 28 weeks' gestation and studied 7 days after birth; PCr/Pi = 0.80.
B: Born at 40 weeks' gestation and studied aged one day; PCr/Pi = 1.27.
For peak-assignments, see text.

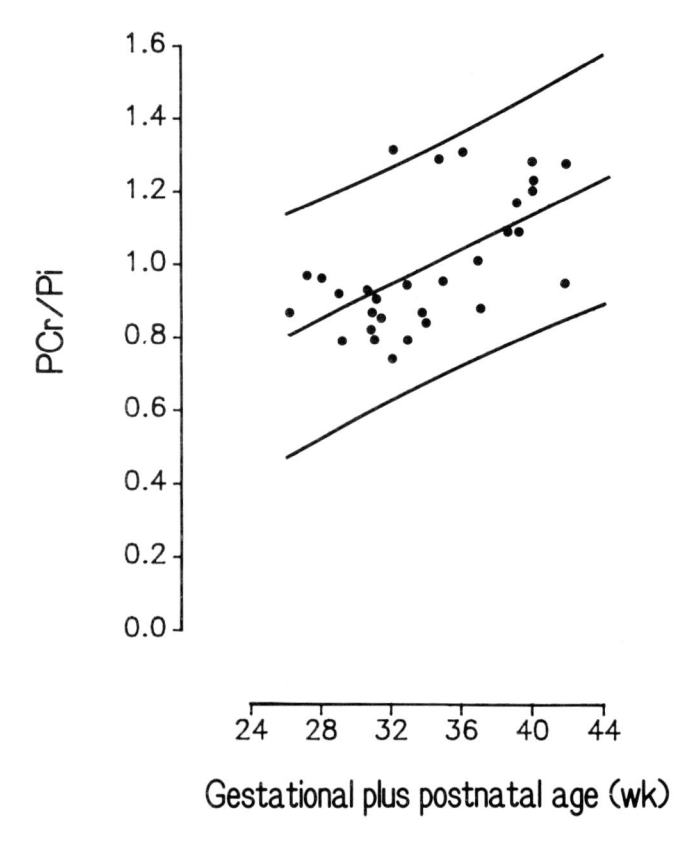

Fig. 3 Relation between PCr/Pi and gestational plus postnatal age in 30 infants with normal brains. The regression line and 95% confidence limits are shown.

tissue increases with maturation of the brain. Data for this and other metabolite concentration ratios are given in Table 1; the demonstration that PCr/total P (total phosphorus signal) and PCr/ATP increase, and Pi/total P and Pi/ATP fall with maturation are consistent with this view. Data from newborn animals show similar changes.[24] By comparison, the newborn human infant seems, in terms of phosphorus energetics, to be at about the same stage of maturation as other altricial animals such as the newborn rat but less so than the guinea pig or lamb[24,25] which are precocious. Table 1 also gives changes in other metabolite ratios. The prominent phosphomonoester (PME) peak has been shown by chemical analysis of the brain in the newborn of several animal species to be almost entirely attributable to phosphoethanolamine,[26] so it must be assumed that the same is true of the newborn

Table 1 Changes in phosphorus metabolite concentration ratios and intracellular pH with gestational plus postnatal age in 30 infants with normal brains[15]

	28 wk	42 wk	r	P
PCr/Pi	0.85 ± 0.33	1.18 ± 0.33	0.58	<0.001
ATP/total P	0.09 ± 0.03	0.10 ± 0.03	0.19	ns
PCr/total P	0.09 ± 0.02	0.11 ± 0.02	0.56	<0.01
Pi/total P	0.10 ± 0.02	0.09 ± 0.02	−0.40	<0.05
PME/total P	0.32 ± 0.04	0.26 ± 0.04	−0.68	<0.001
PDE/total P	0.19 ± 0.04	0.22 ± 0.04	0.47	<0.01
PCr/ATP	0.97 ± 0.42	1.09 ± 0.42	0.20	ns
Pi/ATP	1.13 ± 0.50	0.95 ± 0.50	−0.25	ns
PME/ATP	3.49 ± 1.23	2.79 ± 1.25	−0.37	<0.05
PDE/ATP	2.11 ± 1.03	2.34 ± 1.05	0.15	ns
pH$_i$	7.13 ± 0.39	7.13 ± 0.40	0.00	ns

Mean values ±95% confidence limits from the regression lines are given.
PCr = phosphocreatine, Pi = inorganic orthophosphate, ATP = adenosine triphosphate, total P = total phosphorus, PME = phosphomonoester, PDE = phosphodiester, pH$_i$ = intracellular pH

human infant. Phosphoethanolamine is a major precursor of phospholipid in membranes and myelin. PME/total P and PME/ATP fall with maturation of the brain (see table) and it is known that the PME peak is small in spectra from the brains of adult animals and human subjects.[24,27–29] At the same time as the reduction in PME, phosphodiester (PDE)/total P and PDE/ATP increase. The PDE peak is due mainly to phosphatidylethanolamine and phosphatidylcholine, which are important constituents of membranes and myelin.[30] The fall in PME and rise in PDE with maturity have also been found in newborn animals and appear to reflect myelination and the proliferation of membranes.[24] With current developments in MRS, it will shortly be possible to provide data for absolute rather than relative concentrations of metabolites in brain and other tissue.[31,32]

Small-for-gestational-age (SGA) infants

SGA infants are at increased risk of neurodevelopmental disabilities. In one study, several such infants were found to have evidence of impaired oxidative phosphorylation (low PCr/Pi ratios) in brain tissue in association with increased cerebral echodensities.[19] To find out whether SGA babies had intrinsic abnormalities of ^{31}P spectra indicating abnormal energy metabolism, or defective cell synthesis or myelination (as judged from metabolite ratios) a group of 13 babies with birthweights below the 3rd centile for gestation was studied.[15] Their gestational ages ranged from 28 to 40 weeks (median 34 weeks) and birthweights from 780–2532 g (median 1405 g). The infants were selected because, apart from being SGA, they appeared completely normal as indicated by their clinical features and cranial ultrasound scans. No evidence was found of any difference in metabolite ratios or pH$_i$ between the SGA infants and appropriately grown infants. Derangements of ^{31}P spectra previously found in SGA babies were thought likely, therefore, to have been due to superimposed perinatal events, rather than any intrinsic cerebral abnormality.

Hypoxic-ischaemic brain injury

The ^{31}P spectra have been found to show similar abnormalities in a variety of situations associated with hypoxic-ischaemic injury, for example following birth asphyxia, during the progression of periventricular leucomalacia and other forms of cerebral infarction, and in the presence of intraparenchymal periventricular haemorrhage (Figs 4, 5). The evolution of the abnormalities has been investigated more thoroughly following birth asphyxia than in the other conditions, because birth-asphyxiated infants are often born at term and can be studied repeatedly, whereas this is not possible in small preterm infants.

Birth asphyxia

The evolution of the changes in the ^{31}P spectra following birth asphyxia has been illustrated elsewhere.[14,20] It has been found that the spectra are often normal in the first hours of life. A progressive fall in PCr/Pi then takes place, to a minimum value at about 3 days of age. In the worst-affected babies, when PCr/Pi is very low, ATP/total P then also falls and death is likely to ensue. In surviving infants, PCr/Pi recovers to normal by about two weeks, though the total phosphorus signal may by then be reduced, due to loss of brain tissue. Intracellular pH is often elevated when PCr/Pi is low. The mechanisms responsible for this progression of events are by no means clear. In the newborn lamb[25] (as in adults of various species)[28,29] a severe acute hypoxic-ischaemic episode, analogous to an episode of birth asphyxia, causes immediate changes in the ^{31}P spectra—first a fall in PCr/Pi and then in ATP/total P, as expected from consideration of the creatine kinase reaction (Fig. 1). At the same time, pH$_i$ falls to a very low level, due to the production of lactic acid. When cerebral

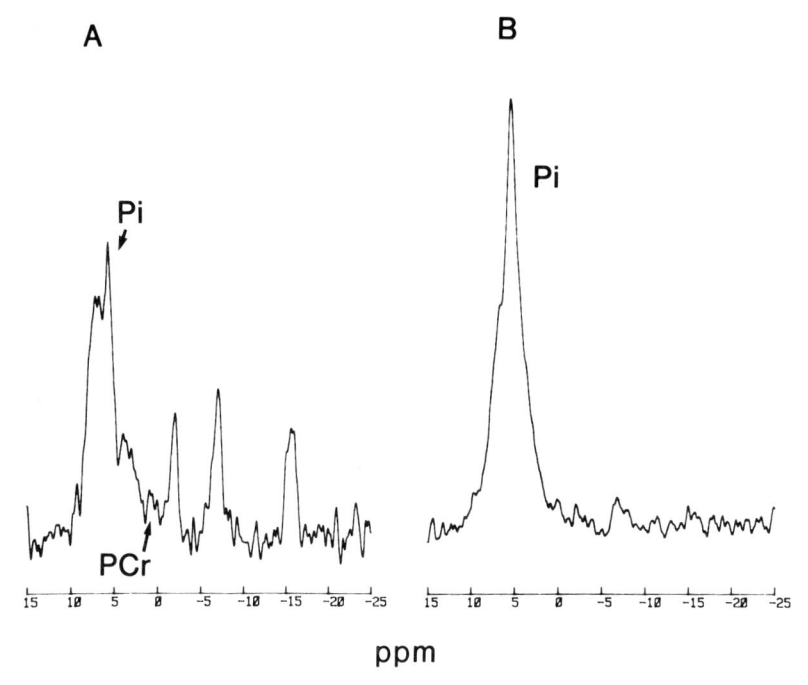

Fig. 4 ^{31}P spectra from two infants with severe brain injury.

A: Born at 25 weeks' gestation and studied aged 3 days (right hemisphere). Bilateral intraventricular haemorrhages and haemorrhagic parenchymal echodensities were present. PCr/Pi = 0.22. Died aged 7 days.

B: Born at 27 weeks' gestation and studied aged 8 days (left hemisphere). He had suffered an extremely severe asphyxial episode aged 5 days. Bilateral intraventricular haemorrhages and diffusely increased parenchymal echodensities were present. PCr and ATP were virtually absent. Died aged 11 days.

oxygenation is restored all the abnormalities can revert to normal within about one hour.[25] It must be assumed that severely birth-asphyxiated babies, when studied during the first hours of life have been through this phase of acute (or primary) energy failure and are often in a state of apparently normal oxidative phosphorylation—possibly due partly to reduced demands for energy associated with cerebral depression. The subsequent development of 'secondary' energy failure is a well-recognized phenomenon of cerebral pathophysiology which is attributable to various imprecisely defined influences associated with reperfusion and reoxygenation of the tissue.[33,34] Which influences are the most important are unknown. Damage to the mitochondrial respiratory electron chain is very likely, following the abnormal entry of calcium ions into the cells, the generation of free radicals and

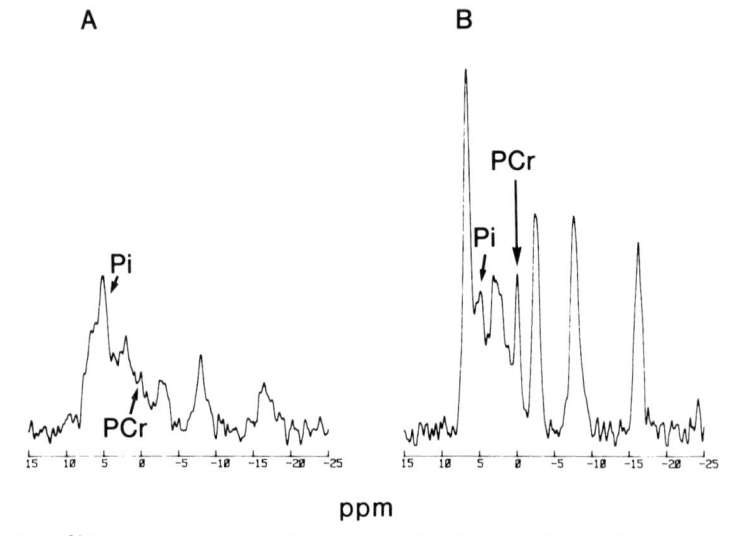

Fig. 5 ^{31}P spectra from the left (**A**) and right (**B**) hemispheres of a baby with infarction of the left hemisphere. He was born at 26 weeks' gestation and studied aged 6 days. Diffusely increased echodensities were present on the left.

The spectrum from the right hemisphere is normal; PCr/Pi 0.93. On the left, PCr/Pi = 0.40, and the total ^{31}P signal is reduced indicating death of cells.

He survived with a large left-sided porencephalic cyst.

the toxic effects of excitatory neurotransmitters.[33-35] Inadequate oxygen supply to the tissue because of capillary stasis and progressive cerebral oedema also probably plays a part. The increase in pH$_i$ above normal may be due to abnormalities of sodium-hydrogen exchange. Further information about these mechanisms is urgently required, so that the effects of rationally based early treatment can be tested. Several investigations by MRS of the effects of an acute reduction in cerebral oxygenation,[25] and of manipulations of arterial carbon dioxide tension in newborn experimental animals, have been reported,[36] and the results of systemic glucose and bicarbonate administration during or immediately after a hypoxic-ischaemic episode have been documented.[37] These studies provide valuable information about brain buffering capacity, glucose consumption and lactate production in response to an acute hypoxic-ischaemic insult. They also show that lactate (measured by ^{1}H MRS) may persist in brain tissue after the phosphorus spectra and pH$_i$ have returned to normal.[25]

Periventricular leucomalacia and other forms of infarction

Periventricular leucomalacia is infarction of the periventricular region of the brain in preterm infants following a hypoxic-ischaemic episode. The localization of the lesion to the periventricular tissue is probably due to the poorly developed blood supply to this region of the immature brain, which therefore sustains damage before other regions.[1] Periventricular leucomalacia may progress to cystic lesions or passive ventricular dilatation and is an extremely important cause of permanent neurodevelopmental disability, notably spastic diplegia. The timing of the initial injury is difficult to define precisely but appears usually to be in the peripartum period, sometimes initiated before delivery and sometimes afterwards. It is quite possible that damage to the periventricular region in very immature ill infants is cumulative, due to repeated episodes of hypotension and hypoxaemia.

Periventricular leucomalacia and other forms of infarction may be suspected before cysts or ventricular dilatation develop, because of the appearance on ultrasound scans of increased periventricular echodensities. However, as indicated earlier, the presence of increased echodensities of this type is not accurately diagnostic. A study with MRS has therefore been done of 27 infants with increased echodensities suggestive of periventricular leucomalacia, as well as of other forms of hypoxic-ischaemic injury—such as middle cerebral artery infarction and birth asphyxia.[19] The aim was to see if evidence of impaired energy metabolism could be found, and if so whether the severity of the impairment was related to subsequent death or loss of brain tissue (cysts or generalized loss) as assessed by ultrasound scans. Fifteen of the 27 infants had PCr/Pi ratios below normal 95% confidence limits, indicating impaired oxidative metabolism. Nine of these 15 died and in all 6 survivors loss of brain tissue developed. By contrast, all 12 infants whose ratios remained within the normal range survived, although loss of brain tissue developed in 3 infants with ratios towards the lower limit of normal. It was concluded that when impaired metabolism was detected in infants with increased echodensities the immediate prognosis was very bad.

Abnormal ^{31}P spectra associated with periventricular leucomalacia have been illustrated previously.[9,19] Figures 4 and 5 show abnormalities in other forms of hypoxic-ischaemic injury. The progression of the abnormalities in different types of injury appears similar. In situations where the eventual outcome is loss of brain tissue, the total ^{31}P signal becomes reduced[17] (Fig. 5).

Neurodevelopmental prognosis

The MRS data have been found to provide prognostic information for neurodevelopmental outcome at one year of age.[21] More recently the brains of 43 infants born at 31–42 weeks of gestation were studied who were known or suspected on various grounds to have suffered hypoxic-ischaemic brain injury. (Ref. 38 and unpublished observations). The surviving infants were examined by independent observers. All 8 infants whose ATP/total P values fell below 95% confidence limits died. Of the 21 infants whose PCr/Pi values fell below 95% confidence limits, 14 died and 6 of the 7 survivors had disabling neurodevelopmental impairments. Only one of the 22 infants with a normal value for PCr/Pi died, and although 5 of the 21 survivors had impairments, these were less serious.

The data from this study and from the study of infants with increased echodensities cited above demonstrate that when severe failure of oxidative phosphorylation following a hypoxic-ischaemic insult is found, death ensues. Less severe, or localized, failure often leads to loss of brain tissue in survivors and is associated with a very high risk of neurodevelopmental disability.

NEAR INFRARED SPECTROSCOPY (NIRS)

NIRS provides continuous cotside information about a wide range of indices of cerebral oxygenation and haemodynamics. The technique therefore shows great promise for the monitoring of ill babies, and it is complementary to MRS in exploring the mechanisms of impaired oxidative phosphorylation.

Background and theory

Spectral analysis of transmitted or reflected visible light is a well-established method for measuring various indices of oxygenation in blood or tissue. However, visible light penetrates tissue very poorly, and information about oxygenation deep inside organs such as the brain cannot be obtained. In 1977 Jobsis showed that if near infrared light with a wavelength of 700–1000 nm was used instead of visible light, penetration of tissue was much greater and spectral measurements could be made across the heads of small animals.[39] At near infrared wavelengths, absorption can be detected due to oxyhaemoglobin (HbO_2), deoxyhaemoglobin (Hb) and the oxidized form of cytochrome aa3, the terminal enzyme of the mitochondrial respiratory electron transport chain, which passes electrons to molecular oxygen. The oxidative (redox) state of this enzyme is an index of intracellular oxygen availability.

Apart from its potential value in enabling brain oxygenation in ill babies to be monitored and regulated, data obtained by the combined use of MRS and NIRS may help elucidate some of the mechanisms of brain damage following a hypoxic-ischaemic episode. Measurements of HbO_2 and Hb in brain tissue give data about the circulating supply of oxygen, and measurement of oxidized cytochrome aa3, about the intracellular availability of oxygen to fuel oxidative phosphorylation. Figure 6 is a very simplified diagram summarizing oxidative phosphorylation. It shows that as a result of the activity of the citric acid cycle, substrate is consumed, and carbon dioxide and electrons are generated. The electrons pass down the respiratory chain, causing protons to be pumped out of the mitochondrial matrix, thereby generating a membrane potential. ATP is synthesized from ADP and Pi when the protons flow back to the matrix through a channel in an ATP-synthesizing complex (mitochondrial ATP-ase). At the end of the chain the electrons reduce cytochrome aa3, which becomes reoxidized when they combine with molecular oxygen:

$$\tfrac{1}{2}O_2 + 2e^- + 2H^+ \rightarrow H_2O$$

This reaction accounts for nearly all of the oxygen uptake of the body.

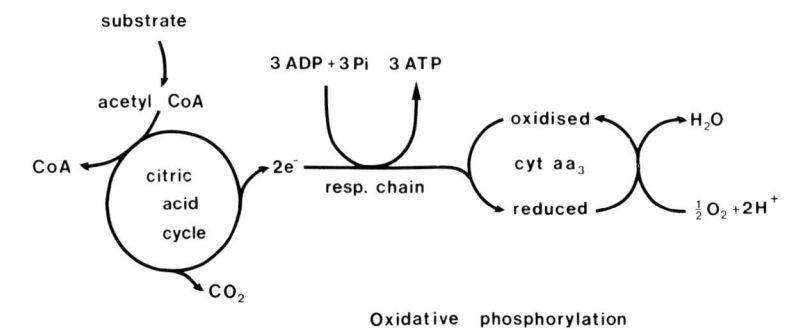

Fig. 6 Simplified diagram to illustrate oxidative phosphorylation. For explanation, see text.

Inadequate oxidative phosphorylation leads first to a fall in the PCr/Pi ratio and then in ATP concentration, as described above. The inadequacy could be due to several different mechanisms which can be investigated by observing the coexisting changes in haemoglobin and cytochrome aa3 oxygenation. For example, if insufficient oxygen supply to tissue was to blame, deoxygenation of haemoglobin and reduction of cytochrome aa3 would be expected, whereas failure of electron transport due to lack of substrate or to mitochondrial disruption would cause cytochrome aa3 to become highly oxidized.

Equipment and methods for studying the brain in newborn infants

Fluctuations in signals from haemoglobin and oxidized cytochrome aa3 have previously been detected from the brains of newborn infants during hypoxaemic episodes[40] and transient elevations of blood pressure,[41] but until very recently quantitation of the data has not been possible.[42]

For quantitation certain variables must be defined. In particular, the spectral absorption properties of the compounds being investigated, and the optical path length (represented by the average distance travelled by photons through the tissue), must be known.

The Beer-Lambert law describing optical absorption in a scattering medium can be expressed as:

$$\text{absorption (in optical densities)} = \alpha cLB$$

where α is the absorption coefficient ($mM^{-1}\,cm^{-1}$), c is concentration (mM), L is the distance between the points where light enters and leaves the tissue (cm), and B is a 'path length factor' which takes account the scattering of light in the tissue (which causes the optical path length to be greater than L). If α, L and B are known, then changes in absorption are directly proportional to changes in concentration.

Because of uncertainty about the absorption spectrum of oxidized cytochrome aa3 in vivo, observations have been made across the heads of rats exchange-transfused with a fluorocarbon blood-substitute, thus removing the signals from haemoglobin.[43] These observations allowed the absorption difference between oxidized and reduced cytochrome aa3 to be defined and, together with in vitro data for the absorption spectra of HbO_2 and Hb provide information for obtaining the necessary values of α. Measurements of optical path length across the head have only recently been made. In initial studies of babies, a path length factor (B) of 1[42,44] or 2[45] was assumed, but recent studies, including those in which the time taken for near infrared light to traverse the head of the rat was measured in picoseconds, suggest a value for B of between 4 and 5.[43,46,47]

Since more than one light-absorbing compound is present in the tissue, several NIR wavelengths must be transmitted and an algorithm is required to convert changes in optical absorption to changes in concentration. The observations described above have enabled a suitable algorithm to be devised.

For current studies, three wavelengths 778, 813 and 867 nm, are employed and the factors for converting changes in optical density at these wavelengths to changes in concentration are given in Table 2. Concentration changes in HbO_2, Hb and oxidized cytochrome aa3 are calculated by summation of absorption changes (measured in optical densities) multiplied by the appropriate factors. The values obtained are expressed in mM l^{-1} cm^{-1} of path length. If a value for tissue density in the light path of 1.05 is assumed, the data can be converted to mM·100 g^{-1}.

To study the brains of newborn infants, portable apparatus has been designed and built.[42,48] Near infrared light at the three wavelengths is emitted from laser diodes and directed into the head through a fibre-optic bundle positioned at a site equidistant from the anterior fontanelle and the external auditory meatus. Light emerging from the opposite side of the head is conveyed through another fibre-optic bundle to a photomultiplier tube operating in photon-counting mode. The ends of the fibres (optodes) are fixed to the scalp with adhesive rings, and optical contact is ensured by means of standard ultrasound contact gel. Background light is excluded by an opaque bonnet.

Table 2 The factors for converting changes in optical density at 778, 813 and 867 nm to changes in concentration

Compound	Multiplying factor		
	778 nm	813 nm	867 nm
HbO_2	0.32	−2.31	2.89
Hb	2.40	−2.67	0.66
Oxidized cytochrome aa3	−0.77	2.28	−1.30

The total light energy emitted by the laser diodes is about half that of a standard cold-light source, and the amount of energy absorbed by brain tissue is several orders of magnitude below British Standards Institute safety limits (BS 4803).

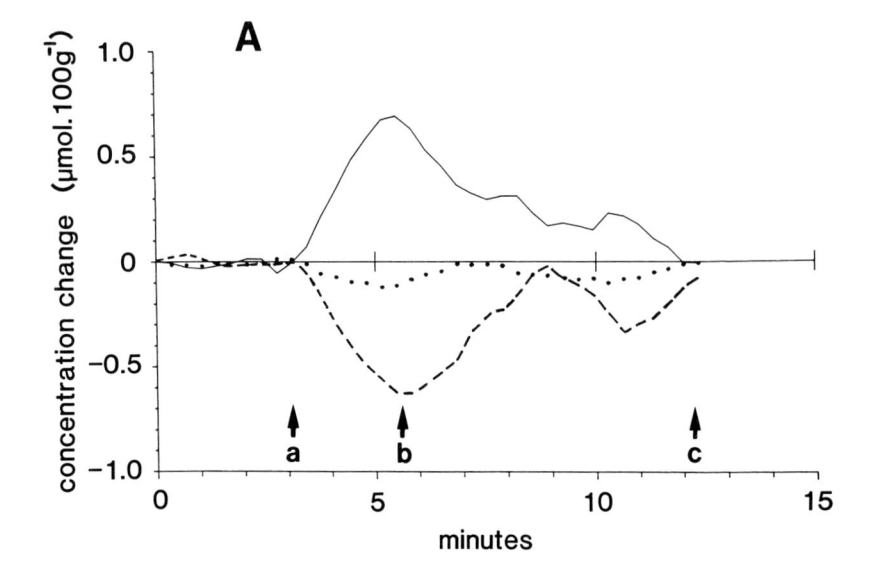

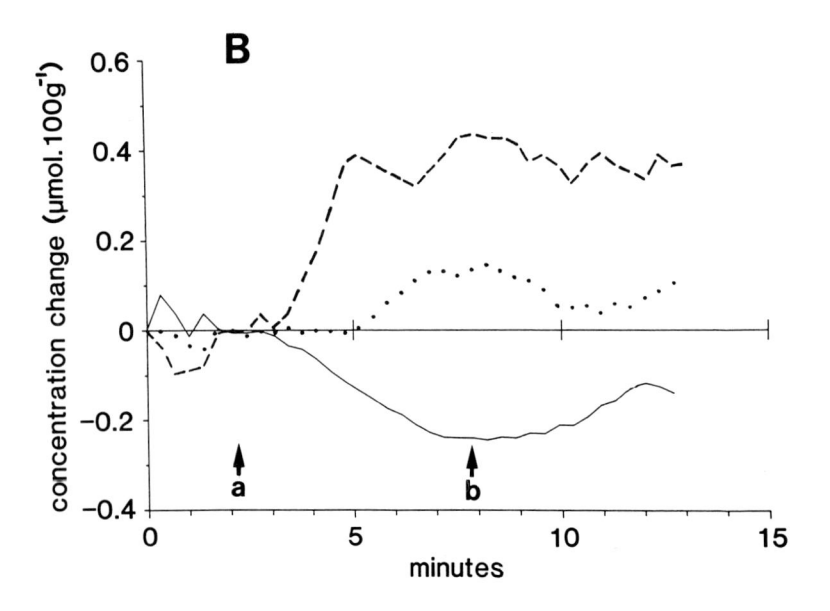

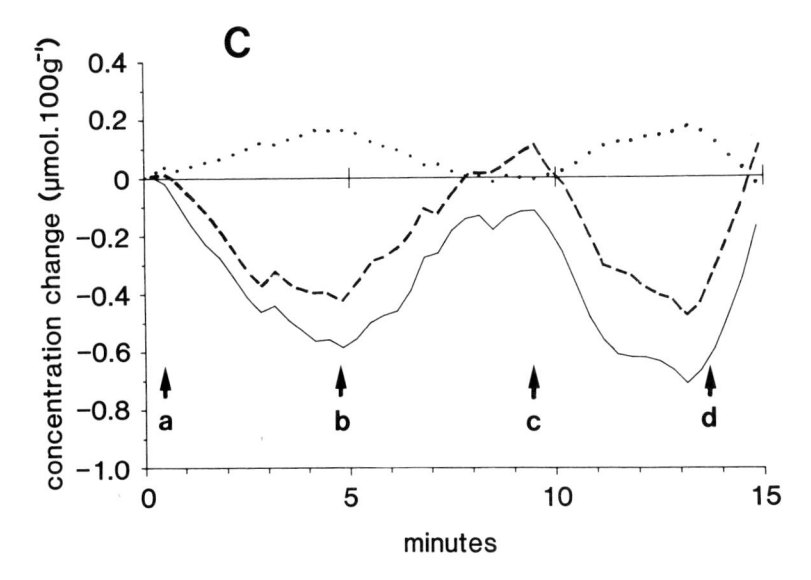

Fig. 7 Changes in the cerebral concentrations of HbO_2 (-----), Hb (—) and oxidized cytochrome aa3 (......) in two infants with normal brains, born at 27 weeks' gestation and studied aged one day (**A** and **B**), and at 25 weeks and studied aged 70 days (**C**).
Changes are shown during:
A: Alterations in S_aO_2, which was 96% at **a** and **c**, and 84% at **b**.
B: Alterations in P_aCO_2 which was 4.6 kPa at **a** and 5.7 kPa at **b**.
C: Head up tilting by 10° at **a** and **c**; and back to level at **b** and **d**.

Figure 7 shows changes in the concentrations of HbO_2, Hb and oxidized cytochrome aa3 in response to small alterations in arterial oxygen saturation (S_aO_2) and carbon dioxide tension (P_aCO_2), and to head-up tilting.

Quantitation of haemodynamic variables

NIRS primarily provides information about **changes** in the concentration of light-absorbing compounds in the brain as shown in Figure 7. In addition, **absolute** values for a number of important haemodynamic variables can be estimated, if the results of various manoeuvres are observed.[42,44,45,49] For example, total cerebral haemoglobin concentration (tHb) in $mM \cdot 100 \text{ g}^{-1}$ of tissue can be derived from the alterations in the concentration difference $[HbO_2] - [Hb]$ which occur during a small transient change in S_aO_2. Provided cerebral blood flow and oxygen consumption remain constant during this change,

$[HbO_2] - [Hb]$ will vary linearly with S_aO_2[42,49] and tHb can be estimated from the expression:

$$tHb = \Delta([HbO_2] - [Hb]) \times 0.5/\Delta(S_aO_2)$$

Cerebral blood volume in ml·100 g^{-1} of tissue can then be obtained if a value for mean cerebral haematocrit is estimated.

It has also been suggested that an estimate of mixed cerebral venous saturation (S_vO_2) can be made from observing the results of a small head-up or head-down tilt (Fig. 7c).[42] The skull of a newborn, particularly preterm, infant is much more compliant than later in life; hence the acute alterations in the cerebral concentrations of HbO_2 and Hb which result from a tilt may reasonably be assumed to be due initially to changes in the size of the intracranial venous compartment. S_vO_2 can then be calculated from the formula:

$$S_vO_2 = \Delta[HbO_2]/\Delta([HbO_2] + [Hb])$$

In the near future it is likely that methods will be described for quantitating a number of other important variables, notably cerebral blood flow and cerebral arterial saturation.

Results in newborn infants

Quantitative results from NIRS of the brain in infants are so far scanty.[42,44,45,49] A number of tentative inferences may however be drawn from the available information. For example, the cerebral blood volume was 2.3 (SD $\pm$ 0.3) ml·100 g^{-1} in 8 babies born at 27–43 weeks of gestation who were thought to have normal brains. By contrast, it was significantly elevated, 4.4 (SD $\pm$ 1.0) ml·100 g^{-1}, when studied in 9 infants 24–42 hours after they had sustained brain injury—hypoxic-ischaemic in 7, and associated with cerebral haemorrhage in 2.[45] (It should be noted that the technique used does not measure blood-clot as part of the cerebral blood volume.) The response of the cerebral blood volume to small alterations in P_aCO_2 was investigated in these same infants. The change in blood volume ranged from 0.2 to 0.8 ml·100 g^{-1}. kPa^{-1} in infants with normal brains, with evidence of reduced sensitivity to changes in P_aCO_2 in the least mature ones. Infants with brain injury showed a significant decrease in response to changes in P_aCO_2. These preliminary findings suggest that fixed vasodilatation of the cerebral circulation and reduction of the responses to changes in P_aCO_2 are common following brain injury.

This situation has been found to precede and be associated with the development of secondary energy failure, as detected by MRS and discussed above. The combined use of MRS and NIRS in experimental animals is beginning to provide further information about this sequence of events.[50]

Alterations in cytochrome aa3 oxidation have been quantified during transient alterations in S_aO_2 and P_aCO_2.[42,43] Changes in the oxidation-state of the enzyme appear to follow those of haemoglobin (Fig. 7) demonstrating the relation between haemoglobin saturation and intracellular oxygen availability.

Repeated observations in five infants with convulsions have shown a fall in cerebral HbO_2 concentration during the fit, together with a rise in that of Hb and a significant increase in cerebral blood volume.[44] At the same time cytochrome aa3 became less oxidized—except in one infant who was muscle-relaxed and showed increased haemoglobin oxygenation and cytochrome oxidation during paroxysmal electrical activity.

These findings all require confirmation in larger studies.

SUMMARY AND CONCLUSIONS

Very preterm infants and other infants who require intensive care are at considerable risk of death or long-term neurodevelopmental disability. Non-invasive methods have therefore been sought for assessing the structure and function of the brain in the immediate newborn period. The availability of these methods allows the prevalence and mechanisms of potentially brain-damaging influences to be explored, preventive strategies and treatment to be tested and the prognosis for the infants to be assigned. Several methods have proved their worth: for example, ultrasound imaging, electroencephalography, including the testing of evoked potentials, and Doppler ultrasonography for measuring flow-velocity in intracerebral vessels.

Ultrasound-imaging is particularly valuable for investigating cerebral haemorrhage in very preterm infants, but is of little use for elucidating the early events of hypoxic-ischaemic brain injury, which is a more important cause than haemorrhage of long-term disability in very preterm and other infants who survive after intensive care. Furthermore, recent evidence suggests that lesser degrees of injury may go unrecognized by current techniques and could account for some of the subtle neurodevelopmental abnormalities that are found at school age in surviving infants. Non-invasive methods have therefore been introduced for studying hypoxic-ischaemic injury. The purpose of this review has been to discuss two new methods, magnetic resonance spectroscopy and near infrared spectroscopy.

Magnetic resonance spectroscopy is used to investigate phosphorus energy metabolism and intracellular pH. Clear evidence of deranged energy metabolism has been found in a range of conditions of hypoxic-ischaemic injury. A latent period of many hours often follows acute injury before energy failure develops, suggesting the possibility of effective early treatment. Abnormalities of oxidative phosphorylation are predictive of a very poor prognosis for normal survival. Many new developments in magnetic resonance spectroscopy are imminent, particularly employing proton (^{1}H) spectroscopy which will enable a wide range of metabolites, including neurotransmitters, to be measured. The combination of magnetic resonance spectroscopy with imaging will allow quantifiable data to be obtained from small selected volumes within the brain, and measurements of blood and cerebrospinal fluid flow are becoming possible.

Near infrared spectroscopy provides continuous information about cerebral oxygenation and haemodynamics at the cotside. Quantitative measurements of oxyhaemoglobin, deoxyhaemoglobin and oxidized cytochrome aa3 can be made, and a range of haemodynamic indices can be derived. The technique is already beginning to provide information about the haemodynamic events occurring in the brain after a hypoxic-ischaemic insult and before overt energy failure develops, both in newborn infants and experimental animals. It is likely eventually to go into routine use for monitoring brain oxygenation in ill babies and guiding therapy. Imaging of brain-oxygenation at the cotside will in the future probably be feasible.

The deployment of non-invasive techniques for examining the brains of very preterm and other ill infants looked after in neonatal intensive care units provides the best hope for achieving the major aim of intensive care, namely to ensure the maximum chances of survival for potentially normal children, but at minimum risk of salvaging hopelessly disabled ones.

ACKNOWLEDGEMENTS

We thank for their help, R Aldridge, Dr AD Edwards, E Eldon, Dr PA Hamilton, Dr PL Hope, Miss C Richardson, and many members of the staff of the Neonatal

Unit and the Departments of Paediatrics, Medical Physics and Bioengineering, and Physiology; and we are grateful to Mrs G Harris for preparing the manuscript. This work was supported by Action Research for the Crippled Child, the DHSS, Hamamatsu Photonics, the MRC and the Wellcome Trust.

REFERENCES

1 Pape KE, Wigglesworth JS. Haemorrhage, ischaemia and the perinatal brain. For: Spastics International Medical Publications, London: Heinemann, 1979
2 Levene MI, Williams JL, Fawer C-L. Ultrasound of the infant brain. Clinics in developmental medicine, No. 92. For: Spastics International Publications, Oxford: Blackwell, 1985
3 Gould S, Howard S, Hope PL, Reynolds EOR. Periventricular intraparenchymal cerebral haemorrhage in preterm infants: the role of venous infarction. J Pathol 1987; 151: 197–202
4 Stewart AL, Thorburn RJ, Hope PL, Goldsmith M, Lipscomb AP, Reynolds EOR. Ultrasound appearance of the brain in very preterm infants and neurodevelopmental outcome at 18 months of age. Arch Dis Child 1983; 58: 598–604
5 De Vries LS, Dubowitz LMS, Dubowitz V et al. Predictive value of cranial ultrasound in the newborn baby: a reappraisal. Lancet 1985; ii: 137–140
6 Sinha SK, Davies JM, Sims DG, Chiswick ML. Relation between periventricular haemorrhage and ischaemic brain lesions diagnosed by ultrasound in very preterm infants. Lancet 1985; ii: 1154–1156
7 Fawer C-L, Calame A, Perentes E, Anderegg A. Periventricular leukomalacia: a correlation study between real-time ultrasound and autopsy findings. Neuroradiology 1985; 27: 292–300
8 Trounce JQ, Fagan D, Levene MI. Intraventricular haemorrhage and periventricular leucomalacia: ultrasound and autopsy correlation. Arch Dis Child 1986; 61: 1203–1207
9 Hope PL, Gould SJ, Howard S et al. Precision of ultrasound diagnosis of pathologically verified lesions in the brains of very preterm infants. Dev Med Child Neurol 1988 (In press)
10 Stewart AL, Reynolds EOR, Hope PL et al. Probability of neuro-developmental disorders estimated from ultrasound appearance of brain in very preterm infants. Dev Med Child Neurol 1987; 29: 3–11
11 Gadian DG. Nuclear magnetic resonance and its application to living systems. Oxford, Clarendon Press, 1982
12 Chu A, Delpy DT, Thalayasingam S. A transport and life support system for newborn infants during NMR spectroscopy. In: Rolfe P, ed. Fetal and neonatal physiological measurements. London: Butterworths, 1986: pp. 409–415
13 Tofts PS, Cady EB, Delpy DT et al. Surface coil NMR spectroscopy of brain. Lancet 1984; i: 459
14 Hope PL, Costello AMdeL, Cady EB et al. Cerebral energy metabolism studied with phosphorus NMR spectroscopy in normal and birth-asphyxiated infants. Lancet 1984; ii: 366–370
15 Azzopardi D, Hamilton PA, Wyatt JS et al. Phosphorus metabolites and intracellular pH in the brains of normal and small-for-gestational age infants investigated by magnetic resonance spectroscopy (Submitted)
16 Petroff OAC, Prichard JW, Behar KL, Alger JR, den Hollander JA, Shulman RG. Cerebral intracellular pH by ^{31}P magnetic resonance spectroscopy. Neurology 1985; 35: 781–788
17 Cady EB, Costello AMdeL, Dawson MJ et al. Non-invasive investigation of cerebral metabolism in newborn infants by phosphorus nuclear magnetic resonance spectroscopy. Lancet 1983; i: 1059–1062
18 Hope PL, Reynolds EOR. Investigation of cerebral energy metabolism in

newborn infants by phosphorus magnetic resonance spectroscopy. Clin Perinatol 1985; 12: 261–275
19 Hamilton PA, Hope PL, Cady EB, Delpy DT, Wyatt JS, Reynolds EOR. Impaired energy metabolism in brains of newborn infants with increased cerebral echodensities. Lancet. 1986; i: 1242–1246
20 Delpy DT, Cope MC, Cady EB et al. Cerebral monitoring in newborn infants by magnetic resonance and near infrared spectroscopy. Scand J Clin Lab Invest 1987; 47 (Suppl 188): 9–17
21 Reynolds EOR, Hamilton PA. Magnetic resonance spectroscopy of the brain and early neurodevelopmental outcome. In: Kubli F, Patel N, Schmidt W, Linderkamp O, eds. Perinatal events and brain damage in surviving children. Berlin: Springer-Verlag, 1987: pp. 247–253
22 Younkin DP, Delivoria-Papadopolous M, Leonard J et al. Unique aspects of human newborn cerebral metabolism evaluated with phosphorus nuclear magnetic resonance spectroscopy. Ann Neurol 1984; 16: 581–586
23 Lawson B, Anday E, Guillet R, Wagerle LC, Chance B, Delivoria-Papadopoulos M. Brain oxidative phosphorylation following alteration in head position in preterm and term infants. Pediatr Res 1987; 22: 302–305
24 Tofts PS, Wray S. Changes in brain phosphorus metabolites during the postnatal development of the rat. J Physiol 1985; 359: 417–429
25 Hope PL, Cady EB, Chu A, Delpy DT, Gardiner RM, Reynolds EOR. Brain metabolism and intracellular pH during ischaemia and hypoxia. An in vivo ^{31}P and ^{1}H nuclear magnetic resonance study in the lamb. J Neurochem 1987; 49: 75–82
26 Gyulai L, Bolinger L, Leigh JS, Barlow C, Chance B. Phosphorylethanolamine—the major constituent of phosphomonoester peak observed by ^{31}P-NMR in developing dog brain. FEBS Lett 1984; 178: 137–142
27 Bottomley PA, Hart HR, Edelstein WA et al. Anatomy and metabolism of the normal human brain studied by magnetic resonance at 1.5 tesla. Radiology 1984; 150: 441–446
28 Delpy DT, Gordon RE, Hope PL et al. Non-invasive detection of cerebral ischemia by phosphorus nuclear magnetic resonance. Pediatrics 1982; 70: 310–313
29 Behar KL, den Hollander JA, Stromski ME et al. High resolution ^{1}H nuclear magnetic resonance study of cerebral hypoxia in vivo. Proc Natl Acad Sci USA 1983; 80: 4945–4948
30 Cerdan S, Subramanian H, Hilberman M et al. ^{31}P NMR detection of mobile dog brain phospholipids. J Mag Res Med 1986; 3: 432–439
31 Wray S, Tofts PS. Direct in vivo measurement of absolute metabolite concentrations using ^{31}P nuclear magnetic resonance spectroscopy. Biochim Biophys Acta 1986; 886: 399–405
32 Tofts PS, Wray S. Non-invasive measurement of molar concentrations of ^{31}P metabolites in vivo using surface coil NMR spectroscopy. J Mag Res Med 1988; 6: 84–86
33 Siesjo BK. Brain energy metabolism. New York: Wiley, 1978
34 Siesjo BK. Cerebral circulation and metabolism. J Neurochem 1984; 60: 883–908
35 Schwarcz R, Meldrum B. Excitatory amino acid antagonists provide a therapeutic approach to neurological disorders. Lancet 1985; ii: 140–143
36 Cady EB, Chu A, Costello AmdeL et al. Brain intracellular pH and metabolism during hypercapnia and hypocapnia in the new-born lamb. J Physiol 1987; 382: 1–14
37 Hope PL, Cady EB, Delpy DT, Ives NK, Gardiner RM, Reynolds EOR. Brain metabolism and intracellular pH during ischaemia: The effects of systemic glucose and bicarbonate administration studied by ^{31}P and ^{1}H nuclear magnetic resonance spectroscopy in vivo in the lamb. J Neurochem 1988; 50: 1394–1402

38 Azzopardi D, Wyatt JS, Cady EB et al. Prognosis of infants with hypoxic-ischaemic brain injury assessed by phosphorus magnetic resonance spectroscopy Pediatr Res 1987; 22: 220
39 Jobsis FF. Non-invasive infrared monitoring of cerebral and myocardial oxygen sufficiency and circulatory parameters. Science 1977; 198: 1264-1267
40 Brazy JE, Lewis DV, Mitnick MH, Jobsis van der Vliet. Non-invasive monitoring of cerebral oxygenation in preterm infants: preliminary observations. Pediatrics 1985; 75: 217-225
41 Brazy JE, Lewis DV. Changes in cerebral blood volume and cytochrome aa3 during hypertensive peaks in preterm infants. J Pediatr 1986; 108: 983-987
42 Wyatt JS, Cope M, Delpy DT, Wray S, Reynolds EOR. Quantitation of cerebral oxygenation and haemodynamics in sick newborn infants by near infrared spectrophotometry. Lancet 1986; ii: 1063-1066
43 Wray S, Cope M, Delpy DT, Wyatt JS, Reynolds EOR. Characterisation of near infrared absorption spectra of cytochrome aa3 and haemoglobin for the non-invasive monitoring of cerebral oxygenation. Biochim Biophys Acta 1988; 933: 184-192
44 Wyatt JS, Cope M, Delpy DT, Wray S, Reynolds EOR. Cerebral oxygen and haemodynamics during neonatal seizures assessed by continuous near infrared spectrophotometry. Early Hum Dev 1987; 15: 307
45 Wyatt JS, Cope M, Delpy DT, Wray S, Richardson C, Reynolds EOR. Responses of cerebral vasculature to changes in arterial carbon dioxide measured by near infrared spectroscopy in newborn infants. Pediatr Res 1987; 22: 230
46 van der Zee P, Delpy DT. Simulation of the point spread function for light in tissue by a Monte Carlo technique. Adv Exp Med Biol 1988; 215: 179-192
47 Cope M, van der Zee P, Arridge SR, Wray S, Wyatt JS, Delpy DT. Direct measurement of optical pathlength during NIR transillumination of the brain. Phys Med Biol (In press)
48 Cope M, Delpy DT. A system for long term measurement of cerebral blood and tissue oxygenation in newborn infants. Med Biol Eng Comput 1988 (In press)
49 Wyatt JS, Cope M, Delpy DT, Richardson C, Edwards AD, Reynolds EOR. Measurement of cerebral blood volume in newborn infants by near infrared spectroscopy (Submitted)
50 Aldridge R, Cady EB, Cope MC et al. Simultaneous measurements of cerebral oxygenation and metabolites by near infrared (nir) and ^{31}P nuclear magnetic resonance (nmr) spectroscopy during hypoxia in rats. J Physiol 1988; 396: 96P

Neurophysiological assessment of the immature central nervous system

J A Eyre
Department of Child Health, University of Newcastle upon Tyne, Newcastle upon Tyne, UK

> During the first trimester of gestaton differentiation and maturation of the cortical neurons occurs and myelination of cortical and subcortical afferent and efferent pathways begins. These processes are reflected in marked changes in the EEG and in sensory evoked potentials. In extremely preterm infants the EEG and evoked potentials are characterized by significant intra and inter subject variability. Prolonged recordings of the EEG in the first few days after birth have, however, been shown to be of prognostic significance. The variability of sensory evoked potentials limits their prognostic significance; recordings in this very high risk group at one month corrected postnatal age are of greater prognostic significance. The recently developed technique of electromagnetic stimulation of the cortex has the potential to provide for the first time an objective measure of corticospinal tract function in these babies who are at very high risk of cerebral palsy.

Perinatal brain damage is the most common cause of life long handicap for the survivors of extremely premature birth. In these infants clinical physical examination is unreliable for the detection of lesions in the central nervous system; emphasis has, therefore, been placed on the diagnosis of structural lesions in the brain by ultrasonography, computerized tomography and magnetic resonance imaging, the study of neural metabolism with nuclear magnetic spectroscopy and the identification of neurophysiological abnormality through the recording of the electroencephalogram (EEG) or sensory evoked potentials.

From 23–24 weeks gestation to term there is rapid growth, maturation and differentiation of neurons and glial cells within the central nervous system. To place normal and abnormal neurphysiological measurements in context it is important to have an overview of the developmental changes occurring within the central nervous system in the final trimester of gestation. It is in a sense an abstraction to consider the neurophysiology of the infant of less than 28 weeks gestation in isolation because this period is but a small window with in a continuing process of development. It is therefore also important to place these neurophysiological observations in the context of those obtained later in gestation and in the older child.

DEVELOPMENT OF THE CENTRAL NERVOUS SYSTEM

The ontogeny of the human central nervous system begins during embryogenesis with the formation of the neural plate and groove followed by the development of the neural tube.[1] This is followed in the second month of gestation by the differentiation of the rostral end of the neural tube into the diencephalon, from which the thalami, the hypothalamus and the optic placodes are formed, and the telencephalon, which gives rise to the basal ganglia, the ventricles and the cerebral hemispheres.[1] Neural proliferation and migration also begin during the second month, and continue until the fifth month of gestation. The cerebral cortical neurons are derived from subependymal cells in the periventricular region and migrate from there to their ultimate destination; the earliest neurons form layer six of the cortex and the later neurons migrate through these cells to form the more superficial layers of the cerebral cortex.[2]

In the final trimester of gestation the differentiation of cortical neurons and the organization of the cerebral cortex into six layers occurs and the mature pattern of sulci and gryi becomes established. During this period there is the elaboration of neuronal dendritic and axonal processes, the formation of synapses between cortical neurons and the establishment of afferent and efferent sub-cortical connections.[3] There has been little detailed study of these processes in man. Purpura and his co-workers have described the progress of dendritic development in the hippocampus and have shown that the maximal rate of development of dendritic spines occurs between 20–28 weeks of gestation.[4] The period for maximal development of dendritic spines in the visual cortex occurs between 25–32 weeks.[5]

The third trimester is also a period of rapid proliferation and differentiation of glial cells, however, glial cell proliferation and differentiation also remain incompletely understood in man. Most is understood concerning the development of myelination in the central nervous system.[6] The studies by Yakovlev and Lecours demonstrate that myelination of central afferent and efferent pathways begins at approximately 24 weeks gestation. Myelination of these pathways proceeds at different rates but in general myelination at afferent sensory pathways precedes that of the ascending and descending motor pathways.

THE ELECTROENCEPHALOGRAM OF THE EXTREMELY PRETERM INFANT

Ontogeny of the normal EEG

There are striking changes in the EEG of the preterm infant with increasing gestational age which probably reflect the differentiation of the cortical neurons and the progressive development of intra-cortical and subcortical interneuronal connections. The appearance of cyclical changes in the pattern of the EEG with sleep and wakefulness and the synchronization of the rhythms with changes in the pattern of other physiological variables correspond with the development of subcortical connections. Repeated recording of the EEG, therefore, can provide a simple and noninvasive means to monitor cerebrocortical maturation.

The systematic study of the EEG of newborn babies began with the pioneering descriptions of Gibbs and Gibbs.[7] The initial description of the cyclical organization of sleep in infants by Askerinsky and his collegues[8] aroused further interest in studies of the EEG in the newborn and in the preterm infant. The healthy full term infant has since been shown to have well developed and easily recognized sleep wake cycles;[9-11] these states can be identified by the characteristic patterns of EEG, the polygraphic and the behavioural criteria defined by Prechtl[10] and Anders and his colleagues.[11] Unlike the term baby the very preterm baby does not have clearly defined states of arousal.[9] The first signs of an organized pattern of sleep states, however, appear at approximately 24–26 weeks of gestational age with the emergence of two distinct patterns of EEG (Fig. 1). The first pattern called 'trace alternant' is characteristic of the pattern of EEG during quiet sleep in the term baby.[9-12] This pattern of EEG comprises bursts of high voltage slow wave activity interspersed between periods of suppressed EEG activity. The second pattern is a precursor of the EEG later associated with wakefulness and active sleep and comprises a continuous EEG of mixed frequencies with a predominance of slow wave activity.[9-12]

It has been thought previously that the EEG of the very preterm baby comprised almost entirely the first, discontinuous, pattern with little or no continuous activity.[9,12] This conclusion, however, has been based either on the findings of early studies when such extremely preterm babies were not viable, or from recordings made from sleeping babies. Recently it has become possible to make continuous prolonged recordings of the EEG over many

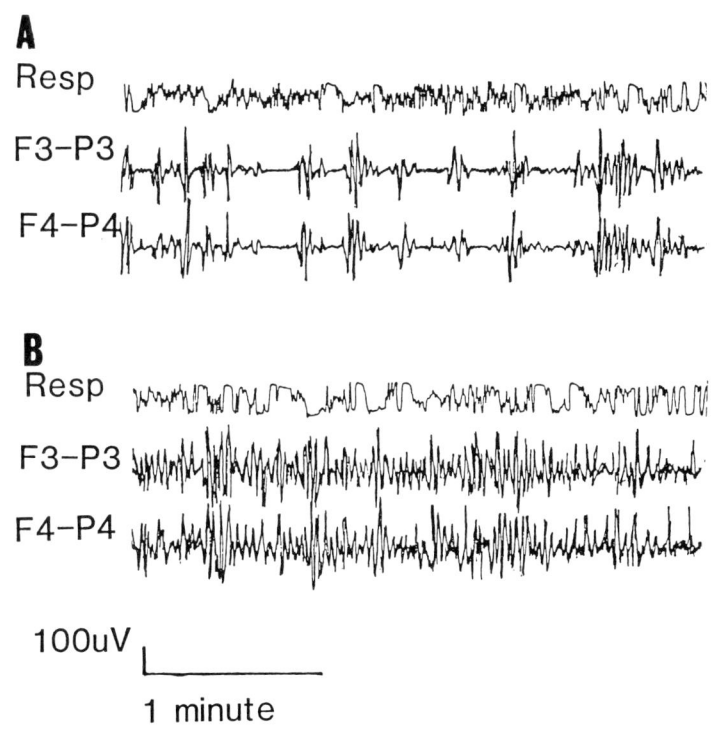

Fig. 1 EEG recorded at 26 weeks gestation showing: **A**, trace alternant activity; and **B**, continuous activity.

days in healthy extremely preterm babies.[13] Such prolonged recordings have demonstrated that although the EEG of babies born as prematurely as 24 weeks gestation is predominantly discontinuous, there are frequent periods of continuous activity particularly during wakefulness.[14,15] The duration of individual epochs of continuous activity and the percentage of the total EEG which is continuous increase progressively as the child matures; thus, the EEG changes rapidly from being predominantly discontinuous at 24 weeks gestation to being predominantly continuous by 28 weeks gestation. This process of maturation continues so that at term the epochs of trace alternant are of 5 minutes or less duration every 45–60 minutes and occur only when the child is sleeping.[14,15] The trace alternant pattern is rarely if every seen in the EEG of healthy children older than 3 months of age.

While the two basic patterns of EEG exist in very preterm babies there is little synchronization of the EEG with the other variables which together define sleep states in the older baby.[9,12] Thus eye movements, body movements, irregularity of respiration and spontaneous fluctuations of the skin resistance can and do occur independently and with either pattern of the EEG. It is not until 32 weeks gestation that the organization of these parameters into recognizable sleep states begins;[9,12] from then until 40 weeks post conceptional age the interrelations between different elements become more clearly defined and organized into the two sleep termed active and quiet sleep. The two sleep states appear to mature independently and studies by Drefus-Brisac show that active sleep is seen in its typical form by 35 weeks and quiet sleep by 37 weeks gestation.[9,12]

In addition to the progressive change in the gross pattern of the EEG there are changes in the background EEG which reflect the increasing maturity of the cerebral cortex. Two variables, the progressive changes with gestation in the trace alternant pattern and the incidence of delta brush (see below), can easily be quantified from relatively short recordings of the EEG and these provide useful indices of cortical maturity.

There are striking changes in the trace alternant pattern with increasing maturation (Fig. 2). First, there is a progressive reduction in the duration of the periods of suppression between the bursts of the high voltage slow waves.[14–16] The mean duration at 26 weeks duration is approximately 26 s and this decreases progressively to be approximately 13 s at 32 weeks gestation and 4 s at term.[14,15] In addition to the longer mean duration of suppression

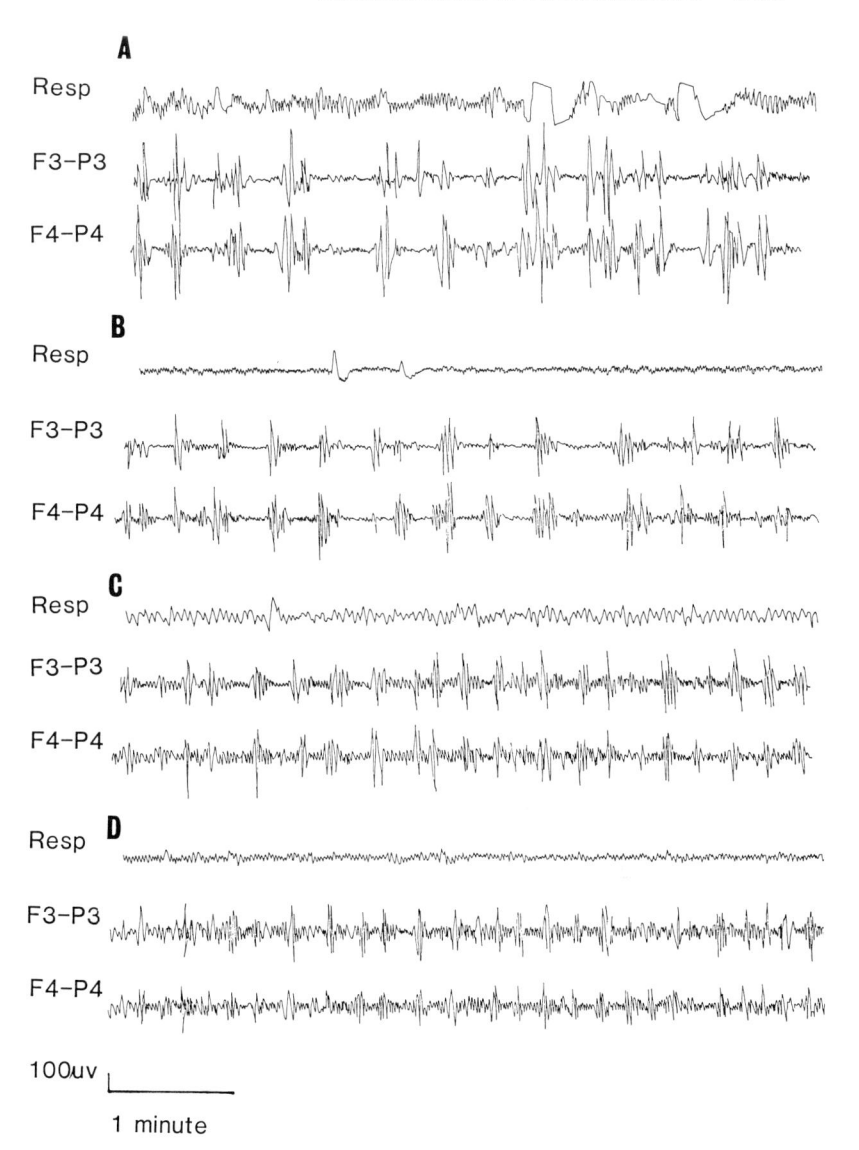

Fig. 2 The progressive changes in the trace alternant activity with increasing gestational age.

between bursts, there is a much greater intra-individual variability of this duration in the extremely preterm infant, thus the standard deviation in the extremely preterm infant, thus the standard deviation for the duration of the suppressed interval is approximately 7 s at 26 weeks gestation, 3 s at 32 weeks and 1.8 s at term.[14,15]

In contrast to the duration of suppression, the duration of each burst of high voltage slow waves does not change with increasing gestation and remains between 2 and 5 s.[14,15] The amplitude of the high voltage slow wave activity during bursts, however, does change with gestational age; between 26–31 weeks the mean voltage remains constant, approximately 440 µV, it decreases to 130 µV at 42 weeks gestation.[14,15] The intra-individual variability of the maximum voltage is much greater in the very preterm babies and this variability also decreases significantly over the same period.[14,15]

Delta brush is the name given to high frequency (8–20 Hz), spindle like activity which is superimposed on delta wave (1–2 Hz) activity (Fig. 3).[9,16,17] Whilst the origin of this activity is unknown, this pattern of activity is recognized to be characteristic of the EEG of extremely preterm babies.[9,16,17] Delta brush is seen only very infrequently, less than once in 5 minutes of EEG record, in babies of 26 or less weeks of gestation, from 27–31 weeks the frequency of its occurrence increases rapidly so that by 31 weeks it occurs as often as 30–50 times in a 5 minute period.[16,17] The incidence of delta brush becomes then progressively less and it is rarely seen in the EEG of a baby of more than 37 weeks gestation.[16,17]

In summary the EEG of the extremely preterm baby is characterized by marked changes with increasing gestational age. There is, however, great intra and inter subject variability in the pattern of the EEG in such immature babies, and thus to characterize

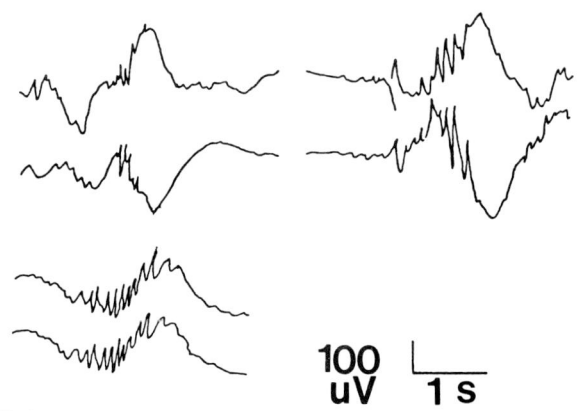

Fig. 3 Delta brush activity recorded at 28 weeks gestation.

adequately the pattern of the EEG long periods of recording are required. Only limited conclusions can be drawn from a single recording but repeated recordings of the EEG with increasing gestational age will allow the rapid maturation of the cerebral cortex to be monitored.

Prognostic significance of abnormality in the EEG

The value of the EEG in the prediction of the long term neurological outcome of newborn babies who have sustained a variety of brain injuries has been assessed repeatedly, e.g.[18,19] Although the prognostic significance of normal and severely abnormal EEGs has been established, mild and moderate abnormalities in the EEG been shown previously to be of little prognostic significance.[18,19] Early recording of the EEG and serial recording during the period of intensive care, however, has been shown to improve the prognostic significance of the EEG.[18,19] Recently it has become possible to make continuous records of the EEG in very sick preterm infants during the period of the intensive care.[13] Such recordings have revealed a high incidence of subclinical seizure activity in very ill preterm babies and the calculation of both the degree and total duration of abnormalities in the EEG improved its prognostic significance.[13,14]

In a recent study[14] of the EEG recorded for the first 5 days after birth in 35 babies of less than 32 weeks gestation (range 25–31 weeks) who were receiving intensive care, electrographic seizure activity occurred in 13 (37%). This study demonstrated that unless EEGs are recorded within the first 24–48 hours after birth the diagnosis of seizure will be missed. Thus, the median time of onset of seizure activity was 10 hours after birth (range 2–63 h) and for all but 2 of the 13 babies the seizures were present for less than 72 hours. In addition the total duration of seizure activity was greatest on the first day after seizure onset and decreased markedly on the second and subsequent days. Nine of the 35 babies died in the perinatal period; a detailed neurological and developmental assessment of all 26 surviving babies was made at 18 months of age. Nine were found to have neurodevelopmental abnormalities and 17 were normal. Both the occurrence and the duration of seizure activity in the first 5 days after birth were found to be strongly predictive of outcome (Table 1). The duration of normal EEG and of mild, moderate and severe abnormality was also found to be strongly predictive of outcome (Table 2).

Table 1 The outcome of 35 preterm babies in relation to the presence and duration of electrographic seizure activity in the first 5 days after birth[13]

Outcome	No Seizure n	Seizure n	Mean total duration of seizure activity h
Died	1	8	3.70
Abnormal	5	4	1.31
Normal	16	1	0.49

Table 2 The outcome of 35 preterm infants in relation to the degree and duration of abnormality in the EEG recorded in the first 5 days after birth[13]

Outcome	Mean % of total EEG record			
	Normal	Mild abn	Moderate abn	Severe abn
Normal	82	13	6	0
Abnormal	45	17	16	17
Died	0	3	34	67

abn = abnormality

Thus prolonged recording of the EEG particularly in the first few days after birth has been found to be of both diagnostic and prognostic value in preterm babies receiving intensive care.[14,19]

EVOKED POTENTIALS

The EEG reflects the integrated function of the cortical neurons, and as such, while abnormality may give an indication of the severity of the injury, the EEG gives only limited information on the localization of cortical lesions. It is not possible from the EEG to determine if there are lesions involving specific subcortical areas or pathways.

An evoked potential represents the brain's response to an external stimulus, for example the visual evoked potential in response to a flash of light can often be seen as a wave in the occipital region of the EEG. The clinical utility of evoked potentials is based on the assumption that they test objectively and quantitatively the maturity and integrity of specific sensory pathways from the sense organ or peripheral nerve to the cortex. Most evoked potentials cannot be seen on a standard EEG because of their low amplitude and they must be extracted from the ongoing EEG activity by computer averaging of the responses to many repeated stimuli.

One or more waves may be present in an evoked potential; the presence or absence of appropriate waves and their latencies are the major features used to assess the majority and integrity of a sensory pathway. There are three types of sensory evoked potential, the auditory, the somatosensory and the visual. The discussion below will consider only auditory and somatosensory evoked potentials in anticipation that visual evoked potentials will be discussed in the subsequent chapter.

Auditory evoked potentials

The brainstem auditory evoked potential (BAEP) represents the electrical activity generated by the auditory nerve, and centres in the pons and midbrain in response to repeated auditory stimulation. Typically in the adult or older child it shows a 7 wave pattern (Fig. 4); wave 1 is thought to be generated in the eight nerve and the 5th wave is assumed to be generated in the rostral part of the pons or the caudal part of the midbrain.[20] Therefore, the waves I to 5 inter-peak latency provides an objective measure of the conduction time within the auditory pathway of the brain stem.

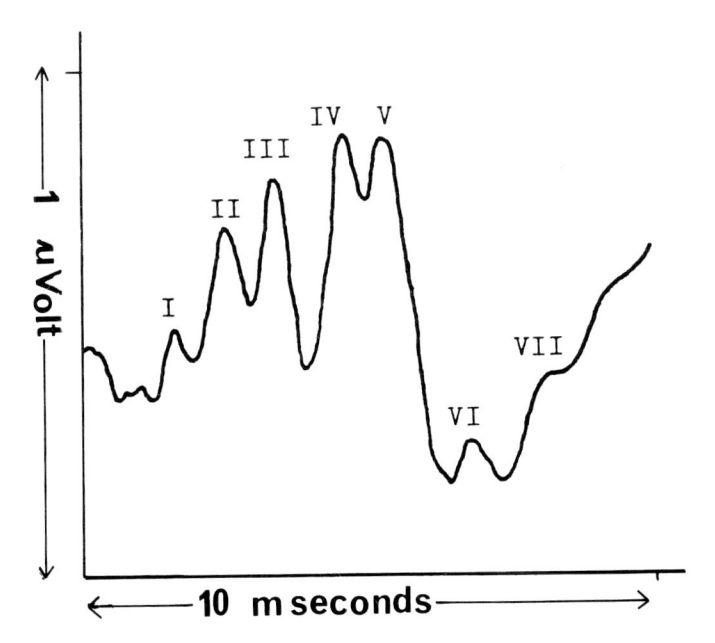

Fig. 4 Brain stem auditory evoked potential recorded in an adult illustrating the 7 waves.

The 8th cranial nerve has been shown to be amongst the first cranial nerves to have myelinated fibres with myelination being demonstrated from the 14th fetal week in the semicircular canals[1] and by the 5th fetal month the roots of both divisions of the eight nerve are myelinated.[6] At the end of the 5th fetal month the medial longitudinal fasciculus, the tectospinal tract, the trapezoid body, the lateral lemniscus and the inferior colliculi begin to show their first myelinated fibres and myelination of the brainstem auditory pathway is completed by the middle of the 9th fetal month.[6]

With such rapid myelination of the brainstem auditory pathways occurring between the 5th and 8th month of gestation, the value of the BAEP has been studied extensively in the preterm infant to assess its value both as an objective measure of gestational age and as an immediate indicator of brainstem damage.

BAEPs have been recorded in response to auditory stimuli from 25 weeks gestation.[21] Such studies have demonstrated that an auditory stimulus of much higher intensity (70–110 dB) is required to elicit BAEPs in babies between 25–28 weeks than in adults.[22] As one would predict from the morphological studies of myelination, the wave 1–5 latency is prolonged in extremely preterm infants and this latency decreases progressively with postconceptional age.[23,24] (Fig. 5) In exremely preterm babies there is, however, a wide inter-individual variability in all parameters studied including wave form, relative amplitudes, and peak and inter-peak latencies.[24] This wide variability makes it impractical to use a single recording of the BAEP to estimate gestation. Recently it has been suggested that serial measurements and the calculation of the rate of change in the wave 1–5 latency may provide a more useful index of healthy brainstem development in extremely preterm infants.[23]

Several investigators have reported considerable test-retest variability in the wave 1–5 latency among sick extremely preterm infants and this clearly limits the prognostic value of measurements made during intensive care. A persisting abnormality, however, once the baby had recovered from the acute illness, or at term and beyond has been shown to be correlated with a poor neurodevelopmental outcome.[25]

Finally, extremely preterm babies are at high risk of subsequent deafness. The correlation in term infants between the BAEP and audiological outcome demonstrated by Galambos and his associates[26] and by others, suggest that BAEPs provide an effective means of detecting hearing impairment. The brainstem auditory

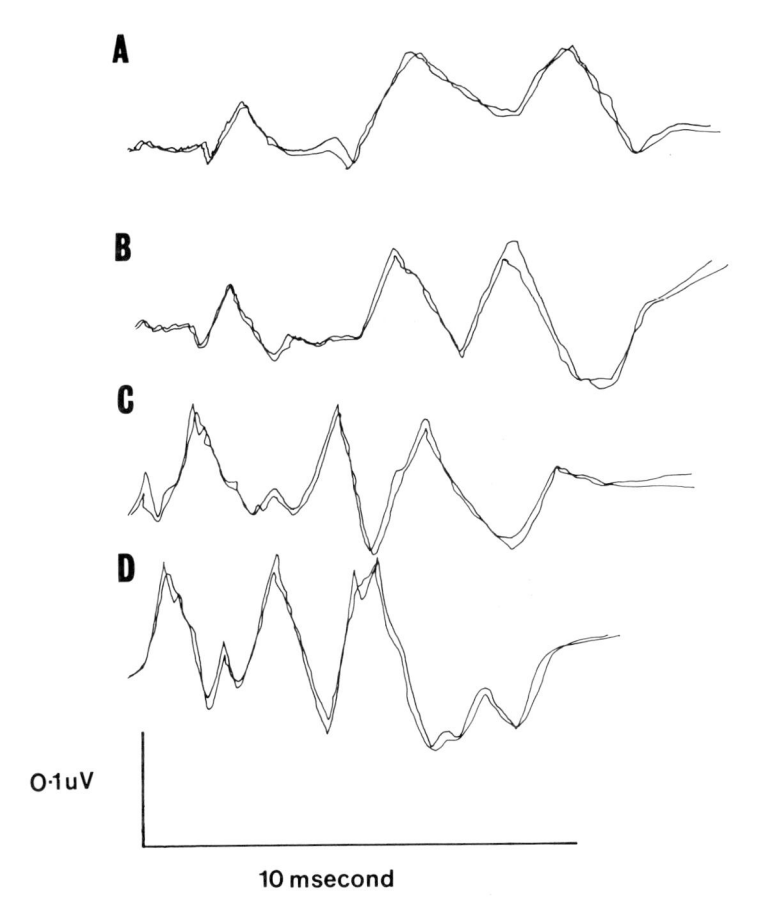

Fig. 5 Serial brain stem auditory evoked potentials recorded in a baby: **A**, 27 weeks; **B**, 30 weeks; **C**, 33 weeks; and **D**, 40 weeks gestation.

evoked potential is not, however, simply a hearing test. Predictions of hearing loss cannot be made from any recorded abnormality in the BAEP where there is clinically evident brainstem damage nor when recordings are made from extremely preterm infants.[25]

Somatosensory evoked potential

Somatosensory evoked potentials (SEPs) are usually evoked by percutaneous stimulation of peripheral nerves. Most commonly, the median nerve is used for stimulation in the upper limb, and the peroneal or posterior tibial nerve for the leg. The SEPs are best recorded in the contralateral parietal somatosensory cortex. Like other evoked potentials the SEP is a complex sequence of waves. With median nerve stimulation the earliest component is a negative wave, N_{20} or N_1, which in adults has a latency of 20 msec. This wave is thought to result from the first arrival of an afferent volley at the somatosensory cortex.

Clinical and experimental observations suggest that the SEP is derived from activity in the dorsal columns, the medial lemniscus, thalamus and the sensory cortex. The SEP has been, therefore, of particular interest to the neonatologist because this afferent sensory pathway passes through areas of particular vulnerability in the periventricular region of the lateral ventricles, and because of its close anatomical proximity in this region to the pyramidal tract. In the absence of an established technique to assess corticospinal tract function the SEP has been used primarily as a means to allow early detection of cerebral palsy in these very high risk babies.

Hrbek and his colleagues[27] have reported obtaining somatosensory evoked potentials in preterm infants of 24 weeks gestation and have demonstrated progressive changes with increasing gestational age. In the premature infant they describe the SEP as comprising a high amplitude and very prolonged slow wave. The latency to the onset of this wave decreased with increasing gestational age as did its amplitude and duration.

There are clearly, however, many difficulties associated with the recording of SEPs in newborn infants and these difficulties are exacerbated in the extremely preterm infant. First, it has been shown to be extremely difficult to record SEPs consistently even in healthy term newborn infants and where recording times are reported each study has taken between 2 and 5 hours. In the papers citing the sucess rate for obtaining SEPs in healthy neonates it has varied from inability to obtain cortical responses in the majority[28] to being able to obtain SEPs in only 80% of healthy newborn subjects at term.[29] No papers as yet have discussed the sucess rate in obtaining SEPs in preterm infants but our own unpublished observations show that the SEPs are evoked progressively less frequently in healthy preterm infants with increasing immaturity.

Second, when SEPs have been successfully evoked, there are reports of significant intra and intersubject variability in the latency and in the morphology of N_1 in newborn infants and young children.[30,31]

Finally, Gorke[32] assessed the value of SEP recording in the detection of motor pathway dysfunction in children aged 1 to 10 months. He found that although abnormality in the SEP was closely associated with abnormal or delayed motor development, there was a high false negative rate with 19 of 38 children with delayed motor development having normal SEP examinations.

These observations must limit the clinical application of SEPs for both the assessment of central nervous system maturity and for the identification of upper motor neuron lesions in the extremely preterm infant.

ELECTROMAGNETIC STIMULATION OF THE MOTOR CORTEX

The periventricular region of the lateral ventricles is the most common site of injury to the brain of extremely preterm infants resulting either from haemorrhage or infarction. Lesions in this area commonly involve damage to the pyramidal tracts or the basal ganglia and there is a very high incidence of cerebral palsy amongst the survivors of extremely preterm birth. An objective neurophysiological measure of the maturity and integrity of the descending motor pathways has not been available until now. The recent development of the technique of electromagnetic stimulation of the motor cortex,[33] provides for the first time the exciting opportunity to assess objectively the integrity of the descending motor pathways, most probably primarily of the corticospinal tracts, in very young children including the extremely preterm infant. This method uses a flat circular stimulating coil through which a brief current is passed. The pulsed magnetic field so generated induces electrical currents in the brain which are assumed to excite the superficial layers of the cortex. When the coil is held above the scalp overlying the motor cortex, activity is evoked in the descending motor pathways including the corticospinal tracts and results in muscle action potentials measurable by skin mounted EMG electrodes. The particular advantages of this technique for use in children are first, the stimulating coil does not need to touch the baby and second, the motor action potential induced is large, with an amplitude in millivolts rather than the microvolts of sensory evoked potentials, and so repeated stimulation and computer averaging is not required. The technique is, therefore, simple, painless and very quick. Prolongation of the latency to evoked muscle action potential following electromagnetic stimulation of the motor cortex has been shown to be a sensitive indicator of motor pathway dysfunction in adults.[33]

Recently, following an evaluation of the safety of the technique in an animal model,[34] electromagnetic stimulation has been applied to the study of corticospinal tract function in children including preterm infants.[35] These studies have demonstrated that it is possible to stimulate the motor cortex and to evoke motor action potentials in biceps brachii in babies of less than 28 weeks gestation. With increasing gestational age there is a progressive reduction in the latency to the evoked muscle action potential and adult values are not achieved in fact until the age of eight years. Studies in children of one month and older with clinical signs of an upper motor neuron lesion have shown that electromagnetic stimulation is a sensitive indicator of motor pathway dysfunction in children (Koh and Eyre, unpublished observations). The findings in extremely preterm infants are only preliminary. Studies are currently in progress to establish whether electromagnetic stimulation of the motor cortex will provide a sensitive method for the early detection of cerebral palsy in this very high risk group of babies even when there are no clinical signs of motor dysfunction.

ACKNOWLEDGEMENTS

The generous support of the following is gratefully acknowledged; the National Fund for Research into Crippling Disorders, the MRC, the Newcastle Health Authority, the Spastics Society.

REFERENCES

1 Lemire RJ, Loeser JD, Leech RW, Alvord EC Jr. Normal and abnormal development of the human nervous system. Maryland: Harper and Row, 1975
2 Sidman RL, Rakic P. Neuronal migration with special reference to developing human brain: a review. Brain Res 1973; 62: 1–15
3 Marin-Padilla M. Prenatal and early postnatal ontogenesis of the human motor cortex: a golgi study II. The basket pyramidal system. Brain Res 1970; 23: 185–191
4 Paldino AM, Purpura DP. Quantitative analysis of the spatial distribution of axon and dendritic terminals of hippocampal pyramidal neurons in immature brain. Exp Neurol 1979; 64: 604–619
5 Takashima S, Chan F, Becker LE, Armstrong DL. Morphology of the visual cortex of the human infant. J Neuropathol Exp Neurol 1980; 39: 488–501
6 Yakovlev PI, Lecours A. The myelogenic cycles of regional maturation of the brain. In: Minkowski A, ed. Regional development of the brain in early life. Oxford: Blackwell, 1967: pp. 3–65
7 Gibbs FA, Gibbs EL. Atlas of encephalography. Reading: Addison-Wesley, 1950
8 Askerinsky KE, Klietman N. Regularly occurring periods of eye mortality and concomitant phenomena during sleep. Science 1953; 118: 273–274
9 Dreyfus-Brisac C. Ontogenesis of brain bioelectrical activity and sleep organis-

ation in neonates and infants. In: Falkner F, Tanner JM, eds. Human Growth, Vol 3. London: Plenum, 1979: pp. 157–182
10 Prechtl HPR. States of the infant. Clin Dev Med 1968; 28: 27–41
11 Anders TF, Emde R, Parmelee AH. A manual of standardised terminology, techniques and criteria for scoring states of sleep and wakefulness in newborn infants. California: UCLA Information Service BRI Publications, 1971
12 Dreyfus-Brisac C. Neonatal electroencephalography. In: Scarpelli EM, Cosmi EV, eds. Reviews in Perinatal Medicine, Vol 3. New York: Raven Press, 1979
13 Eyre JA, Oozeer RC, Wilkinson AR. Diagnosis of neonatal seizure by continuous recording and rapid analysis of the electroencephalogram. Arch Dis Child 1983; 58: 785–790
14 Eyre JA. Neurological disorders: EEG. In Harvey D, Cooke R, Levitt G. eds. The baby under 1000 gms. London: Wright (In press)
15 Eyre JA, Nanei S, Wilkinson AR. Quantification of changes in pattern of normal electroencephalogram in relation to gestational age from continuous five day recordings. Dev Med Child Neurol 1988 (In press)
16 Anderson CM, Torres F, Faoro A. The EEG of the early premature. Electroencephalogr Clin Neurophysiol 1985; 60: 95–105
17 Lombroso CT. Quantified electrographic scales on 10 pre-term healthy newborns followed up to 40–43 weeks of conceptional age by serial polygraphic recording. Electroencephalogr Clin Neurophysiol 1979; 46: 460–471
18 Watanabe K, Miyazaki S, Hara K, Hakamada S. Behavioural state cycles, background EEGs and prognosis of newborns with perinatal asphyxia. Electroencephalogr Clin Neurol 1980; 49: 618–625
19 Tharp BR, Cukier F, Monod N. The prognostic value of the electroencephalogram in premature infants. Electroencephalogr Clin Neurol 1981; 51: 219–236
20 Jewett DL, Romano MN, Williston JS. Human auditory evoked potentials: possible brainstem components detected on the scalp. Science 1970; 167: 1517–1518
21 Marshall RE, Reichert TJ, Kerley SM, Davis H. Auditory function in newborn intensive care unit patients revealed by auditory brain stem evoked potentials. J Pediatr 1980; 96: 731–735
22 Mjoen S, Langslet A, Tangsrud SE, Sundby A. Auditory brainstem responses in high risk neonates. Acta Paediatr Scand 1982; 71: 711–715
23 Vles JSH, Casper P, Kingma H, Swennen C, Daniels H. A longitudinal study of brainstem auditory evoked potentials of preterm infants. Dev Med Child Neurol 1987; 29: 577–585
24 Krumholz A, Jacob KF, Goldstein PJ, McKenzie E. Maturation of the brainstem auditory evoked potential in premature infants. Electroencephalogr Clin Neurol 1985; 62: 124–134
25 Stockard JE, Stockard JJ, Kleinberg F, Westmoreland BF. Prognostic value of brainstem auditory evoked potentials in neonates. Arch Neurol 1983; 40: 360–365
26 Galambos R, Despland P. The auditory brainstem response (ABR) evaluates risk factors for hearing loss in the newborn. Pediatr Res 1980; 14: 154–158
27 Hebek A, Karlberg P, Olsson T. Development of visual and somatosensory evoked responses in preterm newborn infants. Electroencephalogr Clin Neurophysiol 1973; 34: 225–232
28 Platt H, Amlie RN, Starr A. Short latency mechanically evoked peripheral nerve and somatosensory potentials in newborn infants. Pediatr Res 1981; 15: 295–298
29 Cullity P, Franks CI, Duckworth T, Brown BH. Somatosensory evoked cortical responses: detection in normal infants. Dev Med Child Neurol 1976; 18: 11–18
30 Whittle IR, Johnston IH, Besser M. Short latency somatosensory-evoked potentials in children—part I. Surg Neurol 1987; 27: 9–18

31 Blair AW. Sensory examinations using electrically induced somatosensory potentials. Dev Med Child Neurol 1971; 13: 447–455
32 Gorke W. Somatosensory evoked cortical potentials indicating impaired motor development in infancy. Dev Med Child Neurol 1986; 28: 633–641
33 Barker AT, Freestone IL, Jalinous R, Jarratt JA. Magnetic stimulation of the human brain and peripheral nervous sytem: An introduction and the results of an initial clinical evaluation. Neurosurgery 1987; 20: 100–109
34 Eyre JA, Flecknell PA, Kenynon BR, Koh THHG, Miller S. The effects of electromagnetic stimulation of the brain on cortical activity, cortical blood flow, blood pressure, and heart rate in the cat. Proceedings of the Physiological Society, Sept 1987
35 Eyre JA, Koh THHG. Maturation of descending motor pathways in man from birth to adulthood. Proceedings of the Physiological Society, Sept 1987

The immature visual system and premature birth

Alistair R Fielder[1]
Merrick J Moseley[1]
Yin K Ng[1,2]
Departments of Ophthalmology[1] and Child Health,[2] University of Leicester Medical School, Leicester

> At term the eye is at a relatively advanced stage of development, compared to rest of the body, and the period from 28 to 40 weeks gestation is one of particularly active growth. As by this time the very immature infant has already been born, we have first reviewed ocular growth and then considered the effects certain aspects of the neonatal environment, such as light and temperature, may have on the developing visual system. Using a technique orientated approach we discussed the visual development of 'normal' preterm infants, and those who have suffered neurological damage. Finally we considered the incidence of acute and cicatricial retinopahty of prematurity, concluding with a brief discussion of certain aspects of the pathogenesis of this perplexing condition.

The effects preterm birth may have on the visual system have not been systematically investigated, not surprising in view of the relatively recent increase in the survival of this population. To set the scene for the rest of this article a few anatomical aspects of the developing visual system will first be reviewed. This will be followed by consideration of the neonatal environment and the developing visual system, visual development, and finally retinopathy of prematurity. Inevitably the topics covered will reflect the authors' clinical and research activities. Our current dearth of knowledge will soon become apparent, but we hope this article will serve as a review and indicate some of the many important challenges which remain.

THE DEVELOPING VISUAL SYSTEM

Growth of the eyeball

At term the eye is relatively well developed, growing only three times compared to 20 times for the rest of the body to achieve adult size.[1] The most active phase of ocular growth is between six months gestation and term, normally in utero, but at a time when the very immature infant has already been born. Recently Birnholz,[2] using ultrasonography visualised several ocular structures including the lens, iris, pupil and cornea, and measured various ocular parameters during the second and third trimesters of pregnancy. He observed two phases of accelerated growth of eyeball diameter between 12 and 20 weeks, and 28 and 32 weeks gestational age (GA). Transverse ocular diameters at 22.1, 26.8 and 37.8 weeks GA were 9.57 mm, 11.74 mm and 15.82 mm respectively (adult value 24.0 mm). These measurements of the internal ocular diameter are about 90% of those obtained from necropsy material when readings are taken from the external scleral surface.

Corneal diameter increases linearly from three months gestation and has achieved adult dimensions within a month or so after term.[1,3] Prior to approximately 27 weeks GA the cornea is hazy.[4] Retinal surface area doubles between six months and term and a further 50% increase takes place over the ensuing two years.[3] Interestingly this increase in retinal size occurs after cell division in this tissue has ceased[5] and is achieved by shifts of distribution. As growth of the anterior segment of the eye is almost complete at term, most of the subsequent ocular growth involves the posterior segment of the eye, predominantly in the periphery (the anterior region of the retina, just behind the ciliary body) and not in the region of the optic disc and macula.[6]

Vascular development

The hyaloid artery enters the eye posteriorly at about the sixth week of gestation. Over the next few weeks this vascular complex fills the vitreous cavity and forms a network of vessels around both surfaces of the lens, this latter known as the tunica vasculosa lentis (TVL). Atrophy of this transient vascular system commences during the fourth month—the hyaloid artery has usually disappeared by seven months and the anterior portion of the TVL regresses between 28 and 34 weeks GA.[4]

Before the 16th week of gestation the retina is completely avascular, but from this time mesenchymal cells extend out from the optic disc forming a primitive vascular network from which capillaries and later arterioles and veins develop.[7] This process reaches the periphery of the nasal retina at about 8 months gestation but the temporal retina is not fully vascularised until just after term. Before this process has commenced, and in decreasing amounts prior to its completion, the metabolic requirements of the retina are met by the choroid.

Visual pathway

At term the peripheral retina is well developed[8] but this is not so for the central retina. In the adult, the macula is an oval, vessel-free area about 4.0 mm temporal and slightly inferior to the level of the optic disc, it is 4.0 to 5.5 mm across and contains a central 1.5 mm depression the fovea with the foveolar pit in its centre. Ophthalmoscopically, both the fovea and foveolar give rise to visible reflexes. At 22 weeks GA the fovea is flat and contains only one layer of cones. Peripheral migration of the inner retinal layers to form a central foveolar depression commences at 24 weeks and is completed by 15 months post-term. Later there is a central migration of cones, with increased packing into the foveola, so that by 15 months these photoreceptors are 6–8 cells deep and cone density in the centralmost 250 μm has risen from 28 to 47. This high cone density is thought to be necessary for fine resolution.[9] Cones are probably recruited from the immediate surrounding retina, with a corresponding removal of rods towards the periphery, although the total cone density in the foeva changes little. Thus, contrary to standard teaching, the fovea is not fully developed by six months of term, and even at 45 months there are morphological differences from the adult.[9]

Early in development, apart from its absence of retinal vessels, the macular region cannot be distinguished ophthalmoscopically from the rest of the retina. At about 34 weeks this area develops a dark red appearance and an incomplete foveal reflex, which is not complete until 36.3 weeks ($+/-2.2$ weeks) and the foveolar reflex is not observed until almost 42 weeks GA.[10]

The posterior visual pathway also undergoes rapid developmental changes in early postnatal life (review[11]) with the lateral geniculate nucleus and visual cortex both reaching a maximum volume by six months of age.

Myelination of the optic nerve commences between six and eight months gestation but is not completed until the age of two years.[12] Myelination of the posterior geniculostriate visual pathway and superior colliculus commences just before term and is complete within a few months, however, myelination of the extrastriate visual areas takes at least another decade (review[13]).

Gestational age assessment

Regression of the tunica vasculosa lentis (TVL) and the ophthalmoscopic appearance of the fovea can both be used as guides to gestational age. They are however both influenced by retinopathy of prematurity (ROP) and are therefore of value only at birth or in the early neonatal period. The central gap appears in the TVL at 27 to 28 weeks GA and enlarges until only a few peripheral remnants remain at 34 weeks. After this time the appearance of the fovea can be used as a guide to gestational age, as an incomplete foveal reflex is first seen at 34 weeks, which is completed by 36. A foveolar reflex appears at 41 weeks gestation.[10]

Summary

> At 28 weeks gestation the eye is less than half adult size, the retina is only partly vascularised and the transitory tunica vasculosa lentis has yet to atrophy fully. The fovea is very poorly differentiated and myelination of the visual pathway is only just beginning. As, at term, the eye is at a relatively advanced stage of development compared to the rest of the body, the period from 28 to 40 weeks is one of the most active periods of ocular growth.

NEONATAL ENVIRONMENT

Compared to the fetal environment, that into which the preterm infant is placed is relatively harsh, being usually continuously and brightly illuminated, and noisy.[14] Yet knowledge of its effect on the visual system of the very immature, often sick infant is limited; whether it be beneficial, with accelerated visual development, or adverse due to phototoxic retinal damage. In this section we consider two factors, light and temperature, which may influence the developing visual system.

Light

Neonatal exposure to light may be classified according to source and falls into two categories: the ambient environment, and that arising from treatment and examination, such as phototherapy and ophthalmoscopy. Estimates of the amount of light reaching the eye and retina need to be known before considering the effects, beneficial or otherwise, that premature exposure to light may exert on the developing visual system. This, the ocular light dose, depends not only on environmental illumination but also on biological factors such as eyelid opening and the transmission characteristics of the various ocular tissues including the closed eyelid. Having first considered these aspects, the possible effect light may exert on the immature visual system of animals and humans will then be discussed. For a detailed review see Moseley and Fielder.[15]

The environment

The very small premature infant spends the first few weeks or months of life in an environment which is constantly and brightly illuminated. Landry and associates[16] who surveyed eight neonatal units, reported mean levels of illumination ranging from 258 lx to 1485 lx and levels in excess of 10^4 lx have been measured when sunlight is added.[17] Such light levels are capable of causing retinal damage in certain laboratory animals.

Phototherapy. A recent survey[18] found that all eyeshields available in the United Kingdom were effective in reducing the intensity of light reaching the eye to less than 0.1%. But it is also well known that they tend to slip, leaving the eyes unprotected. As yet there is little evidence that phototherapy causes retinal damage in human infants (review[19]), although most investigators (see[19]) have studied carefully patched infants—those least at risk.

Ophthalmic examination. Indirect ophthalmoscopy can produce potentially hazardous retinal irradiance. Kirkness[20] suggests a maximum examination duration of 23 to 80 seconds in adults, and, it would seem prudent that this is also adhered to in the neonate. Unfortunately the origin of these safety levels is not quoted: 23 seconds is an extremely short time to scrutinize the entire retina carefully.

Biological factors influencing the ocular light dose

Eyelid opening. Seemingly a trivial topic, which hitherto has been largely ignored, but knowledge of the duration of eyelid opening is a necessary prerequisite to studying the following: amount of light entering the eye, ocular temperature, and visual experience. Recently, eyelid opening has been studied in 12 well preterm neonates at 33 to 40 weeks postmentstrual age (PMA).[21] Observations were made in a specially allocated cubicle in which illumination was controlled. Eyelid opening was often asymmetric with the eyelid in contact with the mattress opening less than its fellow. Overall, irrespective of state, they were closed for about 80% of the time.[21,22] Recently this investigation has been extended to neonates with gestational ages ranging from 24 to 40 weeks (Robinson, Fielder and Moseley—in preparation), and in contrast to previous studies, factors such as handling and feeding have been taken into account. Observations commenced within the first week of life, with data sampling spread over the 24 hour period. Broadly, these findings confirm the previous finding but with interesting differences: the eyelids of neonates of 27 to 31 weeks GA were closed at least 80% of the time but this figure declines with increasing gestational age (Fig.1). However, for the most immature neonate, the situation is quite different. At 24 weeks GA the eyelids are closed for about 55% of the time, rising to 70% by 26 weeks GA. There is considerable individual variation (Fig. 2) with values ranging from 50% to 90%.

Light transmission through the eyelid and ocular tissues. As the eyelids are closed for a significant proportion of the time the transmission characteristics of the eyelid must be known in order to determine the ocular light dose. This is not known for the neonate but has been determined experimentally in the adult.[23] Light transmission varied as a function of wavelength from approximately 1% at the blue, increasing to 10% at the red end of the spectrum.

Other factors influencing the light dose include transmission through the ocular media, pupil size and retinal surface area. The media of older infants are known to be highly transparent, particularly at the blue and ultraviolet end of the spectrum.[24] Corneal haze, the tunica vasculosa lentis and the relatively opaque vascularised vitreous, will all reduce ocular transmissivity in the very immature infant, depending on postmenstrual age. According to Robinson[25] the pupils are unreactive until 29 to 31 weeks GA. Birnholz[2] using ultrasound observed fetal pupil size to be small (2–3 mm). Measurements recently obtained in our department (Robinson, Fielder and Moseley—in preparation) indicate that preterm pupil-

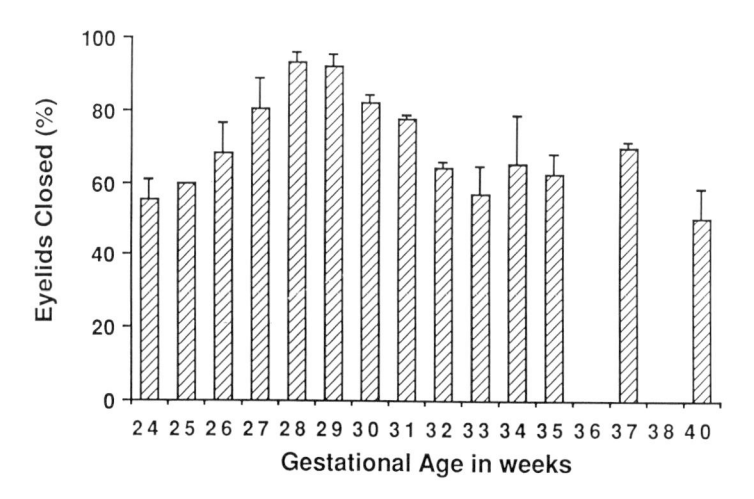

Fig. 1 Eyelid closure: observations taken over a 24 hour period in the first week of life. Infants grouped according to GA, mean of all values ($\pm$ SEM). Infants between 27 and 31 weeks GA have their eyelids closed for at least 80% of the time, those more or less mature open their eyes for longer periods.

lary size is 3.46 mm $\pm$ 0.13 and varies little between about 25 and 30 weeks GA.

Effect of light on the immature visual system

Although the eyelids of preterm infants are often closed for much of the time, even when closed some light predominantly at the red end of the spectrum, reaches the eyes. Moreover the most immature neonate requiring prolonged intensive care tends to keep his eyelids open for longer periods than his relatively older counterpart, thereby greatly increasing his retinal light dose.

Exposure to light has been shown to cause retinal damage in a number of laboratory animals (reviews[15,24,26]) including the rat, pig, and monkey[15] and in some instances at intensities encountered in a neonatal unit. In general, except for the rat[27] the degree of damage is greater in the more immature animal and is increased by elevation of body temperature[28] over a narrow range of 1 to 3°C.[29] Retinal photodamage is also increased by a rise in oxygen tension.[30,31] Photodamage demonstrates 'biological reciprocity', thus short intense exposure can produce the same effect as a less intense exposure of longer duration.[32] Thus both the retinal dose (total radiant exposure) and dose rate (retinal irradiance) are important. The results of animal studies must be translated to

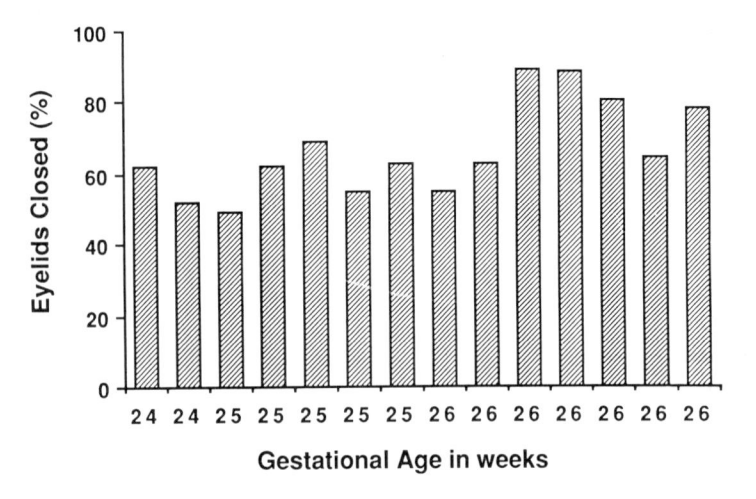

Fig. 2 Eyelid closure: the percentage of time the eyelids are closed over a 24 hour period for individual infants 24–26 weeks GA. Note some very immature babies have their eyelids open for about 50% of the time.

clinical practice with caution, not only because of the species differences but also because laboratory conditions have often been far removed from the clinical situation.[19]

The evidence for premature exposure to light affecting the developing visual system of the human, particularly that of the very immature infant, is sparse. Hamer and associates[17] examined infants (29.5 to 40.0 weeks GA) at three weeks post-term and could not detect any evidence of visual function loss due to exposure to the continuous illumination of the neonatal unit. The authors recognized that subtle defects may have passed undetected, an important caveat as at this age due to the normally low resolution ability of the immature visual system, acuity testing is necessarily a relatively insensitive tool and only a major generalised defect could reduce acuity. The possible retinotoxic effects of phototherapy have been suspected almost since its inception and investigated using the ERG on a number of occasions,[32-34] of which two used preterm infants.[32,33] No abnormality was detected, not entirely surprising as many of the infants had been patched during treatment, and recent evidence points to cone rather than rod damage (see below). Ophthalmic examination of children (not necessarily all ex-prematures) has revealed a high incidence of strabismus (review[15]). The possible causal relationship between this finding and either phototherapy or hyperbilirubinaemia, must be treated with caution in view of the known high incidence of strabismus in preterm infants, particularly if neurologically damaged. Abramov and associates[35] studied the visual performance of seven year-olds who had been born at term, undergone neonatal intensive care, but had not all received phototherapy. They detected subtle deficits in cone-mediated functions, acuity and colour vision, which were not present in controls, and which could not have been identified by the previously mentioned study.[17] These authors[35] suggested that these defects could be due to both the high levels of ambient illumination of the neonatal unit and stray light from phototherapy of neighbouring babies. Two studies, without commenting on the use of phototherapy (or not), reported acuities at the lower end of the normal range in ex-prematures, at three to four years[36] and 10 to 18 years of age.[37]

The suggestion that light may hasten myelination has yet to be determined.[13] Zetterstrom[38] proposed that early exposure to light might hasten the development of the ERG of the preterm, an observation recently supported by results from a few preterm neonates (youngest 29 weeks GA) investigated by Ricci and associates.[39] As already mentioned, ocular growth is at its most active during the third trimester but the possible effect of early exposure to light (predominantly red intermingled with varying periods of white) on this process has not been investigated.

Summary

Although exposure to levels of illumination encountered in the modern neonatal unit have been shown to result in retinal damage in the experimental animal, the evidence for similar damage to the human visual system has been less forthcoming. To date almost all research has been directed at the term or relatively mature preterm infant, but in all probability if damage does occur it is likely to be subtle and affect cone rather than rod mediated function.

TEMPERATURE

Recently the ocular (corneal) temperature of preterm and term neonates has been studied using non-contact infrared radiation thermometry.[40] Mean ocular temperature was 36.54 and 36.8°C for the right and left eyes of preterm infants (mean rectal temperature 36.78°C), whilst for term babies the corresponding values were 36.40 and 36.25°C (mean rectal temperature 37.03°C). Although rectal temperature did not vary in either group with incubation, ocular temperature was significantly higher under the latter condition, this difference being rather greater for the premature baby.

Fetal temperature at 38.1°C is above maternal core temperature.[41] Thus the very immature infant suffers an ocular temperature deficit of approximately 1.5 to 2.0°C, which is never regained, for a period depending on the degree of prematurity. The magnitude of this loss is not known precisely, but the estimate given above is almost certainly an underestimate, as corneal temperature is controlled in part by eyelid opening and environmental temperature, both of which change before term in directions which would reduce corneal temperature further. The possible effect this temperature deficit may have on the eye is unknown, but it is interesting to speculate (and at present it is no more than speculation) that it may retard corneal development and thereby prevent the normal increase in corneal radius (flattening) which occurs around term.[42] This would account for the higher incidence of myopia in ex-prematures noted by Fledelius (discussed by Weale[42]). This is distinct from the myopia associated with retinopathy of prematurity.

Pertinent to this topic are the observations by Glass and associates[43] who reported that infants kept in an environment of 36.5°C grow faster than those at 35.0°C, and that reduction of environmental temperature retards head growth.[44]

VISUAL DEVELOPMENT

This heading has been used loosely to include several aspects of the visual development of the preterm infant which will be discussed on a technique oriented basis.

Electrophysiology

Electroretinogram

As a means of assessing retinal function in the preterm, the electroretinogram (ERG) is almost a forgotten response. Zetterstrom[38] and Horsten and Winkelman[45] have recorded the ERG in preterm neonates, but the youngest infant studied to date has been 29 weeks GA.[39] These investigators were able to record consistently an ERG in the first week of life from this and other slightly more mature preterm infants. They[39] also suggested that early exposure accelerated ERG development.

Visual evoked potential

The visual evoked potential (VEP) to a flash stimulus can be elicited as early as 23,[46] 24,[47] and 25 weeks GA.[48] This response is a useful indicator of visual pathway maturation but, unlike the pattern VEP, cannot be used as a test of acuity. At 24 weeks the response consists of a negative wave appearing after 300 ms. Around 34 weeks a positive wave of latency 200–250 ms appears just preceding the negative peak[49] and by term a well defined negative-positive-negative complex is present. The latency of this response in early infancy decreases rapidly and its morphology becomes more complex between two and three months.[50] Norcia and co-workers[51] have recently used the 'sweep' pattern reversal VEP technique to measure visual acuity in a group of preterm (26 to 37 weeks GA) and term infants between four and 40 weeks post-term. The acuity of healthy preterm infants was found to be about 0.5 octaves higher than that of the term infant at the same corrected age.

Behavioural tests

The blink response has been observed from 28 weeks PMA,[25] and from 30 weeks PMA, there are periods of awareness and fixation.[52] Dubowitz and associates[53] elicited following from 31 weeks and responses to a patterned stimulus have been elicited from about 32 weeks PMA.[49,53,54] These studies have all used preferential looking (PL) based tests of visual acuity measurement.[55,56] Although the visual development of preterm infants at different postnatal ages lags behind that of term infants, when corrected for the degree of prematurity both groups behave similarly,[13,54,57–59] and after about one year of age the difference between postnatal and corrected ages is negligible.[13]

These results from infants who were free of the ocular and neurological complications of preterm birth, leave us with the impression that preterm birth neither hastens nor retards visual development. However there are reports, two using PL based techniques[53,60] and two using the pattern VEP[51,61] which suggest that preterm birth does accelerate visual development, albeit slightly. Thus, although the acuity of preterm versus fullterm infants is lower in early infancy, the former group exhibit more rapid development than the term infant. Corrected for prematurity the acuity of preterms is slightly greater than for fullterm infants and the extremely premature has a slightly better acuity than the less premature infant.[60] It has been suggested[60] that this may represent increased visual experience, but what this constitutes for the preterm neonate on the neonatal intensive care unit has not been defined, and highlights our ignorance of the effect of premature exteriorization on the developing visual system. Many of the factors discussed earlier in this article may be relevant, including light exposure (even through the closed eyelid), eyelid opening and accelerated ERG development. Although there is some evidence to suggest that visual development early on is slightly accelerated the reader is reminded of the findings that children[36] and teenagers[37] who were born prematurely have visual acuities at the lower end of the normal range.

Acuity card procedure

One of the most exciting recent developments in clinical vision science has been the introduction of the acuity card procedure (ACP).[62] This test is an adaptation of preferential looking (PL) technique, but for a number of reasons, unlike formal PL, is eminently suitable for clinical use.[63,64] Within the context of this article, ACP is particularly suitable for use with infants, even when premature, and permits the quantitative evaluation of normal and abnormal visual development.[55,56,64] There are pitfalls[64,65] and some skill is required, but ACP allows for the first time a clinically viable method for obtaining monocular and binocular visual acuity measurements in the preterm infant who may have retinal and/or more posterior visual pathway pathology.

Effects of neurological damage

So far only the visual development of the healthy preterm infant has been considered. Neurologically abnormal preterm infants[51,66,67] may show a delay in visual acuity development and almost certainly form part of the increasingly complex spectrum of delayed visual maturation (DVM). The relatively frequent association of preterm birth and DVM has been noted already, as has the high incidence of neonatal problems.[68,69] In 1974 Bronson (see[70]) proposed that vision in early infancy was predominantly subcortical, using the phylogenetically older second visual system, the extrageniculostriate pathway (colliculus–pulvinar–parietal pathway), with the geniculostriate system becoming increasingly important from about the third month after term birth. In 1984 Atkinson[70] suggested that the relationship between the subcortical and cortical pathways is probably flexible in the first few months of life. Dubowitz and co-workers[71] made the interesting observation that lesions near the thalamus, and not the occipital cortex, are more likely to affect visual behaviour. Although DVM was originally thought to represent an abnormality of cortical maturation the possibility that the defect lies subcortically has recently been discussed.[68] With the advent of the acuity card procedure in clinical practice it has become possible to quantify the severity of the visual deficit in DVM and study its kinetics.[64] It has become apparent that many of these infants have suffered a perinatal neurological insult the consistent exception being DVM associated with albinism (Tressider and Fielder, personal observation). It is now clearly necessary to reconsider the pathogenesis of this intriguing condition and whether the term 'cortical' blindness is correct when applied during infancy.

Periventricular leukomalocia (PVL) is a complication of term and preterm birth, and although visual involvement is common[72-75] our knowledge about its effects on the visual pathway is still scanty. Scher and co-workers[76] have recently studied 10 infants (23 to 40 weeks GA) with PVL (cavitating in one infant). More than half of these infants exhibited delayed visual field development and strabismus was present in four. Two had reduced visual acuity, but interestingly, as had been noted in another study,[74] this was not apparent in the neonatal period. Thus either vision deteriorated or, more likely, is indicative of the insensitivity of grating, or any test of acuity in early infancy, to relatively mild visual defects. This has already been discussed in the section on light toxicity. For instance a defect which would result in a reduced acuity to, say 10.0 c/deg (6/18), would not be identified until visual development had reached this level. The alternative is a proportionate downgrading at all acuity levels. Lambert and associates[75] reported an inverse relationship between the age at hypoxic insult and the visual outcome, thus asphyxia in preterm infants was associated with a poor visual prognosis compared to that occurring in the older child, particularly in the presence of a normal scan of the posterior visual pathway. These cases[75] having been referred because of severe visual impairment constitute one end of a spectrum, which probably consists at one end of DVM and at the other permanent and severe visual impairment.

RETINOPATHY OF PREMATURITY

The past decade or so has seen a resurgence of interest in retinopathy of prematurity (ROP) and there have been a number of excellent review articles (e.g. Refs 77, 78) including at least two books devoted entirely to the subject.[79,80] As another review would serve little purpose here we will discuss topics which we consider of particular interest.

Terminiology and classification

In 1984 the International Classification of ROP was published[81] with several important features: the retina is divided into three zones centred on the optic disc (see section on vascular development), the stages of acute ROP are logical and easy to memorize, and the examination record is computer-compatible. An interesting but important by-product of this scheme is that in order to complete the examination record, the full 360 degrees of the retina have to be scrutinized, the relevance of which will be shortly become apparent. This classification dealt only with acute ROP and it was decided that the term retrolental fibroplasia (RLF) should be confined only to the later cicatricial changes. Recently the late stages of ROP have also been re-classified,[82] the terms cicatricial and RLF have been eliminated and the term ROP is now used to denote all stages. In time, the value of the new late-stage classification will become apparent, but in this article we will continue to use the Reese, King and Owens[83] classification of cicatricial ROP as it remains in common usage.

Incidence

East Midlands study

We have recently undertaken a prospective study in an area of the East Midlands.[84] The criteria for entry were a birthweight of <1700 g and survival for three weeks after birth. A total of 607 infants were enrolled, including 35 heavier siblings of twins who satisfied the birthweight criterion. No supplementary vitamin E was given. Ophthalmic examinations commenced at three weeks and were performed weekly whilst on the neonatal unit, or fortnightly following discharge from hospital, until 12 weeks of age, and thereafter as clincially indicated. A final assessment was undertaken at six months corrected age. Examination methods will not be considered here, except to mention that almost all before the age of 12 weeks were performed using a speculum and scleral indentor (98.5% of 2864 examinations), permitting visualization of the most peripheral retina. Demographic and neonatal data were also collected, but in this article we will present briefly only a few ophthalmic results.

Acute ROP developed in 293 of the 607 infants (48.2%). The maximum stage reached was Stage 1 in 173 (28.5%), Stage 2 in 93 (15.3%), Stage 3 in 25 (4.1%), and Stage 4 in 2 (0.3%). The frequency distribution of acute ROP by gestational age groups is shown in Figure 3 and as most publications have grouped infants according to birthweight this also is shown in Figure 4. Spontaneous resolution occurred in most, but 10 eyes of six infants developed cicatricial ROP, Grade 1 in six eyes, 2 in one, and 3 in three eyes. No infant was blind due to ROP, those with grade 3 in one eye had Grade 1 (2 infants) or 2 (1 infant) in the other eye. Cryotherapy was performed on one eye of one infant, which subsequently developed Grade 3 disease. In this study the incidence of cicatricial ROP was 2.0% of those with acute ROP (n = 293) or 1.0% of the original cohort (n = 607).

Comparison with other studies

Despite an agreed international classification of acute ROP, comparison with other centres is still not without problems as methods and frequency of examination differ, as do referral and neonatal management patterns. Comparison with early studies probably has little value as the nature of the preterm population, diagnostic criteria, and the sensitivity of examination techniques have all changed. Thus the incidence of 7.7% reported by the Medical Research Council in 1953[85] almost certainly represents what would now be considered advanced acute disease, and in relatively large infants who now are largely unaffected by ROP. The prevalence of acute and cicatricial ROP has recently been reviewed by Alberman (in Ref. 79) and here we will only discuss the results of a few recently published articles. Keith and Kitchen[86] (vitamin E given routinely) observed acute changes in 47 of 108 infants (43.5%) of birthweight < 1000 g and the corresponding figure reported by Flynn and co-workers[87] for 214 infants < 1300 g was 55.6% (vitamin E not mentioned). In infants < 1500 g; Reisner and associates[88] reported acute ROP in 34.9% (some given vitamin E), whilst for Schaffer and co-workers[89] this was seen in

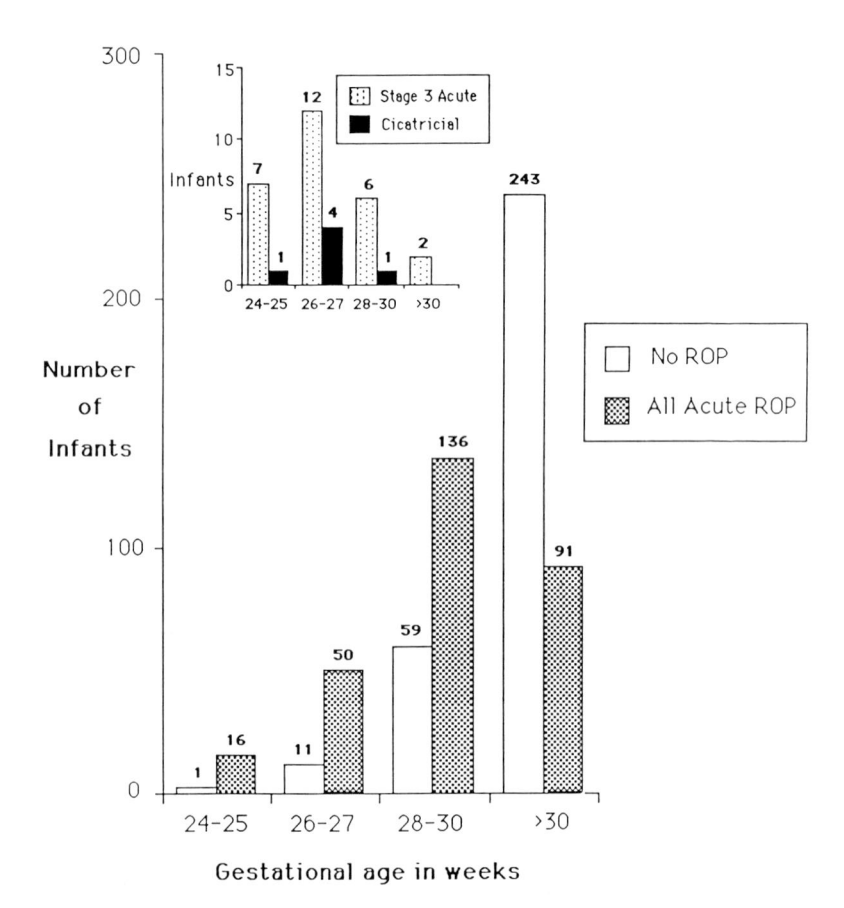

Fig. 3 ROP: East Midlands study. Number of infants who developed acute ROP (all stages). Insert shows the number of infants with stage 3 acute ROP who later developed cicaticial disease. See text for details. Numbers on the histogram bars denote the number of infants.

51.9% of those who received placebo and 50.0% of those who were given vitamin E (n = 328). Results of the East Midlands study for birthweights of < 1000 g, < 1300 g and < 1500 g are 87.0%, 75.4% and 61.7% respectively.

Cicatricial ROP

Most acute ROP undergoes spontaneous resolution, but for those infants in whom it does not, cicatricial, or late-stage, ROP develops, ranging from the visually insignificant to complete

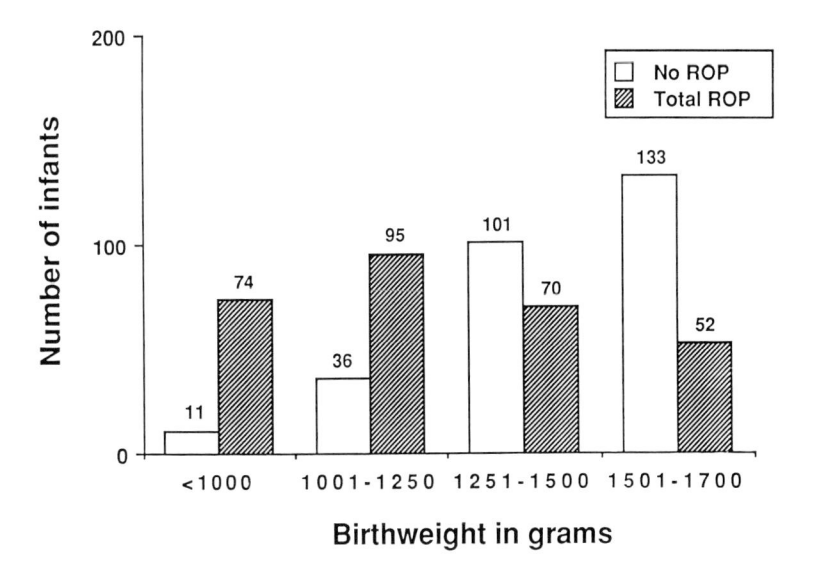

Fig. 4 ROP: East Midlands study. Infants with ROP grouped according to birthweight. Numbers on histogram bars denote the number of infants.

blindness. In the study by Flynn and co-workers[87] no infant received cryotherapy and cicatricial ROP developed in 7.6% of the 119 with acute ROP (4.2% of the original cohort). Schaffer and associated[89] reported cicatricial changes in 6.8% and 7.2% of the placebo and vitamin E treated groups respectively (cryotherapy to one infant). Keith and Kitchen[86] did not employ cryotherapy and reported cicatricial ROP in 19% of the study population, whereas Reisner and co-workers[88] who used cryotherapy on 26% of infants with acute ROP observed relatively mild sequelae in all of them (9.0% of total study population).

Comment

Although the results quoted above vary from centre to centre it is obvious that while acute ROP is extremely common, spontaneous and complete resolution fortunately occurs in the majority. The incidence of acute changes is high in our study yet that of cicatricial disease is low, and less than that reported by others. Why this is so is not known and space does not permit considering the many possibilities, but does indicate the danger of direct comparison between different populations.

At this juncture it is pertinent to consider one of the most enigmatic features of ROP: the relative symmetry of the acute process but the asymmetry of the long term sequelae. This is apparent in published results[87,89] and our own findings, and yet has received little attention. Nevertheless ROP symmetry is one of the basic tenets of the multicentre trial of cryotherapy for ROP, currently under way in the United States of America[90] as it employs treatment to one eye only, with the other eye serving as control. Since the propensity of ROP for resolution is high, unpredictable and often asymmetric, assessing the efficacy of any form of prophylactic or corrective treatment is fraught with difficulty. The results of the cryotherapy trial are eagerly awaited.

Pathogenesis

It is now recognised that the aetiology of ROP in most cases is multifactorial, with increasingly low gestational age being the single most important factor (see Fig. 3). The role of other risk factors, particularly oxygen, has been debated for many years,[77,78] and in all probability their relative importance has changed along with advancements in neonatal management and the nature of the preterm population. In this section we will discuss the age at onset of ROP, the site of initial involvement, factors influencing its severity, and light exposure.

Age at onset

A report by the Medical Research Council in 1955[85] contained the statement: 'the more premature the baby at birth the longer delayed, on the average, will be the onset of the retinopathy.' Three years previously Silverman and co-workers[91] had noted an inverse correlation between birthweight and onset. Recently in a retrospective study[92] a significant negative correlation between GA and the age at onset of ROP was found, with a median postnatal of onset at 51 and 40 days for infants <28 and >28 weeks GA respectively. But when the degree of prematurity was corrected for, the retinopathy became visible over a fairly narrow PMA range with 86% developing between 32.5 and 38.5 weeks. This finding has been confirmed prospectively[93] with 83.4% commencing between 31.0 and 40.0 weeks PMA, the disparity between these two studies being due to a failure of the initial investigation to appreciate that in the very small infant ROP may begin in the nasal retina (see below). Flynn and co-workers[87] reported that 82% ROP was first diagnosed between 35 and 45 weeks PMA, but as their examinations did not commence until 32 weeks PMA or after, and as ROP was present on the first visit in 44 of 119, these results do not indicate precisely the age at onset.

The upper age limit for the onset of acute ROP is governed by the completion of retinal vascular development. But it is the lower limit at which retinopathy is first seen—about 31.5 weeks PMA—which is particularly intriguing. ROP is a condition of the developing retinal vessels, and yet the most premature, often very sick infant does not develop visible retinal changes for several weeks; at a later postnatal age than his less premature counterpart. These observations suggest that although an immature retinal vasculature is an essential prerequisite for the genesis of ROP, immaturity per se cannot be responsible for its timing and it is likely that a certain stage of retinal development has to be reached for this response to develop.

Site of initial retinal involvement

Traditionally it has been accepted that ROP involves first the temporal region of the retina as this is the last region to vascularise (see earlier). Recently the retinal site in which ROP first develops has been investigated prospectively.[92] The results are shown in Figure 5, and indicate that for the infant of 25 to 27 weeks GA the likelihood of ROP developing first in the nasal retina or simultaneously in both the nasal and temporal regions is 68.8%

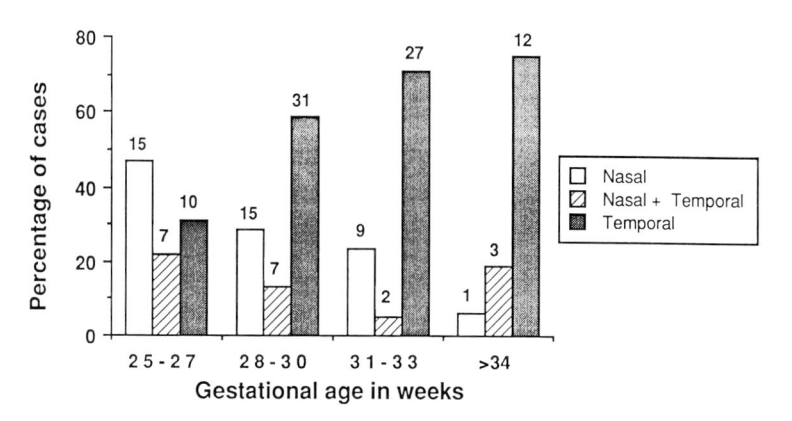

Fig. 5 ROP: East Midlands study. Initial site of retinal involvement. Retinopathy is more likely to involve the nasal retina first in the very immature, but the temporal retina in the more mature infant. ROP commences simultaneously in the nasal and temporal retina in some infants. Numbers of the histogram bars indicate the number of infants.

whereas for those over 31 weeks GA this falls to 28%. It is known that the more immature the infant the more posteriorly (closer to the optic disc) will ROP be situated; proportional to the incompleteness of the outgrowth of the retinal vasculature from the optic disc. However this does not explain the tendency for initial involvement in the nasal retina in the most immature. As discussed in the previous section ROP develops over a relatively narrow postmenstrual age range, suggesting that a certain stage of retinal development has to be reached before the response can become manifest. These results indicate that this stage is reached earlier in the nasal compared to the temporal regions of the retina.

Severity

The very immature infant is the infant most prone to develop ROP, yet clinicians are often perplexed at the seemingly haphazard way in which severe, potentially blinding disease strikes.

The spindle cell hypothesis of ROP has received much attention in recent years (reviews[79,80]) and reactivated the vitamin E controversy, but this has yet to be fully verified and will not be considered here.

At present ROP is generally accepted to have an ischaemic basis,[94,95] as has periventricular leukomalacia (PVL) and recently the association of these two complications of preterm birth has been presented.[96] The basis for this report was the observation that six infants with severe acute ROP and severe PVL accounted for all but one of the most severe ROP cases over a 20 month period. During early fetal life the retina receives its nutrients from the underlying choroidal circulation, although this declines with the development of the retinal vasculature. ROP develops at the junction of the vascularized and non-vascularized retinal, an area particularly vulnerable to changes in blood flow. Although the retinal circulation is capable of autoregulation the choroidal circulation is not, with the consequence that a reduction of flow in the carotid system could render the already ischaemic retina more so. This episode of carotid hypoperfusion could also be responsible for the ischaemic brain lesion—PVL. Lucey and Dangman[77] have considered that severe ROP may be due to cerebral and retinal hypoperfusion, and Brown and associates[97] noted that infants with severe ROP had significantly lower blood pressures than controls. The possible causal relationship between hypoperfusion and PVL is controversial and compounded by the difficulties of continuous blood pressure monitoring.[98,99] It is not proposed that ischaemia due to cerebral hypoperfusion is the sole cause of ROP, but that in some cases it may exacerbate an already ischaemic retina and consequently increase the severity of the retinopathy.

Light

The possibility that light may be a factor in the pathogenesis of acute ROP has been considered for over 45 years (see[15]). Although studies (see[15]) in the ensuing few years failed to substantiate this theory the idea has surfaced again recently.[100] These researchers reported a higher incidence of ROP in infants reared in bright illumination compared to those for whom the illumination was lower, particularly for those with birthweights < 1000 g. (86% versus 54%). This study has stimulated some correspondence (see[15]), but clearly before this aspect can be fully understood further basic research on the light dose to the neonatal eye is mandatory (see earlier).

Summary

It has not been possible to review in detail the pathogenesis of ROP, instead we have concentrated mainly on topics of special interest in this department. To summarize there are four aspects in the development of acute ROP: its occurrence, time of onset, site of initial involvement and severity. The occurrence of ROP is influenced by gestational age and events in the neonatal period such as oxygen therapy, hypercarbia, raised pH and possibly premature exposure to bright light. The age at which ROP is first seen however would appear to be governed, not to a great extent by neonatal events, but mainly by the infant's stage of development, probably at a retinal level, and this is reached earlier in the nasal compared to the temporal retina. Finally, the severity of the response is obviously greatly influenced by the factors responsible for its initiation, as mentioned above, and one of these may be carotid hypoperfusion.

CONCLUSION

A number of topics have been briefly reviewed in this article. Inevitably they reflect the interest of the authors' and also inevitably many of the ideas discussed will subsequently be proven to be incorrect. The effect that premature birth may have on the very immature visual system is largely unknown and as this article indicates this is an area in which much basic and clinical research is needed.

ACKNOWLEDGEMENTS

We are pleased to acknowledge the support of the Wellcome Trust, Medical Research Council and the Royal National Institute for the Blind.

REFERENCES

1. Harayama K, Amemiya T, Nishimura H. Development of the eyeball during fetal life. J Pediatr Ophthalmol Strabismus 1981; 18: 37–40
2. Birnholz JC. Ultrasonic fetal ophthalmology. Early Hum Dev 1985; 12: 198–209
3. Robb RM. Increase in retinal surface area during infancy and childhood. J Pediatr Ophthalmol Strabismus. 1982; 19: 16–20
4. Hittner HM, Hirsch NJ, Rudolph AJ. Assessment of gestational age by examination of the anterior vascular capsule of the lens. J Pediatr 1977; 91: 455–458
5. Hollenberg MJ, Spira AW. Human retinal development: Ultrastructure of the outer retina. Am J Anat 1973; 137: 357–386
6. Streeten BW. Development of the human retinal pigment epithelium and the posterior segment. Arch Ophthalmol 1969; 81: 383–394
7. Ashton N. Retinal angiogenesis in the human embryo. Br Med Bull 1970; 26: 103–106
8. Abramov I, Gordon J, Hendrickson A, Hainline L, Dobson V, LaBossiere E. The retina of the newborn infant. Science 1982; 217: 265–267
9. Yuodelis C, Hendrickson A. A qualitative and quantitative analysis of the human fovea during development. Vision Res. 1986; 26: 847–855
10. Isenberg SJ. Macular development in the premature infant. Am J Ophthalmol 1986; 101: 74–80
11. Garey LJ, De Courten C. Structural development of the lateral geniculate nucleus and visual cortex in monkey and man. Behav Brain Res 1983; 10: 3–13
12. Magoon EH, Robb RM. Development of myelin in human optic nerve and tract. Arch Ophthalmol 1981; 98: 655–659
13. Van Hof-van Duin J, Mohn G. Vision in the preterm infant. In: Prechtl HFR, ed. Continuity of neural functions from prenatal to postnatal life. Clinics in Development Medicine, No. 94. Oxford: Spastics International Medical Publications, 1984; pp. 93–114
14. Wolke D. Environmental neonatalogy. Arch Dis Child 1987; 62: 987–988
15. Moseley MJ, Fielder AR. Light toxicity and the neonatal eye. Clin Vision Sci 1988 (In press)
16. Landry RJ, Scheidt PC, Hammond RW. Ambient light and phototherapy conditions of eight neonatal care units: a summary report. Pediatrics 1985; 75: (suppl) 434–436
17. Hamer RD, Dobson V, Mayer MJ. Absolute thresholds in human infants exposed to continuous illumination. Invest Ophthalmol Vis Sci 1984; 25: 381–388
18. Chin KC, Moseley MJ, Bayliss SC. Light transmission of phototherapy eyeshields. Arch Dis Child 1987; 62: 970–971
19. Moseley MJ, Fielder AR. Phototherapy: an ocular hazard revisited. Arch Dis Child 1988 (In press)

20 Kirkness CM. Do ophthalmic instruments pose a hazard of light-induced damage to the eye? In: Cronly-Dillon J, Rosen ES, Marshall J. Hazards of light, Myths and Realities, Eye and Skin. Oxford: Pergamon Press, 1986: pp. 179–186
21 Moseley MJ, Thompson JR, Levene MI, Fielder AR. Effects of nursery illumination on frequency of eyelid opening. Early Hum Dev 1988 (In press)
22 Berman J, Hutchins R, Gold S, Peli E, Lindsey P. Measurement of light exposure in infants at high risk for developing retinopathy of prematurity. Invest Ophthalmol Vis Sci 1987; 28: (suppl) 119
23 Moseley MJ, Bayliss SC, Fielder AR. Light transmission through the human eyelid: in vivo measurement. Ophthalmic Physiol Opt 1988: 8; 229–230
24 Lerman S. Ocular phototoxicity. In Davidson SI, Fraunfelder FT eds. Recent advances in ophthalmology Edinburgh: Churchill Livingstone, 1985: pp. 109–136
25 Robinson RJ. Assessment of gestational age by neurological examination. Arch Dis Child 1966; 41: 437–447
26 Lanum J. The damaging effects of light on the retina. Empirical findings, theoretical and practical implications. Survey Ophthalmol 1978; 22: 221–249
27 O'Steen WK, Anderson KV, Shear CR. Photoreceptor degeneration in albino rats: dependency on age. Invest Ophthalmol 1974; 13: 334–339
28 Friedman E, Kuwabara T. The retinal pigment epithelium. IV. The damaging effects of radiant energy. Arch Ophthalmol 1968; 80: 265–279
29 Noell WK, Walker VS, Kang BS, Berman S. Retinal damage by light in rats. Invest Ophthalmol 1966; 5: 450–473
30 Sisson TRC, Glauser SC, Glauser EM, Romayanda N, Chan G. Effect of light and various concentrations of oxygen on the retina of the newborn pig. Retinopathy of prematurity conference, Columbus, Ohio, Ross Laboratories. 1981; pp. 581–599
31 Ruffolo JJ, Ham WT, Mueller HA, Millen JE. Photochemical lesions in the primate retina under conditions of elevated blood oxygen. Invest Ophthalmol Vis Sci 1984; 25: 893–898
32 Dobson V, Riggs LA, Siqueland ER. Electroretinographic determination of dark adaptation functions of children exposed to phototherapy as infants. J Pediatr 1974; 85: 25–29
33 Dobson V, Cowett RM, Riggs LA. Long-term effect of phototherapy on visual function. J Pediatr 1975; 86: 555–559
34 Bhupathy K, Sethupathy R, Pildes RS, Constantaras AA, Fournier JH. Electroretinography in neonates treated with phototherapy. Pediatrics 1978; 61: 189–192
35 Abramov I, Hainline L, Lemerise E, Brown AK. Changes in visual functions of children exposed as infants to prolonged illumination. J Am Optom Assoc 1985; 56: 614–619
36 Sebris SL, Dobson V, Hartman EE. Assessment and prediction of visual acuity in 3- and 4-year-old children born prior to term. Hum Neurobiol 1984; 3: 87–92
37 Fledelius HC. Ophthalmic changes from age of 10 to 18 years. A longitudinal study of sequels to low birth weight. II. Visual acuity. Acta Ophthalmol 1981; 59: 64–60
38 Zetterstrom B. The electroretinogram in premature children. Acta Ophthalmol 1952; 30: 405–408
39 Ricci B, Falsini B, Valentini P, Lacerra F, Molle F, Rufi L. Development of the main electroretinographic components in premature infants during the first week of life. Arch Soc Oftal Optom 1983; 17: 159–165
40 Fielder AR, Levene MI, Russell-Eggitt IM, Weale RA. Temperature-a factor in ocular development? Dev Med Child Neurol 1986; 28: 279–284
41 Walker D, Walker A, Wood C. Temperature of the human fetus. J Obstet Gynaecol Br Commonw 1969; 76: 503–511

42 Weale RA. A biography of the eye. London, HK Lewis. 1982
43 Glass L, Silverman WA, Sinclair JC. Effect of the thermal environment on cold resistance and growth of small infants after the first week of life. Pediatrics 1968; 41: 1033–1046
44 Glass L, Lala RV, Jaiswal V, Nigram SK. Effect of thermal environment and caloric intake on head growth of low birthweight infants during late neonatal period. Arch Dis Child 1975; 50: 571–573
45 Horsten GPM, Winkelman JE. Electrical activity of the retina in relation to histological differentiation in infants born prematurely and at full-term. Vision Res 1962; 2: 269–276
46 Chin KC, Taylor MJ, Menzies R, Whyte H. Development of visual evoked potentials in neonates. Arch Dis Child 1985; 60: 1166–1168
47 Hrbek A, Karlberg P, Olsson T. Development of visual and somatosensory evoked responses in pre-term newborn infants. Electroencephalogr Clin Neurophysiol 1973; 34: 225–232
48 Purpura DP. Structure-dysfunction relations in the visual cortex of preterm infants. In: Brazier MAB, Coceani F, eds. Brain dysfunction in infantile febrile convulsions. New York: Raven Press, 1976: pp. 223–240
49 Mushin J, Dubowitz LMS, Arden GB. Visual function in the newborn infant: behavioural and electrophysiological studies. In: Jay B, ed. Detection and measurement of visual impairment in preverbal children. Doc Ophthalmol Proc Series 1986; 45: 119–134
50 Fielder AR, Harper MW, Higgins JE, Clarke CM, Corrigan D. The reliability of the VEP in infancy. Ophthalmic Paediatr Genet 1983; 2: 73–82
51 Norcia AM, Tyler CW, Piecuch R, Clyman R, Grobstein J. Visual acuity development in normal and abnormal preterm human infants. J Pediatr Ophthalmol Strabismus 1987; 24: 70–74
52 Hack M, Muszynski SY, Miranda SB. State of awakeness during visual fixation in preterm infants. Pediatrics 1981; 68: 87–92
53 Dubowitz LMS, Dubowitz V, Morante A, Verghote M. Visual function in the preterm and fullterm newborn infant. Dev Med Child Neurol 1980; 22: 465–475
54 Brown AM, Yamamoto M. Visual acuity in newborn and preterm infants measured with grating acuity cards. Am J Ophthalmol 1986; 102: 245–253
55 Teller DY, McDonald MA, Preston K, Sebris SL, Dobson V. Assessment of visual acuity in infants and children: the acuity card procedure. Dev Med Child Neurol 1986; 28: 779–789
56 Dobson V, Schwartz TL, Sandstrom DJ, Michel L. Binocular visual acuity of neonates: the acuity card procedure. Dev Med Child Neurol 1987; 29: 199–206
57 Dobson V, Mayer L, Lee CL. Visual acuity screening of preterm infants. Invest Ophthalmol Vis Sci 1980; 19: 1498–1505
58 Morante A, Dubowitz LMS, Levene M, Dubowitz V. The development of visual function in normal and neurologically abnormal preterm and fullterm infants. Dev Med Child Neurol 1982; 24: 771–784
59 Van Hof-van Duin J, Mohn G, Fetter WPF, Mettau JW, Baerts W. Preferential looking in preterm infants. Behav Brain Res 1983; 10: 47–50
60 Van Hof-van Duin J, Mohn G. The development of visual acuity in normal fullterm and preterm infants. Vision Res 1986; 26: 909–916
61 Sokol S, Jones K. Implicit time of pattern evoked potentials in infants: an index of maturation of spatial vision. Vision Res 1979; 19: 747–755
62 McDonald MA, Dobson V, Sebris SL, Baitch L, Varner D, Teller DY. The acuity card procedure: a rapid test of infant acuity. Invest Ophthalmol Vis Sci 1985; 26: 1158–1162
63 Preston KL, McDonald MA, Sebris SL, Dobson V, Teller DY. Validation of the acuity card procedure for assessment of infants with ocular disorders. Ophthalmology 1987; 94: 644–653

64 Fielder AR, Moseley MJ. Do we need to measure the vision of children? J R Soc Med 1988: 81; 380–383
65 Robinson J, Moseley MJ, Fielder AR. Grating acuity cards: spurious resolution and the 'edge artifact'. Clin Vision Sci (In press)
66 Dubowitz LMS, Mushin J, Morante A, Placzek M. The maturation of visual acuity in neurologically normal and abnormal newborn infants. Behav Brain Res 1983; 10: 39–45
67 Placzek M, Mushin J, Dubowitz LMS. Maturation of the visual evoked response and its correlation with visual acuity in preterm infants. Dev Med Child Neurol 1985; 27: 448–454
68 Fielder AR, Russell-Eggitt IR, Dodd KL, Mellor DH. Delayed visual maturation. Trans Ophthalmol Soc UK 1985; 104: 653–661
69 Editorial. Delayed visual maturation. Lancet 1984; i: 1158–1159
70 Atkinson J. Human visual development over the first few months of life. A review and a hypothesis. Hum Neurobiol 1984; 3: 61–74
71 Dubowitz LMS, Mushin J, De Vreis L, Arden GB. Visual function in the newborn infant: is it cortically mediated? Lancet 1986; i: 1139–1141
72 Weindling AM, Rochefort MJ, Calvert SA, Folk T-F, Wilkinson A. Development of cerebral palsy after ultrasonographic detection of periventricular cysts in the newborn. Dev Med Child Neurol 1985; 25: 800–806
73 Calvert SA, Hoskins EM, Fong KW, Forsyth SC. Periventricular leukomalacia: ultrasonic diagnosis and neurological outcome. Acta Paediatr Scand 1986; 75: 489–496
74 De Vreis LS, Connell JA, Dubowitz LMS, Oozer RC, Dubowitz V. Neurological electrophysiological and MRI abnormalities in infants with extensive cystic leukomalacia. Neuropediatrics 1987; 18: 61–66
75 Lambert SR, Hoyt CS, Jan JE, Barkovich J, Flodmark O. Visual recovery from hypoxic cortical blindness during childhood. Computed tomographic and magnetic resonance imaging predictors. Arch Ophthalmol 1987; 105: 1371–1377
76 Scher MS, Dobson V, Carpenter NA, Guthrie RD. Visual and neurological outcome of infants with non-cavitary periventricular leukomalacia. Dev Med Child Neurol (In press)
77 Lucey JF, Dangman B. A reexamination of the role of oxygen in retrolental fibroplasia. Pediatrics 1984; 73: 82–96
78 Flynn JT. Retrolental fibroplasia: update. Pediatric Ophthalmology and Strabismus: Transactions of the New Oreleans Academy of Ophthalmology. New York: Raven Press, 1986; 293–325
79 Silverman WA, Flynn JT, eds. Retinopathy of prematurity. Contempary issues in fetal and neonatal medicine 2. Boston: Blackwell Scientific Publications, 1985
80 MacPherson AR, Hittner HM, Kretzer FL, eds. Retinopathy of prematurity. Current concepts and controversies. Toronto: BC Decker, 1986
81 Committee for the classification of retinopathy of prematurity: the international classification of retinopahty of prematurity. Br J Ophthalmol 1984; 68: 690–697
82 Committee for the classification of retinopathy of prematurity. II The classification of retinal detachment. Arch Ophthalmol 1987; 105: 906–912
83 Reese AB, King MJ, Owens WC. A classification of retrolental fibroplasia. Am J Ophthalmol 1953; 36: 1333–1335
84 Fielder AR, Ng YK, Shaw DE, Levene MI. Retinopathy of prematurity: natural history. Invest Ophthalmol Vis Sci 1988; 29: 121 (suppl)
85 Report to the Medical Research Council by their council on retrolental fibroplasia. Retrolental fibroplasia in the United Kingdom. Br Med J 1955; ii: 78–82
86 Keith CG, Kitchen WH. Retinopahty of prematurity in extremely low birthweight infants. Med J Aust 1984; 141: 225–227
87 Flynn JT, Bancalari E, Bachynski BN, et al. Retinopahty of prematurity: diagnosis, severity and natural history. Ophthalmology 1987; 94: 620–629

88 Reisner SH, Amir J, Shohat M, Krikler R, Nissenkorn I, Ben-Sira I. Retinopathy of prematurity: incidence and treatment. Arch Dis Child 1985; 60: 698–701
89 Schaffer DB, Johnson L, Quinn GE, Weston M, Bowen FW. Vitamin E and retinopathy of prematurity: follow-up at one year. Ophthalmology 1985; 92: 1005–1011
90 Palmer EA, Phelps D. Commentary: multicenter trial of cryotherapy for retinopathy of prematurity. Pediatrics 1986; 77: 428–429
91 Silverman WA, Blodi FC, Locke JC, Day RL, Reese AB. Incidence of retrolental fibroplasia in a New York nursery. Arch Ophthalmol 1952; 48: 698–711
92 Fielder AR, Ng YK, Levene MI. Retinopathy of prematurity: age at onset. Arch Dis Child 1986; 61: 774–778
93 Fielder AR, Ng YK, Levene MI, Shaw DE. Retinopathy prematurity: age at onset and the initial site of retinal involvement. A preliminary report. In: Ben Ezra D, Ryan S, Glaser BM, Murphy RP, eds. Ocular circulation and neovascularisation. Dordrecht, Martinus Nijhoff: Dr W Junk Publishers 1987: pp. 147–153
94 Ashton N, Ward B, Serpell G. Role of oxygen in the genesis of retrolental fibroplasia. Br J Ophthalmol 1953; 37: 513–520
95 Ashton N. Oxygen and the retinal blood vessels. Trans Ophthalmol Soc UK 1980; 100: 359–362
96 Ng YK, Fielder AR, Levene MI, Trounce JQ, McLellan N. Are severe acute retinopathy of prematurity and severe periventricular leukomalacia both ischaemic lesions? Br J Ophthalmol 1988 (In press)
97 Brown DR, Milley JR, Ripepi UJ, Biglan AW. Retinopathy of prematurity: risk factors in a five-year cohort of critically ill premature neonates. Am J Dis Child 1987; 141: 154–160
97 Trounce JQ, Shaw DE, Levene MI, Rutter N. Clinical risk factors and periventricular leucomalacia. Arch Dis Child 1988; 63: 17–22
98 Miall-Allen VM, De Vries LS, Whitelaw AGL. Mean arterial blood pressure and neonatal cerebral lesions. Arch Dis Child 1987; 62: 1068–1069
100 Glass P, Avery GB, Kolinjavadi N, et al. Effect of bright light in the hospital nursery on the incidence of retinopathy of prematurity. N Engl J Med 1985; 313: 401–404

Clinical issues

Neil McIntosh
Department of Child Life & Health, University of Edinburgh, Edinburgh, UK

> The personal views that I will express in this chapter are the result firstly of the absence of data relating to this subject in the literature and secondly to the management over a six-year period of 196 such infants at St. George's Hospital, London. In most cases care was provided with one or both of their parents, and extended families were often involved. 117 of the infants were born at St George's Hospital, and in this situation our paediatric contact with the families usually began before delivery at the invitation of our obstetric colleagues. The incidence and mortality over the six-year period are shown in Figure 1 and the breakdown with gestation in Figure 2.

Before the advent of intensive care (ventilatory support or parenteral nutrition) the infant born at less than 28 weeks gestation was very unlikely to survive even if born with signs of life. Historical anecdotes about the survival of extremely small infants almost certainly relate to infants small for gestation where relative maturity has allowed enteral nutrition. The development of ventilation and the provision of full intravenous nutrition in the decade of the sixties provided the potential for support, and experience has now shown that a large proportion of these very immature infants can be saved with relatively less morbidity if the care is provided in a perinatal centre (equivalent to United States level 3 centre).[1]

TO FIGHT OR NOT TO FIGHT

The decision to provide optimal obstetric and neonatal care for the mother with a pregnancy complication before 28 weeks gestation should be considered by both obstetric and paediatric teams taking account of the hopes and fears of the mother or parents. The decision has to be balanced first of all with local mortality and morbidity data for that gestation, secondly with any special features particular to the pregnancy (e.g. prolonged liquor leak and the possibility of hypoplastic lungs) and thirdly, I believe, with less tangible information revolving around the socio-economic circumstances of the family. On rare occasions the socio-economic circumstances may be so extreme that they may tip the balance to inaction: an example might be the case of an unsupported schoolgirl mother where the fetus is the product of an incestuous relationship. Less extreme examples will obviously be less likely to influence treatment decisions. Similarly, socio-economic circumstances may mitigate an invasive, risky (heroic) approach to fight for the survival where there is small chance of success. I feel that this approach is reasonable on occasions for usually it is thoughtless benevolence that more frequently leads to a sad aftermath. At present in the United Kingdom, though not in all countries, national economic circumstances should not influence the decision, but with the continued underfunding of this area it is partly chance whether an appropriately equipped incubator will be available at the time and place required.[2]

I believe that although the parents' feelings and anxieties should be probed regarding fighting for an early gestation infant, these should not necessarily and particularly knowingly dictate the approach to the infant. If religious parents dictate the withdrawal of life support because of their emotional involvement at the time it may be impossible for them to live with the decision months or years later. It is, I believe, far better for the senior paediatrician to make a decision based on extensive experience, taking into account the parents' views though not necessarily colluding with them.

Once the fight is on, it is on to the full unless a decision is made by the paediatric staff in conjunction with the nursing staff that irreparable abnormality or irretrievable damage is present. Again I feel that the hopes and anxieties of the parents should be taken into account, but the parents should not be forced themselves into making the decision. We have never abandoned care ourselves for a primary reason other than gross cerebral damage or multiple lethal abnormality.

Both size and maturity together seem to be important in the outlook though birth weight is possibly more important than gestation (Fig. 1). For the 117 infants born at St George's during this study:
1. 2 out of 15 survived (13%) if the gestation was less than 26 weeks and the birth weight less than 750 g.
2. 2 out of 6 survived (33%) if the gestation was equal to or greater than 26 weeks but the birth weight was less than 750 g.

INFANTS < 28 WEEKS GESTATION, 1981 - 1986

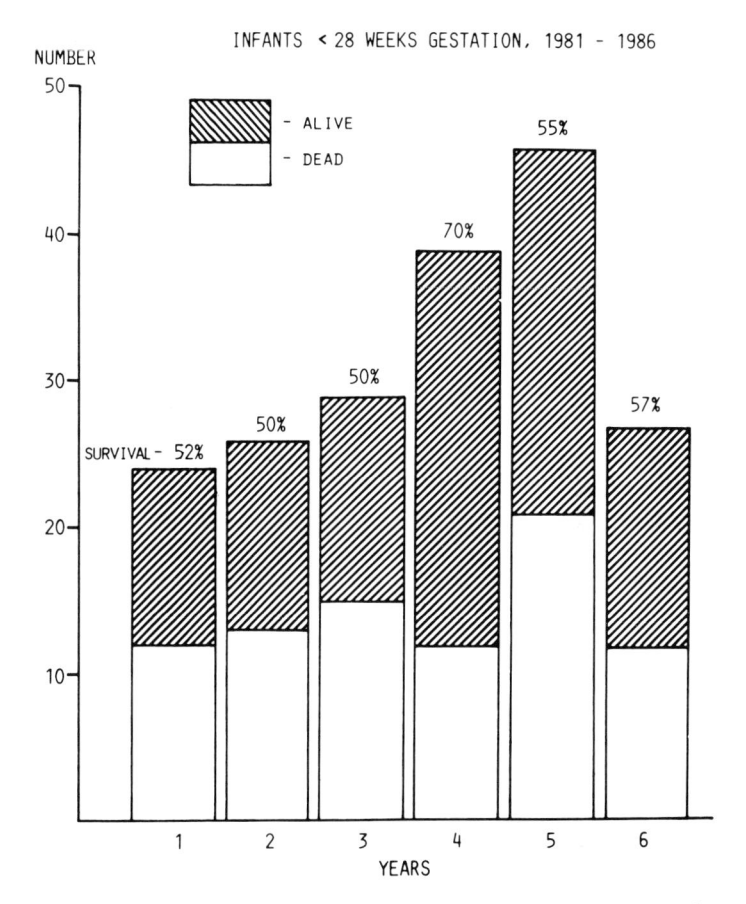

Fig. 1 Number of infants <28 weeks gestation born yearly between 1981 and 1986 inclusive showing percentage mortalities over the 6 years.

3. 7 out of 15 survived (47%) if the gestation was less than 26 weeks but the birth weight was more than 750 g.
4. 53 out of 81 survived (65%) if the gestation was equal to or greater than 26 weeks and the birth weight was more than 750 g.

An accurate knowledge of gestation and the estimated fetal weight is likely to improve our ability statistically to predict survival. The ultrasound estimated fetal weight has an accuracy of $\pm 10\%$ in prospective studies published by enthusiastic experts[3,4] although the smaller the infant the less the accuracy. More relevant, when these measurements are performed as a routine the accuracy is less again. From January 1985 to June 1987 the fetal weight estimates at St George's Hospital for infants less than 28 weeks gestation were frequently more than 30% out (unpublished observations).

Over the six years of this study our own approach has changed. Although I believe this is due to an improved outlook, it is difficult to demonstrate this. The overall survival of liveborn neonates born at less than 28 weeks gestation has not improved over the six years (Fig. 2) but these figures take no account of the increase in the number of elective caesarian sections where the infants might otherwise be intrauterine deaths. The obstetricians' belief that the outlook has improved is reflected in the number of elective sections they are prepared to carry out. There has been a highly significant increase from 10% in the first three years to 32% in the second three years of the study (χ^2 $P<0.001$) of extremely preterm infants delivered at St George's Hospital. Resuscitation has also changed; from 1981–1983 only 60% of these infants were electively ventilated from the time of resuscitation, but in the period 1984–1986 this has increased to 84% (χ^2 $P<0.01$).

MONITORING

As neonatal intensive care developed it was observed that handling immature infants was likely to provoke problems. Falls in body

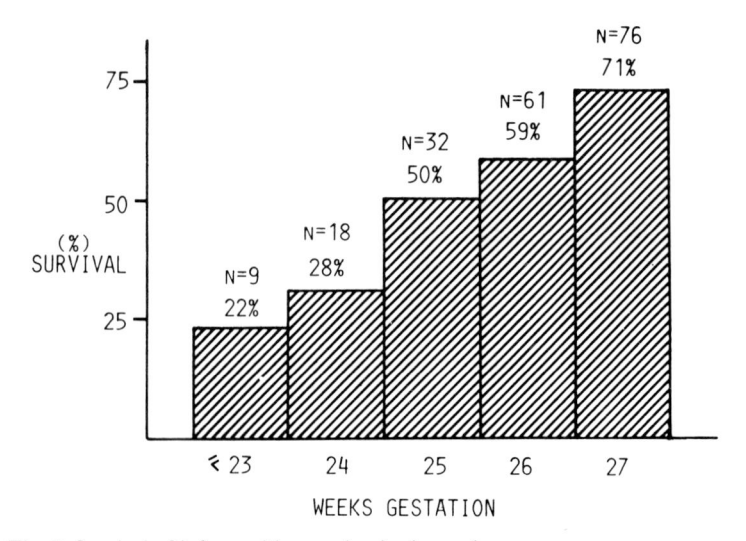

Fig. 2 Survival of infants with gestation in the study.

temperature, apnoea and bradycardia were more common with handling and this could lead to a deteriorating physiological spiral. The resulting 'minimal handling' approach improved the care as soon as it was appreciated that this was not an excuse for lack of observation. The privacy of the plastic womb (incubator) and the development of monitors to allow continuous observation without handling have improved survival and, more importantly, have reduced the incidence of physical and intellectual deficit in the newborn.[5] Initially monitors were designed to identify spontaneously occurring events, such as apnoea and bradycardia. These repeated esisodes, impossible to anticipate because of their irregular occurrence, may result in central nervous system damage after some minutes if undiagnosed. More recently it has been recognised that care procedures themselves can cause deterioration,[6] and the fallacy of intermittent measurements of parameters such as the P_aO_2 may account for some of the morbidity seen in immature babies at follow-up (e.g. retinopathy of prematurity).

Most monitors identify these events and, if alarms are used appropriately, will alert the staff to them. The nurse, however, is still needed both to initiate appropriate action and to transpose the incident to charts. The development of computerised cot-monitoring systems allows not only continuous monitoring but also the storage of monitored data with the ability to examine several different physiological and environmental parameters together.[7] At St George's we initially utilised such a system to show conclusively that air mode incubator temperature control led to far less temperature variation in the very low birth weight infant than did those incubators on servo control.[8] This was opposite to what most had predicted and, we believe, is likely to indicate that incubator servo control is more stressful. More recently we have networked all our intensive care cots to a computerised monitoring system[9] and are finding that care procedures are frequently disturbing to the small infant's physiology. This disturbance is more the smaller and more immature the baby. In a baby < 1500 g in the first week of life, the routine four-hourly 'all care' procedure (consisting of changing nappy, cleaning eyes and mouth, changing the baby's position if sedated or paralysed, and sucking out the endotracheal tube if intubated) leads to a fall of 0.6°C in the central abdominal temperature and 1.1°C in the peripheral temperature, increasing the toe core temperature difference by 0.5°C. Recovery of these temperatures back to baseline may take several hours and is likely to require considerable energy expenditure.[10]

The temperature instability is sometimes accompanied by dramatic changes in heart rate and blood pressure (Fig. 3) and our anxiety that these routines may lead to the development or extension of intraventricular haemorrhage is now being prospectively evaluated. We now feel that all the components of these traditional care procedures must be critically examined and their necessity questioned. An example—does the position of the baby need to be physically altered every four hours? This manoeuvre was designed to prevent the development of bedsores in bedridden adults. Personally I have never seen a bedsore on a premature infant and I suspect this is not due to their positions being changed with such care. Preliminary data suggests that it is position-changing that is most upsetting to the infant's physiological

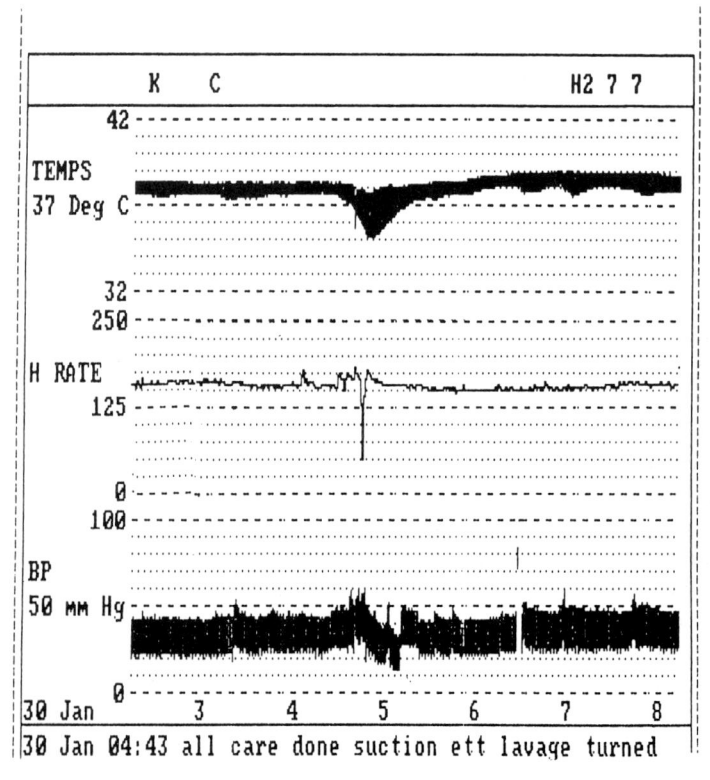

Fig. 3 Computer screen dump of 6-hour period of toe/core temperature difference, heart rate and systolic/diastolic blood pressure difference showing the effect of an all-care procedure on these physiological parameters.

stability, particularly if he is on a ventilator. Endotracheal suction without changing the infant's position did not lead to an increase in blood pressure, but straightening the infant to the midline before performing physio caused elevations as high as 20 mmHg (McIntosh & Williams—unpublished observations).

A considerable anxiety when monitoring the infant of less than 28 weeks gestation is the immaturity of the skin over the first few weeks of life. The epidermal barrier is thin and poorly keratinised, leading to large transepidermal fluid losses (*see* Rutter, this issue). The use of adhesive tape and adhesive electrodes damages the skin and causes even greater fluid losses with colloid exudation similar to that seen in a patient with extensive burns. The use of wrap-on ECG electrodes and temperature probes and umbilical arterial catheters with indwelling oxygen electrodes reduces skin trauma. A simulated ECG trace can be easily developed electronically by means of the blood pressure wave form from the arterial transducer.[11] If transcutaneous oxygen monitoring is required, there is some evidence that a layer of plastic spray dressing (trademark Opsite) prevents the skin being damaged but does not restrict the transcutaneous movement of blood gases.[12]

TREATMENT

It is usual for an infant of less than 28 weeks gestation to require ventilatory support. 111 out of 117 (95%) newborn infants of less than 28 weeks gestation required ventilatory support, 83 of these for surfactant deficiency respiratory distress, and the majority of the remainder for apnoea and hypoventilation. As a consequence there is a large amount of iatrogenic disease, 47 infants (40%) developed air leaks and 23 of the 64 babies who later went home (36%) had an oxygen requirement for more than 28 days, with 19 of these having chest X-ray changes compatible with bronchopulmonary dysplasia. 38 babies (32%) were given total parenteral nutrition for part of their courses even though our unit has a policy of very early feeding. This very early enteral feeding may account for the fact that only 4 babies developed jaundice of intravenous nutrition.

PAIN AND STRESS

99% of infants from our six-year study required intensive care. It cannot be denied that this is highly distressing for the infants and their parents. The sicker the infant and the more frequent the handling, the greater is the disturbance, and this is reflected in our physiological monitoring observations mentioned above. Whether pain is remembered is open to philosophical discussion and whether it leads to short- or long-term benefit or harm is unknown. Reluctance to provide analgesia and sedation for newborn infants stems from doubts about whether pain is felt to the same extent in this group and from concerns regarding the harmful effects of the drugs. Physiologists have theoretically equated reduced myelination of pain fibres and the immature receptors with a reduced perception of pain.[13] In addition, the high circulating levels of beta endorphins and the relative immaturity of the bloodbrain barrier could lead to higher analgesic concentrations in the brain.[14] This theory does not convince the neonatologist or the parents (nor, I suspect, the infant) that pain is not felt.

In contrast, our own data suggests that the extremely immature infant is supersensitive to pain. We have investigated the cutaneous flexor reflex threshold in 75 premature infants, some as early as 24 weeks gestation. This reflex is well correlated with sensory input and is evoked only to noxious stimuli, acting as a defence mechanism whereby the limb is withdrawn from the offending stimulant. The threshold for this reflex in adults parallels pain perception. Figure 4 shows our data suggesting that the earlier the gestation of the infant the lower the sensory threshold (more sensitive) to the stimulus.[15] Others have previously demonstrated exaggerated reflexes in newborn infants[16] but our data would suggest that when tested at threshold the reflexes are not exaggerated but since the threshold is so low and sensitisation is so prominent, stimuli suitable for an adult clearly produced an augmented response.

The further unanswered point is whether pain is harmful or beneficial. It has recently been shown that the endocrine responses to surgical stress of ductal ligation are reduced by the use of Fentanyl anaesthesia. Catecholamines, glucose, mineralocorticoids, insulin, lactate and pyruvate are all disturbed less in the Fentanyl-treated group.[17] This indicates that endocrine and metabolic stress responses can at least be modified in early gestation. If the very immature infant is supersensitive to pain and these and other stimuli lead to endocrine and physiological changes, it is appropriate to investigate this area further in the future. Endocrine and other physiological and behavioural responses must be evaluated in the well and unwell infant at varying gestation and

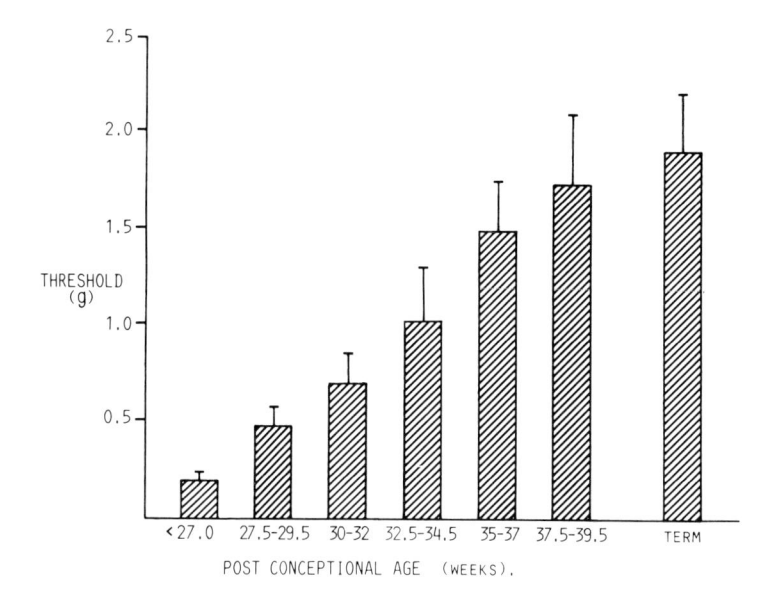

Fig. 4 The postnatal development of the cutaneous flexor reflex. The threshold response ±1 S.D. is shown to stimulus with von Frey hairs at different gestations in 103 infants, 75 of whom were premature.

postnatal age, and the effects of analgesia and sedation must be carefully reviewed. Eventually within the equation of 'care given and outcome' it may be appropriate to consider whether we are truly acting for the baby and the parents in all cases or whether we may sometimes be caught up in the advancement of an emotive area where our inability to measure the stresses that we are causing is too easily offset by an improved mortality outcome. As clinicians we are hopeful of our abilities in each specific case and certain generally about scientific progress. It is thus easy within the highly technological environment of the neonatal unit to raise parental hopes and expectations to a level more appropriate to our own aspirations than to reality.

STIMULATION

Noxious stimuli have been shown to have a physiological, behavioural and endocrine effect (see above) and it is presumed that these effects are not beneficial and may be harmful. On the other hand, adults undoubtedly find some forms of stimuli pleasant and even sensual.

- Is it possible to identify pleasant stimuli for the premature infant, and is it possible to identify whether a pleasant stimulus is beneficial and if the infant is subjected to such stimuli will there be either short- or long-term benefit?
- If a little of a particular form of stimulation is shown to be beneficial, will a lot of it be even more beneficial, and will it be beneficial to all or just some infants?
- Is it possible to equate certain responses with benefit even in the short term?

Good science is scarce in this area of study and the literature is clouded by anecdote:

> I walked into a premature nursery and all the nurses and other personnel were wanting to see a demonstration of the treatment. I felt that I really had to make an impact since this was the first time they were going to see it. So I looked around the nursery for the tiniest and what I thought was the sickest baby. I selected a little 900 g infant who was all wired up to an incubator. He was 46 hours old and no-one had seen him open his eyes and he had not moved. So I began to stroke the baby. In about 10 minutes his colour improved and the nurses standing around were saying, 'Oh look, he's getting pink'. Then he began to urinate. He yawned, opened his eyes, moved around and was trying very much to interact with his environment. I felt he had become alive as a result of some stimulation.[18]

This almost biblical laying-on of hands not surprisingly irritates neonatologists and neonatal nurses who spend all their work shifts looking after these infants to the best of their ability. However, it is too easy to ignore the possibility that certains forms of sensory stimulation may be of benefit. In other slightly more critical though not entirely blameless studies music[19] and rocking waterbeds[20] have been shown to reduce apnoeic attacks in small infants, and tactile stimulation in the form of stroking (?=caressing) has also been shown to improve survival.[21]

There is dispute in this area even about the basic premise: is the preterm infant subject to sensory deprivation—no gently rolling experience as in the womb but a fixed position on a hard mattress within an incubator with no nicely muffled uterine sounds—or is he after birth subject to sensory bombardment and overload with intense light situations, incubator noise, handling and painful procedures? The stimulation postnatally is undoubtedly different. Sensory overload is certainly possible in the older child post-term, and the effect of an early birth probably compounds this. In an extremely good study by Field with infants three months after the expected data of delivery, visual avoidance occurred in both full-term and preterm infants with certian degrees of stimulation, and the threshold for this avoidance was lower in the preterm infants.[22] At St George's the physiological cot-monitoring system has allowed Dr Adamson-Macedo (1986) to investigate the effect of selected stimuli on parameters such as heart rate, respiratory rate and $P_{a}O_{2}$. Ten-second stimulation periods of different tactile manoeuvres (stroking) have been bracketed with ten-second pre- and post-stimulation control periods. These have been linked with video studies identifying behavioural responses. This rather more critical evaluation of the effect of stimulation may allow recommendation of better handling in the future.

PARENTAL RIGHTS

My comments regarding active parental decisions involved in the withdrawal of care in an earlier section will undoubtedly have antagonised many readers. My general feelings about parents in neonatal units are that they should have full and free access. Parents having a child less than 28 weeks gestation know that the odds are stacked against them. Despite this they must make a relationship with their infant which will allow their hopes to come to fruition or at least allow them to provide dignity for a small human being with a short painful life. Parents' anxieties can only be dealt with by frequent honest consultation, I believe, by all members of the team not just a consultant or head nurse. In this way we aim to maintain an appropriate anxiety to the reality of the medical context. In our unit we have wall paintings, mobiles, coloured blinds and colourful floors trying to turn our high technology intensive care unit into a more nursery-like setting. Within the incubator we have pretty coloured sheets and blankets not routine institutional white. The babies are usually clothed even when they are very sick and on ventilators, unless they are receiving phototherapy, and toys are allowed in the incubators, again to individualise the baby as a specific early-born human being. If the mother is unable to visit her infant because she herself is sick and has just had a caesarian section, we have a closed-circuit video ststem which can give her pictures of her infant on a 24-inch colour TV screen in her room.[22]

In these small ways we hope to turn the awfulness of the experience into a rather more dignified situation where the family can all partake in caring for the new member however sick.

DEATH AND DYING

12–15% of admissions to our neonatal unit die annually and over the six years of this study 35% of infants less than 28 weeks gestation have died. It is appropriate and, I feel, important to consider how best to deal with this tragedy. The death of a baby in a neonatal unit can be an undignified event both for the baby and the family, especially when rescue therapy is applied by medical staff until the last moment. In the intensive care unit it is difficult for the parents to express their true emotions when the staff are busy with other critically ill patients. It is difficult for the staff on the one hand to cope with rescue care for some patients and still provide sensitivity for grieving parents in the same nursery, and it is particularly difficult for the parents of the other babies in a unit with an open visiting policy. It is likely that bereavement proceeds most benignly firstly with recognition and understanding of the reasons behind the death and secondly by memories of the time. Memories can be best provided by the full involvement of the parents caring for their infants during their time in the neonatal nursery. They should not be excluded when the going becomes tough in a mistaken attempt to protect them.

In an attempt to dissociate death from the urgency of the intensive care unit we have set aside for the parents a room in the unit which can be used for terminal care as suggested by Whitfield et al.[24] This room has wallpaper, curtains, a rug and easy chairs provided by parents of babies that have died. Full supportive care can be given in this room but the parents can also give care more of the hospice type to their infants in the last hours or occasionally days. In this way we hope that they will come to terms more easily with the impending death. The privacy of this room allows culturally important rituals both during and after the death which would be both difficult and disturbing to other parents and staff on the main unit. We suggest to parents that they may like to hold or groom their dead infant. This is usually met with agitation and a certain degree of horror, particularly by Caucasian parents, but after a short time many request such involvement.

I believe that all parents should be pressed for an autospy, no matter how clear the apparent diagnosis. Porter & Keeling[25] have shown that the neonatal autopsy will reveal new information with implications for counselling in 44% of cases. Conversely, the fact that an autopsy has not revealed anything amiss can be very helpful to parents. The information from the autopsy is best given to the parents as soon as possible, probably before the funeral, and it is (I think) appropriate to see them again 4–6 weeks later when the acute emotional experience is settling and the fuller discussion of all the available information is possible. It is my own practice to give parents both a copy of their infant's summary and the autopsy findings.

ACKNOWLEDGEMENTS

I would like to thank the team of midwives, obstetricians, neonatal nurses and paediatricians at St George's Hospital for the dedicated care of these families during their crises. Also Dr Ian Laing for helpful comments and Miss Elaine Forbes for secretarial assistance.

REFERENCES

1. Watkinson M, McIntosh N. Outcome of neonatal intensive care: obstetric implications for a regional service. Br J Obstet Gynaecol 1986; 93: 711–716
2. British Association of Perinatal Medicine. United Kingdom study of neonatal referrals and refusals. To be published 1988
3. Campbell S, Wilkin D. Ultrasonic measurement of fetal abdomen circumference in the estimation of fetal weight. Br J Obstet Gynaecol 1975; 82: 689–697
4. Shepard MJ, Richards VA, Berkowitz RL, Warsof SL, Hobbins JC. An evaluation of 2 equations for predicting fetal weight by ultrasound. Am J Obstet Gynaecol 1977; 142: 47–54
5. McIntosh N. The monitoring of critically ill neonates. J Med Eng Technol 1983; 7: 121–129
6. Speidel B. Adverse effects of routine procedures in preterm infants. Lancet 1978; 1: 864–866
7. Bass CA, Smith JS, Ducker DA. The use of a computer linked monitoring system for the continuous collection of physiological and environmental data from neonates undergoing intensive care. In: Rolfe P ed. Proceedings of the 2nd International Conference on fetal and neonatal physiological measurement. London: Butterworth, 1984
8. Ducker DA, Lyon AJ, Ross Russell R, Bass CA, McIntosh N. Incubator temperature control: effects on the very low birth weight infant. Arch Dis Child 1985; 60: 902–907
9. Bass CA, McIntosh N, Ducker DA. A cot monitoring system for neonatal intensive care. Intensive Care Med 1987; 13: 436 (Abstract 25)
10. Bass CA, Ducker DA, Mok Q, McIntosh N. Thermal instability in infants less than 1500 g birth weight. Paediatr Res 1987; 22: 225 (Abstract 49)
11. Ducker DA, Wheeler K, McIntosh N. Use of arterial blood pressure wave form to give heart rate readings with audible signal. Biol Neonate 1984; 45: 153
12. Evans NJ, Rutter N. Reduction of skin damage from transcutaneous oxygen electrodes using a spray on dressing. Arch Dis Child 1986; 61: 881–884
13. Editorial. Can a fetus feel pain. BMJ 1985; 291: 1220–1221
14. Fachinetti F, Bagnoli F, Bracci R et al. Plasma opioeds in the first hours of life. Paediatr Res 1982; 16: 95–98
15. Fitzgerald M, Shaw A, McIntosh N. The postnatal development of the cutaneous flexor reflex: a comparative study in premature infants and newborn rat pups. Dev Med Child Neurol 1988; 29: (in press)

16 Issler H, Stephens JA. The maturation of cutaneous reflexes studied in the upper limb in man. J Physiol 1983; 335: 643–654
17 Anand KJS, Sippell WG, Aynsley-Green A. Randomised trial of Fentanyl anaesthesia in preterm babies undergoing surgery: effects of stress response. Lancet 1987; 1: 243–247
18 Rice RD. The effects of the Rice Infant Sensorimotor stimulatin treatment on the development of high risk infants. Birth Defects. Original Article Series 1978; Vol. XV: 7–26
19 Katz V. Auditory stimulation and developmental behaviour of the premature infant. Nurs Res 1971; 20: 196–198
20 Kramer LI, Pierpont ME. Rocking waterbed and auditory stimuli to enhance growth of preterm infants. J Pediatr 1976; 88: 297–299
21 Adamson-Macedo EN. The effects of tactile stimulation on low and very low birth weight infants during the first week of life. Curr Psychol Res Rev 1986; 86: 305–308
22 Field TM. The effects of early separation and manipulation on face/face interaction. Child Dev 1977; 48: 763–770
23 McIntosh N, Berger M, Jays L. Facilitating attachment by television. Matern Child Health 1985; 10: 74–76
24 Whitfield JM, Siegel RE, Glicken AD, Harmon RJ, Powers LK, Goldson EJ. The application of hospice concepts of neonatal care. Am J Dis Child 1982; 136: 421–424
25 Porter HJ, Keeling JW. Value of perinatal necropsy examination. J Clin Pathol 1987; 40: 180–184

Outcome and costs of care for the very immature infant

Richard W I Cooke
Department of Child Health, University of Liverpool, Liverpool Maternity Hospital, Liverpool, UK

> The survival of infants with a gestational age of 27 weeks or less has only recently become commonplace, and little detailed information is available about their longterm outcome. Many methodological differences make the follow-up studies available difficult to compare. Survival below 25 weeks is still exceptional, but from 25 weeks onwards can exceed 50%. The use of antenatal steroids and referral to a regional centre improves the chances of survival. Late deaths after discharge are unfortunately common. Neurodevelopmental assessment of survivors shows a high rate of major impairment ranging from 20–50%. Multiple impairments are commoner in those of lowest gestational age. Neonatal cranial ultrasonography shows cerebral lesions to be present in 40% of these infants at discharge from hospital and these appearances correlate with neurodevelopmental outcome. At school age, minor motor and attentional deficits persist in many of those without major impairments. The costs of providing care to this group are very high, but methods for cost-benefit evaluation remain inadequate at present.

Twenty-eight weeks of gestation has long been seen as the practical limit of viability for the human baby born prematurely, and indeed until the advent of neonatal intensive care this was the case. During the past two decades, however, the survival of such infants has changed from being a comparative rarity to a commonplace event, at least in those centres practising modern intensive care techniques. These results have been tempered in the minds of the profession and the public alike by the fear that this improved survival has been at the cost of a significant increase in impairments both major and minor, and that in crude economic terms the limits of cost-effective neonatal care have been reached. This chapter will explore the problems and methods of assessing outcome for tiny infants, review some of the published results to date for both major and minor impairments, and discuss their economic implications.

METHODOLOGY OF FOLLOW-UP

Neonatologists have until recently used birthweight rather than gestational age to define follow-up groups in the past, mainly because it is easier to determine, particularly in tiny infants. ELBW infants (infants with birthweight below 1000 g) are more often born to mothers with uncertain menstrual dates, and postnatal assessment scoring systems have never been adequately defined for infants of less than 28 weeks. Nevertheless, it has long been recognized that gestational age and birthweight have independent though similar relationships to outcome, at least as far as mortality is concerned. As a greater proportion of women are now examined early in pregnancy by ultrasound for dating purposes, uncertain gestational age is becoming less of a problem. Most follow-up studies of small infants represent hospital series of infants under 1500 g, 1000 g or 800 g, none of which more than approximates to less than 28 weeks. Only a few more recent studies use gestational age as a defining variable, and even fewer do so when a geographically defined rather than a hospital based population is being reported.

In the short term, outcome is defined in terms of survival, but even this variable is variously interpreted as survival to one week, 28 days, discharge from hospital or to the end of the first or even second year of life. Because of the small but real effect of neonatal intensive care to defer death for weeks or even months in occasional cases, a longer term view is preferable if a realistic estimate of the true value of neonatal intensive care is to be obtained.

Most follow-up studies concentrate on neurological and developmental aspects using the presence of neurological problems such as cerebral palsy and delay in motor and social development to assess outcome. Abnormalities thought at the time of assessment to be affecting overall development are defined as 'major' and those not affecting general development as 'minor'. These categories are far from well defined and are very subjective. Furthermore, the assessment of even the presence of major abnormalities can vary as the child matures, with infants assessed as having cerebral palsy at the age of 2 years or less, being considered as normal some years later. In an attempt to make the comparative assessment of infants more objective, standardized scales are widely used such as the Bayley in North America, and the Griffith and the McCarthy in the UK. Even with these systems, however, the predictive value of early assessments is poor. Because of these problems it is important that in any study of outcome, particularly when comparisons are being made, that all infants are of the same post-term age at the time of assessment.

Adequate testing of vision and hearing form a vital part of any follow-up programme because of the marked influence that even minor abnormalities of either may have on overall development. There is again a lack of agreement as to the severity of defects worth reporting. Hearing loss sufficient to delay speech development or to require aids is clearly of significance, but minor degrees of hearing loss due to middle ear disease are also common in ELBW survivors. Severe visual defects are relatively easy to detect and define but lesser problems such as refractive errors may be missed yet have an important effect on later progress at school.

ELBW infants frequently show poor growth on follow-up. This may simply reflect the ongoing effects of neonatal illness on growth through such problems as chronic lung disease following ventilation, or severely *in utero* growth retarded infants showing poor catch-up growth after delivery. The rate of head growth may be affected by neonatal brain injury particularly if cerebral atrophy results. Linear growth may be reduced in those infants showing neonatal rickets. Death after discharge from hospital remains much commoner in these infants, and although much of this is recorded as 'sudden infant death syndrome', residual respiratory disease, neurological deficits and an increased liability to infections are likely to play a role.

Other questions which may be addressed in long term follow-up relate to ongoing use of hospital, general practitioner and social services. This is particularly relevant when the total or lifetime costs of providing care for the very preterm are being considered. However, because of the very small number of tiny survivors, the proportion of such services used by these babies remains small.

SURVIVAL

Recent developments in neonatal intensive care, but in particular mechanical ventilation, have made survival below 28 weeks less of a rarity. Nevertheless 15/127 long-term survivors of 27 weeks or less admitted to Mersey Regional NICU between 1980 and 1985, survived without ventilation.[1] Three decades ago, the UK records indicate a period with no survivors under 1000 g,[2] and so factors other than simply mechanical ventilation may be responsible for recent improvements in survival. Representative examples of reported survival for infants of 28 weeks or less during the last decade are given in Table 1.[1, 3-8] Survival at less than 24 weeks is still a rarity. At 24 weeks of gestation rates of between 0 and 39%

Table 1 Percentage survival by gestational age in weeks

Place, year Study type Reference no. (n=)	Gestational age in weeks					
	23	24	25	26	27	28
Netherlands 1983 National Ref. 3 (375)	0	0	14.6	37.7	49.5	66.2
Liverpool 1980–85 Hospital Ref. 1 (490)	0	9.7	37.7	35.7	56.1	70.6
Merseyside 1979–81 Geographical Ref. 4 (266)	0		8.5		53.9	
Melbourne 1977–84 Hospital Ref. 5 (356)	7	33	25	56	72	72
Boston 1977–80 Hospital Ref. 6 (136)	0	28.6	10.7	44.7	60.5	92
Toronto 1979–82 Hospital Ref. 7 (267)	14.3	39.1	63.6	75	75	80.7
Vermont 1976–79 Hospital Ref. 8 (171)			10.5	35.7	47.2	62.3

Figures lying in between columns indicate combined values for adjacent gestational ages.

are quoted, the lowest rates being in European regional studies and the highest in North American and Australian tertiary centres. Survival improves with each week of gestational age and at 27 weeks ranges from about 50 to 75%. Goldenberg et al.[9] have combined 13 studies derived from the literature between 1978 and 1984 to show the increase in survival to be expected from one day or one week's delay in delivery at each gestational age. This averaged 2–3% per day depending on the gestational age.

Clinical factors and survival

A number of authors have attempted to analyse factors which influence survival of very immature infants apart from gestational age alone. Kitchen et al.[10] showed that maternal hypertension and singleton pregnancy were associated with a decrease and increase in survival below 28 weeks respectively. The only controllable variable shown to be significantly associated with an improved outcome was antenatal steroid administration to reduce the risk of hyaline membrane disease. Earlier studies had not found an effect on the very immature infant as there were too few subjects in this group for any such effect to be statistically detected. Delivery by Caesarian section has been advocated in numerous small and uncontrolled studies as beneficial to survival or quality of survival in these babies. When confounding variables were controlled for both Kitchen et al. and Olshan et al.[11] could find no benefit, even if the infant was presenting by the breech.

Effect of referral on survival

It is assumed in a number of studies that the use of a referral centre with specialist resources is of benefit in high risk infants, but little evidence exists to show that this is so. Usually *in utero* or postnatally referred patients are compared with booked and in-born patients in the same institution, but these represent different groups of patients with different medical problems, and such comparisons are invalid. In the Mersey region and North Wales the 28 day survival of all infants of less than 1000 g registered as born alive was examined over a 4 year period (1980–83) for each of 8 geographically defined areas which comprised the region.[12] The proportion of these infants referred either before or after birth to the regional neonatal intensive care unit was calculated for each area. The survival rate to 28 days for each area was shown to relate directly to the proportion of ELBW infants referred either *in utero* or after birth. Factors such as the distance from the regional unit (1–75 miles, i.e. 2–125 km) or the variation in the proportion of all livebirths weighing less than 1000 g did not appear to affect referral rate.

MERSEY REGIONAL NICU FOLLOW-UP STUDY

Hospital based follow-up studies have many limitations due to patient selection and other factors which have already been discussed. Nevertheless there are certain advantages and these include a more consistent approach to patient management, data collection, and availability of data relating to treatment such as mechanical ventilation and to investigations such as cerebral ultrasound.

Bias due to patient selection in hospital based studies has a greater effect on survival statistics than the 'quality of survival'. In the Mersey Regional NICU follow-up study,[1] 310 infants of 27 weeks and less were admitted to the unit over a period of 6 years. These patients represent 70% of infants of less than 28 weeks born alive in the region over this period, but include 97% of the known survivors. They represented 10% of total admissions to the regional unit. 40% were transferred postnatally, 37% *in utero*, and the remainder were booked and inborn.

Their survival to discharge home is detailed in Table 1 and Figure 1. When annual survival rates were examined over the 6 year period in this group a small but not statistically significant trend to improved survival was seen with time.

Duration of ventilation

Much of the cost of care for very immature infants in the immediate neonatal period relates to the use of mechanical ventilation and the duration of stay on the unit. 2910 days of ventilator care were used for the 310 infants admitted, an average of 9.4 days each. The actual number of days varied from 0–82 days, with the median length of ventilation being longer in survivors (Table 2). There was a trend to shorter median ventilation times in the maturer infants, but over this narrow gestational age range the effect of the presence or absence of factors such as birth asphyxia and surfactant deficiency are likely to be more critical determinants of duration of ventilation. It is interesting to note, and a

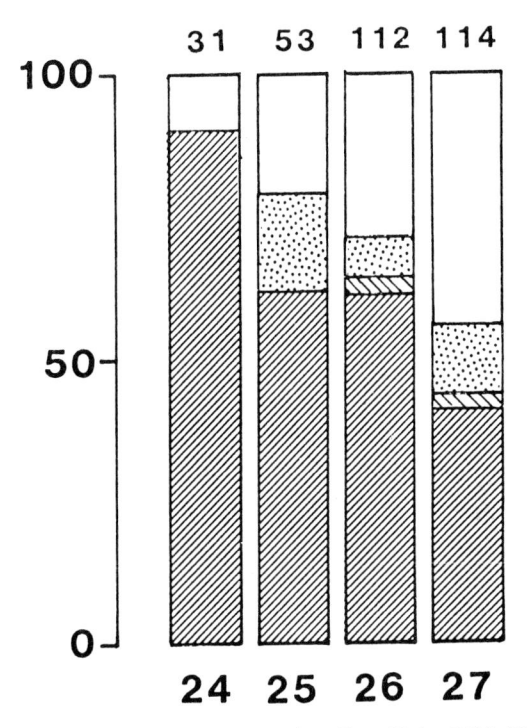

Fig. 1 Mersey Regional Neonatal Intensive Care Unit, 1980–85. Percentage survival and outcome of infants of 27 weeks and below. Histogram represents from below upwards: (1) mortality on unit; (2) mortality after discharge; (3) major impairment; (4) normal.

Table 2 Mersey Regional Neonatal Intensive Care Unit, 1980–85. Days of mechanical ventilation given to infants of 27 weeks and below according to survival (total, median, range)

Gestational age	Lived	Died	Total
24	42	327	369
	8 (7–27)	2 (1–91)	
25	488	186	674
	21 (1–76)	1 (0–30)	
26	476	759	1235
	6 (0–50)	3 (1–82)	
27	416	216	632
	2 (0–70)	2 (1–25)	
Total	1422	1488	2910

problem for economists, that the number of ventilator days used for survivors and non-survivors was similar. This is not always so, and reflects very much the intensity or 'aggressiveness' of the approach to care that is taken by the physician when faced with an infant with a low probability of survival.

Late deaths

There were 6 deaths after discharge from the unit amongst the 133 babies who survived initially. Three of these related to chronic disease from the neonatal period, but the others were considered to be doing well shortly before they died, and were classified as 'sudden infant deaths'.

Developmental assessment

For follow-up purposes, and for developmental assessment, 85% of these infants were seen at a consultant clinic at the regional centre at 3, 6 and 12 months of age, and then anually until the age of 5 years. The remainder were seen regularly at their district child development centre (10%), or in a few cases follow-up was by the general practitioner or a parental questionnaire (5%). When major impairments were identified, appropriate referral to specialist units was made. All the infants in this group have been followed to a minimum age of 2 years, and 50% of them to 5 years of age. No major impairments were detected in this group after the age of 2 years, but in 15% of cases there was a change in the diagnosis of cerebral palsy classification, or in the apparent severity of developmental delay. Major impairment was defined as cerebral palsy, developmental delay with the developmental quotient (DQ) less than 70 (moderate) or 50 (severe), visual or hearing loss severe enough to impair development or to require aids, and epilepsy (not including isolated febrile convulsions). Not all estimates of DQ were made using the same methods, although the majority were using the Griffith's developmental assessment scales.

The proportions of infants with major disabilities and their types are shown in Table 3 and Figure 1. Although these are shown as a proportion of liveborn infants (Fig. 1), this is of course a proportion of liveborn infants admitted to the unit, and will exclude delivery room and other very early deaths, particularly from outside hospitals. The effect of this bias is to increase the apparent incidence of subsequent impairment amongst liveborn infants. It does not affect the rate of impairment in survivors (Table 3). When the annual rate of impairment was examined for the group, it appeared to fall over the 6 years of the study, whether

Table 3 Mersey Regional Neonatal Intensive Care Unit, 1980–85. Impairments in survivors at 2 years of age by gestational age

Impairment	Gestational age in weeks				
	24	25	26	27	All
No. survivors	3	20	40	64	127
Impaired	0	9 (45%)	9 (23%)	18 (28%)	36 (28%)
Cerebral palsy	0	5	3	9	17
Developmental delay, moderate	0	2	3	6	11
severe	0	4	1	2	7
Visual loss	0	4	2	2	8
Hearing loss	0	2	2	2	6
Epilepsy	0	1	1	3	5
Multiple impairments	0	5 (25%)	3 (7.5%)	7 (11%)	15 (12%)

the impairments were considered as a proportion of liveborn infants or as a proportion of the survivors. Care must be taken with the interpretation of such findings however, as the infants had not all reached the same age at assessment, and the possibility of an ascertainment bias could not be excluded. The same result could also have been produced by chance with the relatively small numbers involved, or there could have been a change in the mix of patient type admitted over the 6 year period, i.e. more *in utero* transfers with a better chance of survival because of their growth retardation. Table 4 compares 4 recently published studies of developmental outcome in very immature infants in which outcome is given by each week of gestational age.[1,5,7,10] All except for the Mersey study include inborn infants only, although they

Table 4 Major impairments in survivors of gestational age of 27 weeks or less

Gestation (weeks)	Centre			
	Toronto 1979–82 Ref. 7	Melbourne 1977–82 Ref. 10	Melbourne 1977–84 Ref. 5	Mersey 1980–85 Ref. 1
23	0 (0/1)		50 (1/2)	
24	37 (3/8)	50 (1/2)	8 (1/13)	0 (0/3)
25	15 (4/27)	50 (3/6)	27 (3/11)	45 (9/20)
26	11 (3/27)	33 (7/21)	20 (7/35)	23 (9/40)
27	26 (9/35)	36 (11/30)	10 (6/63)	28 (18/64)

include *in utero* transfers. Each centre has used different definitions of impairment, although they are broadly similar. Also the age at assessment varies from 6 months to 5 years. At a gestational age of 24 weeks or less, all the studies have so few survivors that it is difficult to draw any conclusions as to the rate of impairment in survivors. At 25 weeks and above there is a suggestion in some of the centres that outcome improves with gestational age. When the results of these 4 reports are combined, however, little relationship with gestational age is apparent, although if there is a break in the data it lies between 25 and 26 weeks.

Specific impairments

Consideration of specific impairments by gestational age has not been made in previously published reports of very immature survivors. Yu et al.[5] in a series of 197 survivors between 23 and 28 weeks gestation found a 19% incidence of impairment. The impairments were cerebral palsy (11%), mainly hemiplegias, developmental delay (7%), visual loss (6%), and deafness (3%). About 5% of the infants had multiple impairments. For the Mersey follow-up study,[1] specific impairments by each week of gestational age are shown in Table 3. No impairments were seen in the three 24 week survivors, reflecting the very high mortality in this group and the relatively mild neonatal illnesses they sustained. Cerebral palsy was the commonest impairment occurring in 13.3%. Hemiplegia and bilateral hemiplegia (quadriplegia) made up 14 of 17 (82%) of the cases. This is in contrast with previous studies of low birthweight infants where the most prevalent form of cerebral palsy in survivors was a diplegia. Most of these reports refer to a decade or more ago when the infants being considered here would not have survived.[13] More recent follow-up of very low birthweight survivors of intensive care has shown a similar picture to that seen in this series.[14] No particular relationship between cerebral palsy and gestational age was seen.

Developmental delay as defined occurred in 8.6%, and was more likely to occur in 25 week survivors, and was more likely to be severe. Severe developmental delay only occurred in infants with cerebral palsy. Visual and hearing loss of a severe degree was also more likely in the 25 week survivor. Only half of the cases of blindness were due to retinopathy of prematurity, the others being from cortical blindness in association with extensive cortical atrophy. Severe degrees of hearing loss were often an isolated impairment. De Vries et al.[15] have suggested that such hearing loss is due to hyperbilirubinaemia in association with acidosis which is very common in these infants. Intraventricular haemorrhage with extension to the inner ear might also play a role.[16] Perhaps the most significant finding was the high prevalence of multiple impairment in the group as a whole, and particularly in the 25 week survivors. These infants are likely to develop severe lifelong handicap and to involve longterm medical and nursing care.

Neonatal cranial ultrasonography and outcome

A large number of original papers and reviews of cranial ultrasound in the newborn have been published over the last 10 years and it is not proposed to review them all here. Most of them report findings in the under 1500 g infant, and little reference is made to gestational age except for the rising incidence with shorter gestation. Follow-up studies have shown a clear correlation between the extent of intracranial haemorrhage (and more recently leucomalacia), and neurodevelopmental outcome.[17-19] Cranial ultrasonography was performed daily during the first week of life and weekly thereafter until discharge on all the infants in the Mersey follow-up study. An ATL 850A sector scanner was used with 5 or 7.5 MHz transducers. A simple classification of the early and late appearances was employed, which has been previously described.[18] The first week appearances are mainly those of periventricular haemorrhage and infarction, while the later appearances are those of cerebral atrophy, periventricular leucomalacia and porencephaly.

Table 5 shows the early ultrasound findings in the 127 infants of 27 weeks or less surviving to follow-up. More than half of the infants showed some degree of periventricular haemorrhage. The extent of the haemorrhage tended to be greater in the less mature infants with the exception of the 24 week survivors. It is likely that infants with large periventricular haemorrhage at this gestation die. Even at 25 weeks only one infant with a parenchymal haemorrhage in the first week survived. There is also a trend toward bilateral major haemorrhage in the less mature infants.

Table 6 shows the late ultrasound appearances in a similar format for the same group of infants. Again there is a likelihood for less mature infants to have parenchymal lesions, and more extensive ones. Nearly 40% of the whole group still had ultrasound

Table 5 Mersey Regional Neonatal Intensive Care Unit, 1980–85. Early cranial ultrasound appearances by gestational age in weeks

Grade	Gestational age				
	24 n = 3	25 n = 20	26 n = 40	27 n = 64	24/27 n = 127
0 Normal	2	6 (30%)	15 (37%)	30 (47%)	53 (42%)
1 SEH	1	2 (10%)	7 (17%)	16 (25%)	25 (20%)
2 IVH	0	11 (55%)	13 (33%)	12 (19%)	36 (28%)
3 PH	0	1 (5%)	5 (12%)	6 (9%)	12 (9%)
Unilateral 2 or 3	0	5 (25%)	7 (18%)	7 (11%)	19 (15%)
Bilateral 2 or 3	0	7 (35%)	11 (28%)	11 (17%)	29 (23%)

SEH = subependymal haemorrhage.
IVH = intraventricular haemorrhage.
PH = parenchymal extension of IVH or infarction.

Table 6 Mersey Regional Neonatal Intensive Care Unit, 1980–85. Late cranial ultrasound appearances by gestational age in weeks

Grade	Gestational age				
	24 n = 3	25 n = 20	26 n = 40	27 n = 64	24/27 n = 127
0 Normal	3	9 (45%)	24 (60%)	44 (69%)	80 (63%)
1 PVE	0	3 (15%)	5 (12%)	7 (11%)	15 (12%)
2 PVL	0	6 (30%)	9 (23%)	6 (9%)	21 (17%)
3 PC	0	2 (10%)	2 (5%)	7 (11%)	11 (9%)
Unilateral 2 or 3	0	4 (20%)	7 (18%)	8 (12%)	19 (15%)
Bilateral 2 or 3	0	4 (20%)	4 (10%)	5 (8%)	13 (10%)

PVE = persistent ventricular enlargement (cerebral atrophy).
PVL = periventricular leucomalacia.
PC = porencephalic cysts.

evidence of cerebral injury at discharge from hospital. Periventricular leucomalacia was the most frequent finding, and was more common with shorter gestational age occurring in 30% of the 25 week survivors to some degree.

Both the early and late ultrasound appearances relate to later neurodevelopmental impairments, although it is generally accepted that the later appearances are more specific. Table 7 shows the impairments noted at 2 years of age in the group together with their ultrasound appearances at discharge from hospital. The extent of the lesion noted on ultrasound scan relates broadly to the likelihood of later impairment, although the correlation is not as close as when series of larger infants are examined.[18] Extensive bilateral lesions are more likely to be associated with cerebral palsy, severe developmental delay and multiple impairments. More recently the importance of more minor but persistent ultrasound detected lesions such as 'periventricular flares' have been emphasized, and it is likely that in the near future a more

Table 7 Mersey Regional Neonatal Intensive Care Unit, 1980–85. Impairments in 2 year old survivors of gestational age 24–27 weeks at birth, by late ultrasound appearances

Impairment	Grade					
	0 Normal n=80	1 PVE n=15	2 PVL n=21	3 PC n=11	Unilat. 2 or 3 n=19	Bilat. 2 or 3 n=13
Impaired	13 (16%)	5 (33%)	13 (62%)	6 (55%)	11 (58%)	9 (69%)
CP	2 (2.5%)	2 (13%)	5 (24%)	8 (73%)	6 (32%)	7 (54%)
DD moderate	3 (3%)	1 (7%)	5 (24%)	2 (18%)	4 (21%)	3 (23%)
severe	2 (2.5%)	0	4 (19%)	1 (9%)	1 (5%)	4 (31%)
Visual loss	2 (2.5%)	0	5 (24%)	1 (9%)	2 (11%)	4 (31%)
Hearing loss	1 (1%)	2 (13%)	3 (14%)	0	2 (11%)	1 (8%)
Epilepsy	2 (2.5%)	0	0	3 (27%)	2 (11%)	1 (8%)
Multiple impairments	5 (6%)	1 (7%)	6 (29%)	3 (27%)	2 (11%)	7 (54%)

CP = cerebral palsy.
DD = developmental delay.
PVE = persistent ventricular enlargement.
PVL = periventricular leucomalacia.
PC = porencephalic cysts.

accurate picture of the precise extent of cerebral injury in these infants will be obtained. It is also possible that at least part of the poor neurodevelopmental outcome in these infants relates to lesions at a cellular level which are not visible on ultrasound scans.

THE VERY IMMATURE SURVIVOR AT SCHOOL

While it has been long recognized that low birthweight infants perform less well than their term peers at school age, the differences are often small and become less marked as the influences of environment and culture become more dominant with increasing age. The few very long term studies however, do show that certain groups of low birthweight infants such as those with marked clumsiness, have difficulties which may still be evident in their late teens.[20] By nature of their length of follow-up, these reports concern infants born 20 or more years ago, well before the intensive care used today was widely available, and when the infant of 27 weeks or less rarely survived. Although very immature survivors have a high prevalence of major developmental disorders which may prevent them receiving a normal education, 80% will attend a normal school. In order to assess how these children were coping, Marlow et al. have recently completed a study of 53 six year old children with birthweights of less than 1250 g and who were in normal schools.[21] Half of these children were of less than 28 weeks gestation at birth in 1980 and 1981. The children were compared with age and sex matched controls from the same school class, and were given a test of general intelligence (Wechsler Preschool and Primary Scales), a test of minor motor impairment (Test of Motor Impairment, 'TOMI', Henderson Revision) and a neurological examination. The parents and class teachers also were asked to complete a behavioural questionnaire and a detailed social history was taken.

When asked to rate the classroom performance of the children, the school teachers thought that the low birthweight infants performed similarly to the term controls, although 2 of the index children were in remedial classes. The index children had significantly lower IQ than the controls, although all were within normal limits. Minor neurological signs or so-called 'soft signs' were significantly more frequent in the low birthweight infants. The TOMI also showed an excess of minor impairment in the index children. When the effect of a range of potential confounding variables such as IQ and social factors was examined using a multiple regression analysis, the excess of minor impairments was shown to be largely independent of these and related best to birthweight. Finally, both teachers and parents independently agreed that the low birthweight infants were more clumsy, overactive, more easily frightened, and fidgety than term controls.

Minor motor impairments and poor attention span are associated in other studies with poor educational performance. Longer term follow-up and educational assessment of these children is needed to determine the extent to which their immaturity at birth remains a handicap in later life, and to what extent this may be ameliorated by appropriate interventions at school.

COSTS OF NEONATAL INTENSIVE CARE

It is appropriate to consider the cost of intensive care for the very immature infant here, as it is the outcome of the care which in the long term must form any justification for the not inconsiderable expense of providing it. In the early days of neonatal intensive care, the very immature infant was not considered viable, and since no care was offered costs were negligible. Baumgartner's estimate of the day costs of neonatal care in the US of $24 per day did not include any under 28 week infants.[22]

By the late 1970's the escalating costs of care for premature infants, and more particularly the inability of hospitals to collect these from their parents caused a reappraisal of neonatal intensive care costs. Pomerance et al.[23] showed that the costs were $450 a day for survivors and $825 for non-survivors. The total costs were lower for non-survivors than survivors. The high rate of impairment in these infants was recognized in that the authors also produced a total cost for a 'normal' survivor of $88 058. They concluded that 'the cost of living for infants weighing less than 1000 g at birth is justifiable. Society, however, must be the ultimate judge, for society must pay the bill and reap the benefits and heartaches as well.' The authors of this paper did not try to take into account the long term costs of care of disabled survivors, i.e. loss of income and increased hospital and institutional usage in later years.

In a later article, Pomerance et al,[24] looking for ways to contain hospital costs for tiny infants, examined the theoretical reductions in costs that might be produced by the extension of gestation by the admission of mothers in premature labour and the use of tocolysis. By identifying hospital costs for preterm infants they noted a linear relationship between the cost of survival and gestational age. Between 29 and 34 weeks this cost averaged $772 a day. The cost of admitting the mother to hospital was $310 per day. If the admission resulted in a prolongation of gestation, the difference in costs of $462 a day represented a saving the authors termed 'womb-rent'. However it was also pointed out that if such an admission resulted in a 24 week gestation infant being born at 25 weeks the effect would in all probability be in the opposite direction. The 24 week infant would almost certainly die within a short time, but the 25 week infant was likely to survive at considerable expense and with a high chance of later neurodevelopmental sequelae. This argument has been used elsewhere, despite the lack of evidence that tocolysis is effective or even desirable in very preterm labour.

Sinclair et al.[25] in a review in 1981 made the point that although the individual interventions that went to make up intensive care had often been evaluated, the overall effectiveness of intensive care programmes had not. Such evidence that existed from individual units did not describe the effect on the population served. In calling for a full economic evaluation of care of the very low birthweight infant, they observed that 'there was no firm evidence that measures of the use of neonatal intensive care adequately reflect the desire, need, or demand for these services. Indeed it is possible that the supply of neonatal intensive care determines its use rather than the converse'.

Recently, Hack and Fanaroff in Cleveland, Ohio, have recorded their anxieties about the costs, morbidity and outcome of infants of less than 750 g at birth.[26] They noted that changes in their approach to the very immature infant at birth had resulted in increasing numbers of very immature infants with prolonged and complex courses and with a poor outcome. Average care costs of $158 800 (range $72 110–$524 110) were encountered. Many of the mothers were young, unsupported, black and socially disadvantaged. Some were unable or did not wish to care for their infants after discharge, and there were a number of late deaths. The authors concluded that the implications and cost-benefit ratios of extending the trend whereby intensive care is applied to progressively smaller immature infants must be seriously considered in order for definitive guidelines to be devised.

Interest in the costs of care for very preterm infants developed later in the UK probably as the provision for such care also developed more slowly. In 1984 Newns et al.[27] published day costs of £235 for intensive care, £122 for high dependency care, and £43 for special care. The average cost per survivor of less than 1000 g was £10 000, but for a non-survivor of similar weight only £800. More intensive efforts with the most immature infants has resulted in increased costs for those that eventually die in a way similar to the experience of Hack and Fanaroff. Sandhu et al.[28] from Liverpool, UK, showed similar day costs for intensive care to the study of Newns et al, when corrected for inflation, but much higher costs for non-survivors. Medical policies concerning the approach to the tiniest babies may greatly alter costs without substantially altering outcome. Factors such as the medical 'philosophy' employed need to be taken into account when comparisons of costings are made. Most studies of costs have found a significant negative correlation between the cost of care and birthweight. Sandhu et al.[28] also found such a correlation, but were able to show that it was a very weak one and that it only accounted for 4% of the variance of cost. If variables such as the presence or absence of hyaline membrane disease, periventricular haemorrhage, necrotising enterocolitis or septicaemia were included in the model, 60% of the variance could be accounted for.[29] It seems that it is the illness rather than the size of the infant which is critical in the cost of providing care.

Of the full cost-benefit analyses of neonatal intensive care for very preterm infants made to date, that of Boyle et al.[30] from Ontario in Canada is the most comprehensive. Economic aspects of care were evaluated using the outcomes and cost of care before and after the introduction of a regional neonatal intensive care programme in Hamilton-Wentworth County. Two periods, 1964–69 and 1973–77 were compared. Outcomes were expressed in terms of life years gained and quality adjusted life years (QUALY) gained. For infants weighing less than 1000 g, each additional survivor cost C$102 500 and C$9300 per life year gained. When utility values were included, a cost of C$22 400 per QUALY was derived. The net economic loss produced by intensive care for each livebirth under 1000 g was C$16 100. Examination of subgroups by weight below 1000 g showed progressively greater economic losses for each 100 g reduction in birthweight. Similar results have been shown in two studies by Walker et al. from Rhode Island.[31,32] In the first where estimates of lifetime earnings in addition to neonatal costs were made for survivors under 1000 g, only in the 900–999 g group did lifetime earnings exceed costs of care. In their second study the effects of intensive care for very low birthweight infants in a geographically defined area were compared before and after its introduction. The costs per survivor over the two periods remained essentially the same, but lifetime earnings increased, largely because of an increase in normal survivors. When the subgroups under 1000 g were examined however, the findings were of a net loss in a similar way to those of Boyle et al.[30]

Even if the cost of care for the very immature infant were known with great precision, most clinicians feel that it would not help them to make their daily decisions about these babies. The consequentialist approach that QUALY's seem to require, is seen to legitimize discrimination between patient groups. The QUALY may be a useful tool to determine cost-effectiveness, but is a relatively poor one for determining cost-benefit. The clinician sees his problem not so much as one of provision of resource but of that of coping with the effects of its restrictions at individual patient level. He has the problem of balancing equity with efficiency in resource allocation. Clinical decision making involves these balances, and the knowledge of costs may help the clinician in the assessment of the efficiency side of the equation.

REFERENCES

1 Weindling AM, Cooke RWI. The outcome for infants of less than 28 weeks gestation. Arch Dis Child 1988; 63: 697
2 Douglas JWB, Gear R. Children of low birthweight in the 1946 national cohort. Arch Dis Child 1976; 51: 820–827
3 Verloove-Vanhorick SP, Verwey RA, Ebeling MCA, Brand R, Ruys JH. Mortality in very preterm and very low birthweight infants according to place of birth and level of care: Results of a national collaborative survey of preterm and very low birthweight infants in the Netherlands. Pediatrics 1988; 81: 404–411
4 Powell TG, Pharoah POD, Cooke RWI. Survival and morbidity in a geographically defined population of low birthweight infants. Lancet 1986; 1: 539–544
5 Yu VYH, Loke HL, Bajuk B, Szymonowicz W, Orgill AA, Astbury J. Prognosis for infants born at 23 to 28 weeks gestation. Br Med J 1986; 293: 1200–1203
6 Herschel M, Kennedy JL, Kayne HL, Henry M, Cetrulo CL. Survival of infants born at 24–28 weeks gestation. Obstet Gynecol 1982; 60: 154–158
7 Milligan JE, Shennan AT, Hoskins EM. Perinatal intensive care: Where and how to draw the line. Am J Obstet Gynecol 1984; 148: 499–503
8 Philip AGS, Little GA, Polivy DR, Lucey JF. Neonatal Mortality Risk for the Eighties: The importance of birthweight/gestational age groups. Pediatrics 1981; 68: 122–130
9 Goldenberg RL, Nelson KG, Davis RO, Koski J. Delay in delivery: Influence of gestational age and the duration of delay on perinatal outcome. Obstet Gynecol 1984; 64: 480–484
10 Kitchen W, Ford GW, Doyle LW et al. Cesarean section or vaginal delivery at 24

to 28 weeks gestation: Comparison of survival and neonatal and 2-year morbidity. Obstet Gynecol 1985; 66: 149–157
11 Olshan AF, Shy KK, Luthy DA et al. Cesarean birth and neonatal mortality in very low birthweight infants. Obstet Gynecol 1984; 64: 267–270
12 Cooke RWI. Referral to a regional centre improves outcome in extremely low birthweight infants. Arch Dis Child 1987; 62: 619–621
13 Pharoah POD, Cooke TER, Rosenbloom L, Cooke RWI. Effects of birthweight, gestational age, and maternal obstetric history on birth prevalence of cerebral palsy. Arch Dis Child 1987; 62: 1035–1040
14 Marlow N, Chiswick ML. Neurodevelopmental outcome in extremely low birthweight survivors. In: Chiswick ML, ed. Recent Advances in Perinatal Medicine. Edinburgh: Churchill Livingstone, 1985
15 deVries LS, Lary S, Dubowitz LMS. Relationship of serum bilirubin levels to ototoxicity and deafness in high-risk low birthweight infants. Pediatrics 1985; 75: 351–354
16 Spector GJ, Pettit WJ, Davis G, Strauss M, Rausbach E. Fatal respiratory distress causing CNS and inner ear hemorrhage. Laryngoscope 1978; 88: 764–784
17 Thorburn RJ, Lipscomb AP, Stewart AL, Reynolds EOR, Hope PL, Pape KE. Prediction of death and major handicap in very preterm infants by brain ultrasound. Lancet 1981; 1: 1119–1121
18 Cooke RWI. Early and late cranial ultrasonographic appearances and outcome in very low birthweight infants. Arch Dis Child 1987; 62: 931–937
19 deVries LS, Dubowitz LMS, Dubowitz V. Predictive value of cranial ultrasound in the newborn baby; a reappraisal. Lancet 1985; 2: 137–140
20 Dunn HG. Sequelae of low birthweight: The Vancouver study. Clinics in Developmental Medicine No. 95/96. London: Blackwell Scientific, 1986
21 Marlow N, Roberts BL, Cooke RWI. Minor motor impairments in extremely low birthweight survivors. Arch Dis Child 1988 (In press)
22 Baumgartener L, Jacobziner H, Pakter J. A critical survey of the New York program for the care of premature infants. J Pediatr 1959; 54: 725–729
23 Pomerance JJ, Ukrainski CT, Ukra T, Henderson DH, Nash AH, Meredith JL. Cost of living for infants weighing 1000 grams or less at birth. Pediatrics 1978; 61: 908–910
24 Pomerance JJ, Schifrin BS, Meredith JL. Womb rent. Am J Obstet Gynecol 1980; 137: 486–490
25 Sinclair JC, Torrance GW, Boyle MH, Horwood SP, Saigal S, Sackett DL. Evaluation of neonatal intensive care programs. N Engl J Med 1981; 305: 489–493
26 Hack M, Fanaroff AA. Changes in the delivery room care of the extremely small infant (<750 grams) Effects on morbidity and outcome. N Engl J Med 1986; 314: 660–664
27 Newns B, Drummond MF, Durbin GM, Culley P. Costs and outcomes in a regional neonatal intensive care unit. Arch Dis Child 1984; 59: 1064–1067
28 Sandhu B, Stevenson RC, Cooke RWI, Pharoah POD. Cost of neonatal intensive care for very low birthweight infants. Lancet 1986; 1: 600–602
29 Stevenson RC, Pharoah POD, Cooke RWI, Sandhu B. Costs and benefits of neonatal intensive care. Arch Dis Child 1988; 63, 715–718.
30 Boyle MH, Torrance GW, Sinclair JC, Horwood SP. Economic evaluation of neonatal intensive care of very low birthweight infants. N Engl J Med 1983; 308: 1330–1337
31 Walker D-JB, Feldman A, Vohr BR, Oh W. Cost-benefit analysis of neonatal intensive care for infants weighing less than 1000 grams at birth. Pediatrics 1984; 74: 20–25
32 Walker D-JB, Vohr BR, Oh W. Economic analysis of regionalised neonatal care for very low birthweight infants in the State of Rhode Island. Pediatrics 1985; 76: 69–74

Index

A

Acid-base balance, 834–837
    Base Excess, 835
Active Respiratory Reflex (ARR), 914–915
Adaptation of the respiratory system, 909–918
ARR *see* Active Respiratory Reflex
Aldosterone, 937, 946–947, 1022
Alkalosis, 1002
Alloimmunization, feto-maternal Rh, 829, 833–834, 847
Alphafetoprotein levels, 843, 845, 855
Amniocentesis, 829, 901
Amniotic fluid
    lung growth, 829–830, 840, 938, 900
    prostaglandins levels, 856
    swallowing, 829, 938
    urine production, 829
Anencephaly, 902
Angiotensin II, 852–853, 946
ANP *see* atrial natriuretic peptide
Apnoea, 838, 909
    and respiratory control, 916–917
Asphyxia, 989, 1030, 1032, 1054, 1060
Atrial natriuretic peptide (ANP), 941, 946–948, 990
AZZOPARDI D *see* REYNOLDS E O R

B

BAEP *see* evoked potentials
BCG vaccine, 1040–1041
BENNETT P R & ELDER M G: Extreme prematurity: The aetiology of preterm delivery, 850–860
Beta-methasone, maternal treatment, 1019
Birthweight and gestational age, 870–873
BISSET W M *see* MILLA P J
Blood, fetal, 841–846
    biochemistry, 843–846
    coagulation, 842–843
    flow, 826, 831–833, 852, 854
    haematology, 841–842
Bone disease, 997–1000
BOTTING B *see* MacFARLANE A

Brain imaging and function, 1052–1075
    non-invasive methods (new) for assessing
    haemodynamics, 1052–1075
    oxygenation, 1052–1075
Braxton-Hicks contractions, 857
Broncho-pulmonary dysplasia, 912–913, 919, 929–930
Brown adipose tissue, 973–976

C

C reactive protein, 1046
CADY E B *see* REYNOLDS E O R
Calcium and phosphate, 844, 949, 996–1000
    formulae milk, 999–1000
Calmodulin, 1021
Cardiotocography, 826, 831
Cardiovascular adaptation in the very immature infant, 1025–1036
Cardiovascular system, 830–839
    blood flow, 831–833, 854
    blood pressure, 833–834
    blood volume, 834
    heart rate, 830–831
Catecholamine release, 833, 1031, 1046
Central nervous system (CNS), immature development 1077–1078
    neurophysiological assessment, 1076–1092
Cerebral palsy, 1076
    early detection, 1089–1090
Cervical incompetence, 857–858
Chloridorrhoea, 1021
Chlorothiazide, 938, 1033
Chorioamnionitis, 856
Circulation studies, fetal and placental, 826, 831–833, 854
    blood flow and control, 1026–1029
    perinatal changes, 1029–1031
Clinical issues, 1119–1132
    death and dying, 1130–1131
    fight or not to fight, 1119–1120
    monitoring, 1122–1125
    mortality, 1119–1122
    pain and stress, 1125–1127

parental rights, 1129
  stimulation, 1127–1129
  treatment, 1125
COLE S *see* MacFARLANE A
Congenital defects
  prenatal diagnosis, 826, 829
Congenital disorders, 902
Congenital malformations, 856, 938
COOKE R W I: Outcome and costs of care for the very immature infant, 1133–1151
COPE M *see* REYNOLDS E O R
Copper, 1004–1006
Costs of care, 1133–1151
Creatinine, 952–953
  urinary, 838
Cryptophthalmos-syndactyly (Fraser) syndrome, 905

D

Dating, fetal
  methods of, 1020
Delivery, aetiology of preterm, 850–860
DELPY D T *see* REYNOLDS E O R
Development of immunity, 1037–1051
Development of renal function, 935–956
Diabetes, maternal, 938
Diagnosis and management of fetal disorders, 826
Dopamine, 1030
Doppler blood flow studies of fetal and placental circulation, 826, 831–833, 854, 1071
Ductus arteriosus, patency of (PDA), 1031–1034
Dwarfism, thanatophoric, 902

E

Echocardiography, 1028, 1033
Eclampsia, 851
ELDER M G *see* BENNETT P R
Electroencephalography (EEG) or sensory evoked potentials, 1071, 1076, 1078–1089
  abnormal, 1083–1084
  normal, 1078–1083
  prognostic significance, 1083–1084
Electromagnetic stimulation of the motor cortex, 1089–1090
Emphysema, pulmonary interstitial, 911, 941
Endometritis, maternal, 856
Enzymes, 1020–1022

Epidemiology of birth before 28 weeks of gestation, 861–893
European Society of Paediatric Gastroenterology and Nutrition, Committee on Nutrition (ESPGAN), 984, 998
Evoked potentials, sensory, 1084–1089
  auditory, brainstem (BAEPs), 1085–1087
  somatosensory (SEPs), 1087–1089
  visual 1085
Exchange, feto-maternal, 829–830, 835
Exomphalos, 902
Extreme prematurity: The aetiology of preterm delivery, 850–860
Eyes, preterm birth, 1093–1118
EYRE J A: Neurophysiology of the immature CNS, 1076–1092

F

Fentanyl anaesthesia, 1126
Fetal therapy, 826
Fetoscopy, 841
FIELDER A R, MOSELEY M J & NG Y K: The immature visual system and premature birth, 1093–1118
Folate deficiency, 854–855
Fraser syndrome, 905
Frusemide, 937, 1033

G

Gastrointestinal tract, 1010–1024
  development of function, 1014–1022
  development of structure, 1011–1014
Glucocorticoids, 1046
Glucose, 844, 949–950
  kinetics, 1021
GREENOUGH A *see* MILNER A D
Growth, fetal, 827–829
  factors, 899
  retardation due to pre-eclampsia, 850–854
  very preterm infant, 984–1009

H

Haematocrit, 833–834, 841
  cerebral, 1079
Haemorrhage
  antepartum, 854–855
  cerebral, 1070–1071
  intracranial, 1031
  intraparenchymal, 1053
  intraventricular, 932

periventricular, 854–855, 924, 951, 989, 1058
Head's paradoxical reflex, 913–914
Hering Breuer response, 914
HES *see* Maternity Hospital Episode System
HIPE *see* Maternity Hospital In-patient Enquiry
Histocompatibility antigens, 851–852
HULL D
   Introduction, 821–825
   Thermal control of very immature infants, 971–983
Hyaline membrane disease, 946, 1030
Hydramnios, 1021
Hydratidiform mole, 851
Hydrocephalus, post-haemorrhagic, 1053
Hydrocortisone, 1032
Hypercapnia, 946
Hyperglycaemia, 950
Hypernatraemia, 951
Hyperplasia, 829
Hypertension, 851, 853, 855, 966, 1031
Hypertrophy, 829
Hyponatraemia, 938, 941–942, 951, 990
Hypoplasia
   causes of lung, 899, 902–904
Hypotension, 1031
Hypoxaemia, 966
Hypoxia, 833, 951, 1033, 1044
Hypoxic-ischaemic injury, 902, 1052–1054, 1060–1065, 1070–1072
   periventricular leucomalacia (PVL), 1052–1054, 1060, 1063–1064, 1105, 1112

I

Imaging
   brain function, 1052–1075
Immunisation, 1038, 1047
Immunity
   B lymphocyte development, 1038
   complement, 1042–1044
   human breast milk, 1046–1047
   immunoglobulin synthesis, 1038–1039
   neutrophil numbers, 1044–1046
   opsonisation, 1043–1045
   phagocyte function, 1041–1042
   T lymphocyte development, 1040–1041
Immunity, 902
   development of, 1037–1051

Immunological support therapies, 1038, 1047–1049
   granulocyte replacement, 1048–1049
   immunoglobulin, intravenous, 1048
   plasma, fresh frozen, 1048
   transfusion, exchange, 1048
Indomethacin, 856, 1033–1034
Iniencephaly, 902
Introduction, 821–825

J

JOHNSON A *see* MacFARLANE A

K

Keratinization, 829
Kidneys, 838–841

L

Labour, preterm, 855–858
Laryngeal atresia
   lung development, 904–905
Leukotrienes, 856–857, 1032
Liver immaturity
   coagulation, 843
Lungs, 837–840
   adaptation of, 909–918
   development in the second trimester, 894–908
   growth
      functional aspects, 898–899
      oligohydramnios, 894, 900–901
      other factors, 900
      quantitative, 898
      structural development, 894–898
      vulnerability, 900–906
   L/S ratio for maturity assessment, 829
   volume and mechanics, 912–913
Lupus, systemic, 854

M

MacFARLANE A, COLE S, JOHNSON A & BOTTING B: Epidemiology of birth before 28 weeks of gestation, 861–893
Magnetic resonance spectroscopy (MRS), 1052, 1054–1064, 1071–1072
   equipment and theory, 1054–1056
   neurodevelopmental prognosis, 1064, 1070–1071
   normal changes with brain maturation, 1057–1059

small-for-gestational age (SGA), 1059–1060
Mantoux reaction, 1041
Maternity Hospital Episode System (HES), 863–891
Maternity Hospital In-patient Enquiry (HIPE), 862–891
McINTOSH N: Clinical issues, 1119–1132
Meckel-Gruber syndrome, 902
Mid-trimester fetus, Physiology of, 826–849
Milk
  human breast, 990–1006
    immunity, 1038, 1046–1047
  infant formulae, 990–1006
MILLA P J & BISSET W M: The gastrointestinal tract, 1010–1024
MILNER A D & GREENOUGH A: Adaptation of the respiratory system, 909–918
MODI N: Development of renal function, 935–956
Morbidity, 883–886
MORLEY C J: Surfactant therapy for very premature babies, 919–934
Mortality, 876–882
MOSELEY M J see FIELDER A R.
Muscular dystrophy, 902
Mydriatics, 1031

N

NB see non-metabolisable base
Near infrared spectroscopy (NIRS), 1052, 1071–1072
  results, 1070–1072
  theory and equipment, 1064–1070
Neurophysiological assessment of the immature CNS, 1076–1092
Neutrophil storage pool (NSP) exhaustion, 1048
NG Y K see FIELDER A R
NICOLINI U see RODECK C H
Non-invasive methods (new) for assessing brain oxygenation and haemodynamics, 1052–1075
Non-metabolisable base (net base, NB), 1000–1002
Nutrition and growth
  very preterm infant, 984–1009
Nutrition, parenteral, 1119

O

Oligohydramnios, 936, 938
  lung growth, 894
Oscillometry, 1030

Osteogenesis imperfecta, 902
Osteopenia, 998–999
Outcomes and costs
  costs 1147–1150
  developmental assessment, 1140–1146
  duration of ventilation, 1139–1140
  methodology of follow-up, 1134–1135
  quality adjusted life years (QUALY), 1149–1150
  survival, 1136–1139
  survivors at school, 1146–1147
Outcomes and costs of care for the very immature infant, 1133–1151
Oxford Region Child Development Project, 888
Oxford Region Low Birthweight Study, 863–891

P

Pancuronium, paralysis with, 1031
Parenteral nutrition, total (TPN), 1006
PARKIN J see WHITELAW A
Patent ductus arteriosus (PDA), 926, 989–990
Percutaneous absorption and toxicity, 963–964
Periventricular leucomalacia
  see hypoxic-ischaemic injury
pH, vaginal
  preterm labour, 858
  see also acid-base balance
Phosphate depletion syndrome, 998
Photon absorptiometry, 999–1000
Phrenic nerve section, 899
Physiology of the mid-trimester fetus, 826–849
Phytohaemagglutinin responses, 1040
Placenta praevia, 854–855
Placental abruption, 854–855
Platelet behaviour, 852
Plethysmography, 912, 917
Pneumotachography, 916
Pneumothoraces, 914–915, 919, 926, 941, 951, 989
Potassium, 844, 949
Pre-eclampsia
  aetiology, 851–852, 855
  growth retardation, and, 850–854
Preterm delivery, aetiology of, 850–860
Pre-viable infant, discussion of, 821–822
Prostacyclin, 853–854

Prostaglandins, 853, 946, 951, 1031–1033
    preterm labour, 856–858
Pulsatility Index, 832

Q

Quality adjusted life years (QUALY), 1149–1150

R

RAAS *see* renin-angiotensin-aldosterone system
Reference standards
    growth and nutrition, 985–987
Regional Perinatal Unit in Toronto, 864
Renal agenesis, 901, 902, 905
Renal cystic dysplasia, 902
Renal function
    development of, 935–956
    intrauterine, 936–940
    neonatal, 943–953
    perinatal homeostasis, 940–942
Renin, 946
Renin-angiotensin-aldosterone system (RAAS), 946–948
Respiratory control
    apnoea, 916–917
Respiratory Distress Syndrome (RDS), 900, 910–913, 921, 931–932
    diuretic phase, 941
    prophylaxis, 919
Respiratory reflexes, 913–915
Respiratory system
    adaptation of the, 909–918
    surfactant therapy, 919–934
Resuscitation, 913
Retinopathy of prematurity (ROP), 1106–1113
    cicatricial, 1108–1110
    pathogenesis, 1110–1113
    vitamin E, 1106–1108
Retrolental fibroplasia (RLF), 1106
REYNOLDS E O R, WYATT J S, AZZOPARDI D, DELPY D T, CADY E B, COPE M & WRAY S: New non-invasive methods for assessing brain oxygenation and haemodynamics, 1052–1075
Rhesus
    haemolytic disease, 850
    isoimmunisation, 1040
Rheumatoid arthritis, 856
RODECK C H & NICOLINI U: Physiology of the mid-trimester fetus, 826–849

RUTTER N: The immature skin, 957–970

S

Scottish Morbidity Records system (SMR2), 861–891
Scottish Stillbirth and Neonatal Mortality Survey, 861–891
Sensory evoked potentials *see* electroencephalography
SEPs *see* evoked potentials
Sepsis, neonatal, 856, 1046
SHAW J C L: Growth and nutrition of the very preterm infant, 984–1009
Skin
    function, 960–969
    hazards to, 964–969
    immature, 957–970
    keratinization, 829–830
    structure, 957–960
SMR2 *see* Scottish Morbidity Records system
Sodium, 993–995
    balance, 946–949
Spectrophotometry, 829
Surfactant, 897, 899
    clinical trials, 921–923
    deficiency, 910, 1032
    doses, 930–931
    outcomes, 923–931
    preparations, 920–921
    therapy for very premature babies, 919–934

T

T cell growth factor (TCGF), 1040
Temperature regulation, 971–983
TEWL *see* transepidermal water loss
Thermal control
    very immature infants, 971–983
Thermogenesis, 973–974, 976
Thermoregulatory
    control, 971–983
    responses, 973–976, 988–989
Thrombocytopaenia, 852
Thromboxane, 853–854, 1032
TPN *see* parenteral nutrition, total
Transepidermal water loss (TEWL), 960–966

U

Ultrasound, 1071
    pulsed Doppler, 1028, 1030, 1033
    real-time, 826, 827–829, 831–833, 837

bladder volume, 837
lung dimensions, 837
pre-eclampsia, 852
transabdominal needling, 841
urine production, 939
Ultrasound and hypoxic-ischaemic injury, 1053
Urine production, 937–940

V

Vasopressin, 937–938, 951
 arginine (AVP), 951, 984, 989–990
Ventilation, mechanical, 1119, 1125, 1139–1140
 effects on lung development, 905–906
 intermittent positive pressure, 913–915, 929, 932
Visual system, immature, 1093–1118
 development of system, 1094–1096
 effect of preterm birth, 1093–1118
 neonatal environment, 1096–1101
 retinopathy of prematurity (ROP), 1106–1113
 temperature, 1101–1102
 visual development, 1102–1105
 effects of neurological damage, 1104–1105
Vitamin D efficiency, 998–9999
Vitamin E, 1106–1108

W

Water balance, 950–951
WHITELAW A & PARKIN J: Development of immunity, 1037–1051
WIGGLESWORTH J S: Lung development in the second trimester, 894–908
WILKINSON A R: Cardiovascular adaptation in the very immature infant, 1025–1036
Wilson-Mikity Syndrome, 913
WRAY S *see* REYNOLDS E O R
WYATT J S *see* REYNOLDS E O R

Z

Zinc, 1002–1003

BRITISH MEDICAL BULLETIN

Single issues available
(price £22.50 UK, £28.25/$49.25 overseas)

Vol. 39 (1983)

Issue 2: Chlaydial Disease (*Darougar*)
Issue 4: Early prenatal Diagnosis (*Ferguson-Smith*)

Vol. 40 (1984)

Issue 2: Nuclear Magnetic Resonance and its Clinical Applications (*Steiner & Radda*)
Issue 3: Clinical Applications of Monoclonal Antibodies (*Lennox*)
Issue 4: The Geography of Disease (*Doll*)

Vol. 41 (1985)

Issue 1: Virus Immunity and Pathogenesis (*Mims*)
Issue 2: Trypanosomiasis (*Newton*)
Issue 3: Trauma and its Metabolic Problems (*Barton*)
Issue 4: Antiviral Chemotherapy and Interferon (*Tyrrell & Oxford*)

Vol. 42 (1986)

Issue 1: Alzheimer's Disease and Related Disorders (*Roth & Iversen*)
Issue 2: Childhood Epidemiology (*Alberman & Peckham*)
Issue 3: Endoscopic Surgery (*Miller & Wickham*)
Issue 4: Calcium, Drugs & Hormones (*Baker & Metcalfe*)

Vol. 43 (1987)

Issue 1: H.L.A. in Medicine (*Crumpton*)
Issue 2: Inflammation–Mediators and Mechanisms (*Willoughby*)
Issue 3: The Functional Psychoses (*Crow*)
Issue 4: Hearing (*Haggard & Evans*)

Please send cheque with order to
Sales Dept., Churchill Livingstone,
1–3 Baxters' Place, Leith Walk, Edinburgh EH1 3AF

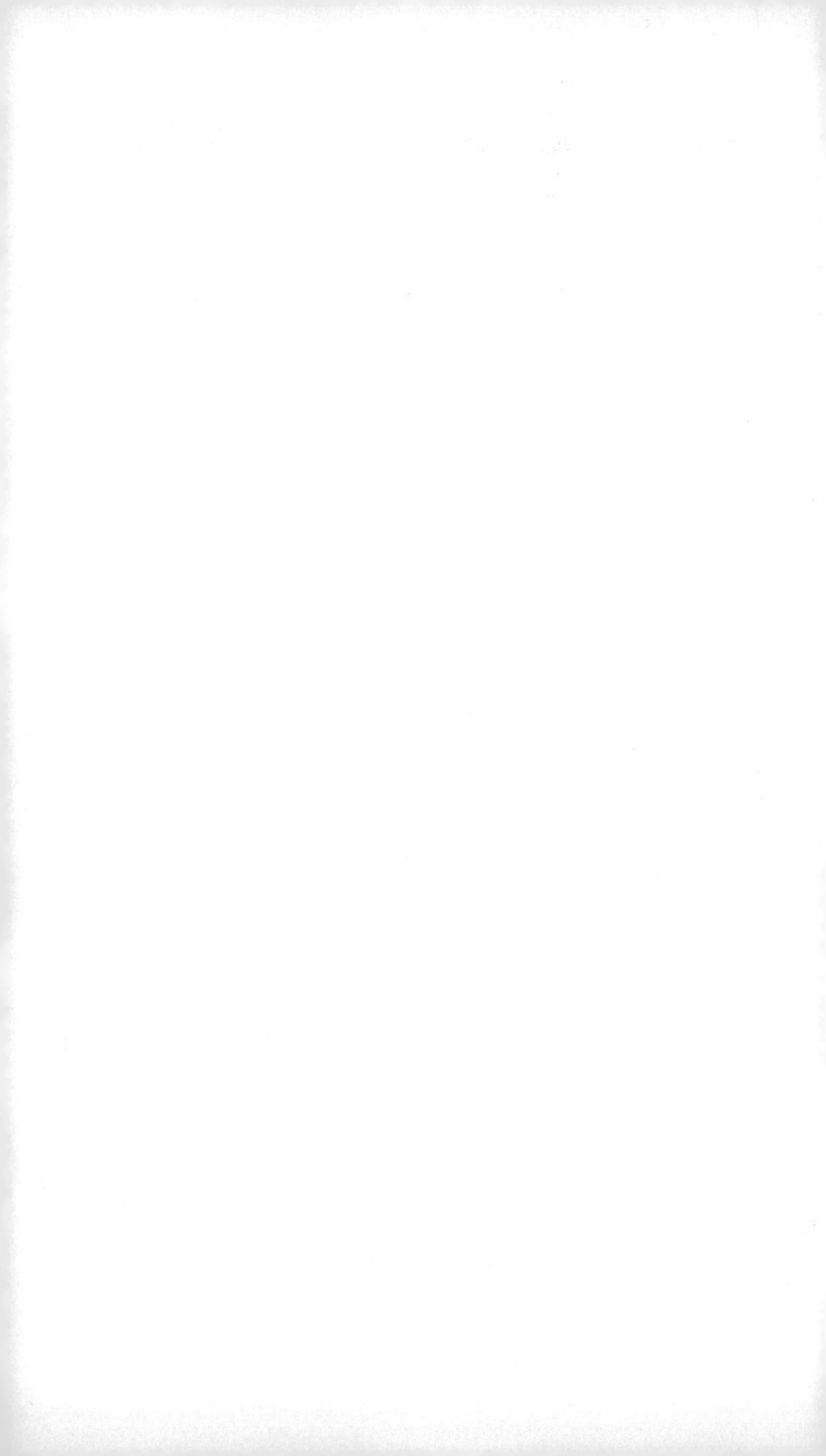

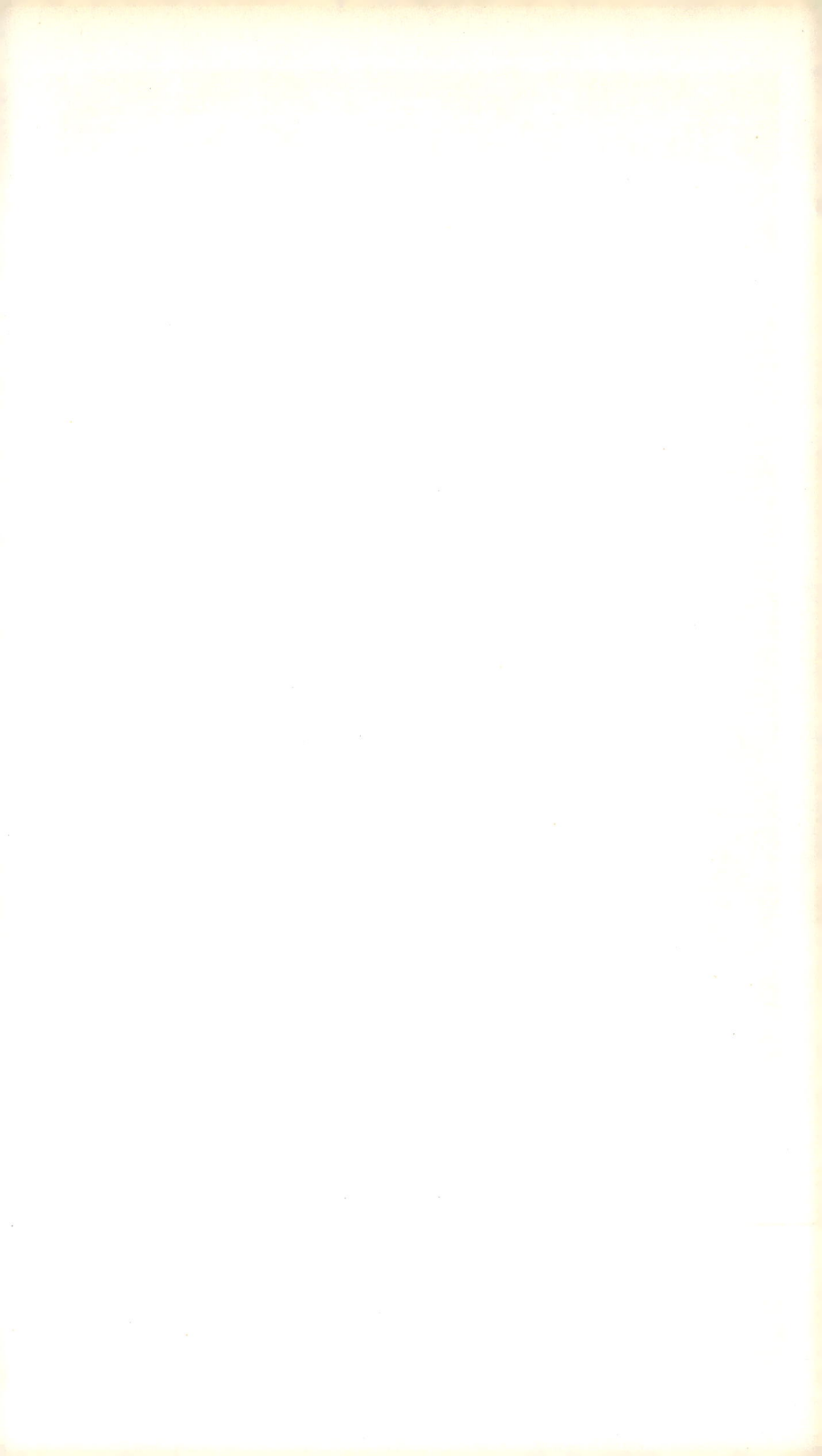